ULTIMATE FOODS FOR ULTIMATE HEALTH

...and don't forget the chocolate!

ULTIMATE FOODS FOR ULTIMATE HEALTH

...and don't forget the chocolate!

Liz Pearson R.D. and Mairlyn Smith H.Ec.

whitecap

This book is dedicated to three very special
people in my life: my daughter Chelsea, who once
explained to her classmates that the reason her
lunch looked like it did was because her mother
was a dietitian; my daughter Shannon, who
wonders why everything that's bad for you tastes
so good; and to my husband Rick, who may not be
a master chef in the kitchen but is the best man
you'll ever find for the clean-up crew.

LIZ PEARSON

www.lizpearson.com

To my parents, Jack and Roberta, who let me
create recipes at the age of 12, ate most of them,
and never got too mad when I broke a kitchen
appliance. Cooking and creating are all about love.

MAIRLYN SMITH

www.mairlynsmith.com

Copyright © 2007 by Liz Pearson and Mairlyn Smith
Seventh printing, 2011
Whitecap Books

Whitecap Books is known for its expertise in the cookbook
market, and has produced some of the most innovative
and familiar titles found in kitchens across North America.
Visit our website at www.whitecap.ca.

Edited by NADINE BOYD
Proofread by BEN D'ANDREA
Cover design by MICHELLE MAYNE & FIVE SEVENTEEN
Interior design by STACEY NOYES / LUZFORM DESIGN
Typesetting by MICHELLE MAYNE
Front cover photographs by MICHELLE MAYNE
Back cover photograph by JENNIFER PEARSON

Library and Archives Canada Cataloguing in Publication

Pearson, Liz, 1962–

  Ultimate foods for ultimate health / Liz Pearson,
Mairlyn Smith.

Includes bibliographical references and index.

ISBN-13: 978-1-55285-845-5
ISBN-10: 1-55285-845-6

  1. Nutrition. 2. Cookery. I. Smith, Mairlyn II. Title.

TX355.P418 2007   613.2   C2006-904994-7

The publisher acknowledges the financial support of the
Government of Canada through the Canada Book Fund
(CBF) and the Province of British Columbia through the Book
Publishing Tax Credit.

Printed and bound in Canada by Friesens

Contents

Acknowledgements
   7

Ultimate Foods for Ultimate Health
   8   **Introduction**
   13   **Good Fats, Bad Fats**
   20   **Phenomenal Fruits & Vegetables**
   32   **Spice Up Your Life**
   38   **A "Whole" Lot More with Whole Grains**
   47   **Low-Fat Milk Makes Sense**
   56   **More Beans, Please!**
   63   **Fatty Fish Is Fabulous**
   72   **More Chicken, Less Beef, & Eggs Are Okay**
   79   **Go Nuts!**
   85   **Fantastic Flax**
   90   **Ditch the Soft Drinks, Drink Water, & Take Time for Tea**
   96   **Red Wine for Good Health?**
   100 **Don't Forget the Chocolate!**
   105 **Pill Popping for Ultimate Health**
   114 **Get Off the Couch!**

Putting It All Together
   124 **Ultimate Eating Plan Checklist**
   130 **Seven-Day Eating Plan for Ultimate Health**
   132 **Life in the Fast Lane**
   137 **Using Food Labels to Make Healthier Choices**

Super Nutritious, Incredibly Delicious Recipes

141 **Pantry List & Kitchen Toys**

143 **Salads & Salad Dressings**

155 **Soups**

164 **Vegetables**

180 **Grains**

195 **Pasta & Sauces**

202 **Beans**

224 **Salmon & Shrimp**

241 **Poultry**

250 **Beef & Pork**

256 **Eggs**

259 **Fruit**

265 **Beverages**

276 **Muffins, Pancakes, & French Toast**

295 **Cookies & Treats**

Appendix

312 **Healthy Weight, Blood Pressure, & Blood Cholesterol Levels**

313 **Healthy Weight Guidelines**

Bibliography

314

Index

323 **Nutrition Information Index**

327 **Recipe Index**

About the Authors

336

Acknowledgements

After the last book I vowed that I'd never again gain tons of weight writing a cookbook. I figured the only way to avoid a calorie catastrophe was to test the recipes over a longer period of time and incorporate my new creations into my family's everyday life. It worked. This time I only bumped the scale up by five pounds, and that included the six weeks I was in a walking cast recovering from ligament reconstruction surgery on my right foot. Portion control is my new favourite buzz phrase.

No one writes a book alone, so here's to my army of friends, family, and tasters.

Thanks to my partner Scott, who ate his way through this book while offering support and encouragement; to my son Andrew, who helped me during crunch time; to my friend Michale, who helped me test the recipes and input nutritional info as well as support me during my surgery; to my girlfriends Jann, Maggie, Vivien, Cathy, Carol, Jill, and Jo, who were there to listen, cook, or just share a cup of tea and a good laugh; to my wonderful assistant Tracey, who helped triple test the recipes and would "un-crabby" me with her sense of fun; to my home economist mentor, friend, and fabulous recipe editor Barb Holland, who saved me many a time; to the Whitecap team (love you, Robert), and finally to my fabulous, fit, and fun co-author Liz, who became more than a friend, wrote her heart out, listened and laughed with me, and helped create a new book that will help you change your health. Cheers.

Mairlyn Smith

Thanks first and foremost to my co-author and friend Mairlyn for exceeding all expectations. Each and every recipe she created was a masterpiece in both nutrition and taste. I especially enjoyed the weekly taste tests at her place or mine.

Thanks to Laureen Fisher for her insightful review of the manuscript.

Thanks to the entire Whitecap team, including Robert, Nadine, Five, Michelle, Ben, Nick, and Aydin for pulling this project together and making it such a success.

Thanks to the many researchers, including those from Harvard, Tufts, Berkeley, and Cornell University for sharing their time and expertise with me. Ongoing research is absolutely critical to understanding the ever-changing, complex world of nutrition.

Last, but certainly not least, thanks always to my mom, dad, sister, brother, husband, and kids for their ever present love and support.

Liz Pearson

ULTIMATE FOODS FOR ULTIMATE HEALTH
. . . and don't forget the chocolate!

Liz Pearson is a registered dietitian with a passion for peanut butter sandwiches and an undying love for chocolate. Mairlyn Smith is a multi-talented home economist who creates recipes that are super nutritious and incredibly delicious. Together these two wrote *The Ultimate Healthy Eating Plan . . . that still leaves room for chocolate*, an award-winning national bestseller. *Ultimate Foods for Ultimate Health . . . and don't forget the chocolate!* is the next level—the next generation. It answers more questions, gives more advice, and highlights more disease-fighting powerhouse foods. And that's not all! In addition to containing 50 "best of the best" recipes from the original book, it contains 90 brand new, tasty, nutrition-packed recipes. Here are 10 ways that *Ultimate Foods for Ultimate Health* is certain to boost your health and well-being:

1 How to Eat Healthy in an Unhealthy World
We live in an unhealthy world. We're bombarded with high-calorie, fat-laden, sugar-loaded, nutritionally-barren foods at every turn. Obesity is considered one of today's most visible—yet most neglected—public health problems. The prevalence of type 2 diabetes is predicted to get worse before it gets better. Our children may be the first generation with a lower life expectancy than their parents. If ever there was a time to take action, that time is now. *Ultimate Foods for Ultimate Health* is designed to help you make healthy choices in an unhealthy world. Whether dining out, grabbing food on the run, or making meals at home, we provide specific, realistic, and achievable advice on your best food choices.

2 Dispels Myths & Clarifies Misconceptions
If you're confused, discouraged, or disheartened about what you should or shouldn't eat, join the crowd. Nutrition headlines seem to change with the weather. One day, a particular food is good for

---

QUOTE OF THE DAY
"When you enter a grocery store today, you see more high-calorie, high-fat choices in three minutes than our ancestors saw in a lifetime."
—David Sobel, MD, Director of Patient Education & Health Promotion, Kaiser Permanente

RESEARCH HIGHLIGHT
Researchers from the Harvard School of Public Health estimate that healthy food choices, together with regular physical activity and not smoking, can prevent over 80% of coronary heart disease, 70% of strokes, and 90% of type 2 diabetes.

you, the next day it's harmful to your health. One person says eat it, the next says don't. *Ultimate Foods for Ultimate Health* does its best to make sense of the complex and ever-changing world of nutrition. Our recommendations are based on the best evidence available from our extensive review of the research and interviews with leading scientists in the field. These questions and more are answered:

» Can you get all you need from food or must you pop a pill?

» Is soy a miracle food or have we been misled?

» Do canned fruits and vegetables really deliver?

» Fish is supposed to be good for you, but is it safe to eat?

» Should we build our bones with milk, or is there a better way?

» Are organic foods worth the money?

Ultimate Foods for Ultimate Health simplifies complex issues, tackles controversial subjects, and provides specific advice.

3 Packed with Super Nutritious, Disease Fighting Foods

Twenty-five hundred years ago Hippocrates said, "Let food be thy medicine and medicine be thy food." Today, research confirms that certain foods and food combinations have the ability to slash your risk of heart disease and cancer, protect against diabetes and osteoporosis, shield against aging and Alzheimer's, cut your risk of eye diseases such as macular degeneration and cataracts, and alleviate inflammatory disorders like arthritis. *Ultimate Foods for Ultimate Health* highlights foods that are the most potent disease fighters—like pomegranate juice, cinnamon, green tea, broccoli, berries, extra virgin olive oil, and almonds. Foods are ranked based on their overall nutrient contribution as well as their health-protecting ability. How much of these foods do you need to eat

RESEARCH HIGHLIGHT
Researchers from Michigan State University list the following four health habits as providing the most benefit: don't smoke, maintain a healthy body weight, eat at least five servings of fruits and vegetables daily, and get at least 30 minutes of physical activity five days a week.

RESEARCH HIGHLIGHT
Researchers estimate that life expectancy would rise by seven years if all forms of major cardiovascular disease were eliminated.

to significantly reduce your risk of disease? Does it matter whether you eat them raw, cooked, peeled, or chopped? Are some foods more beneficial when eaten alongside other foods? *Ultimate Foods for Ultimate Health* gives you the goods on the nutritional world superstars.

4 Highlights Dietary Villains You Need to Avoid

Sugar consumption is skyrocketing around the world. Artery-clogging trans fats and saturated fats lurk in unlikely places. Refined grains, like white bread, can be harmful to your health. Too much red meat can significantly boost your risk of colon cancer. Soft drinks or "liquid candy" are tied to ballooning waistlines and a higher rate of type 2 diabetes. Some specialty coffees made with whole milk, syrups, and whipped cream have enough calories and fat to sink a small ship. Portion sizes are out of control. Most fast foods are a landmine of sodium. *Ultimate Foods for Ultimate Health* helps you avoid the worst of the worst—the foods most harmful to your health. It also provides healthy alternatives that satisfy. Does it get any better?

5 Helps You Lose Pounds & Maintain a Healthy Body Weight

Maintaining a healthy body weight is one of the most important things you can do for your health. You lower your risk of heart attack, stroke, high blood pressure, diabetes, cancer, and osteoarthritis.

Yet in the 21st century, managing a healthy weight is more challenging than ever before. *Ultimate Foods for Ultimate Health* is designed for reducing waistlines and satisfying hunger. It's loaded with great tasting ideas that are low in fat, low in calories, and high in fibre. It will please your taste buds, keep you on track, and motivate you. Great taste, wholesome eating, and healthy weight loss—all in one.

6 Super Nutritious, Incredibly Delicious Recipes!

Fact: people don't want to compromise taste when it comes to eating healthy. Fact: you don't have to. Mairlyn makes it possible to enjoy every single bite of a very healthy day. The Rotini with Feta and Tomatoes tastes like summer. The Grilled Salmon with Raspberries is divine. The Orange Avocado Black Bean Salsa Salad overflows with flavour. The Awesome Lentil and Rice Salad should win a prize. The Jamaican Spiced Marinade with Pork Tenderloin simply couldn't be better. And the lemon-zest sugar topping on the Wild Blueberry Muffins is to die for. When it comes to recipe creation, Mairlyn is the master. There are kid-friendly recipes, impressive-enough-for-entertaining recipes, and, most importantly, tons of super-fast and easy recipes. *Ultimate Foods for Ultimate Health*—super tasty, super nutritious, super wonderful!

QUOTE OF THE DAY

"Obesity is now so common within the world's population that it is beginning to replace undernutrition and infectious diseases as the most significant contributor to ill health. It is an epidemic that threatens global well-being for adults and children alike."
—Peter Kopelman, Professor, Royal London School of Medicine

RESEARCH HIGHLIGHT

Based on a study from the Karolinska Institute in Stockholm involving over 44,000 pairs of twins, genetic makeup and family history were found to contribute minimally to the risk of developing most types of cancer. Researchers concluded that the environment, which includes diet, is the principal cause of most cancers.

7 Realistic & Achievable (includes Seven-Day Meal Plan)

You know you should eat more fruits and vegetables, but you don't. "Top Ten Tips for Meeting Your Fruit & Veggie Quota" (page 23) is guaranteed to help you get there. You've heard that beans are good for you, but how do you eat more of them? "Ten Great Ways to Say Hello to Beans" (pages 60–62) will guide you. The cereal aisle is overflowing with options, but what cereal should you choose? "Ten Terrific Tips for Building a Beautiful Bowl of Cereal"(page 43) makes it easy to pick the best. *Ultimate Foods for Ultimate Health* is loaded with top 10 lists, best of the best lists, and how-to-get-more lists. The ideas are practical and doable. There's even a Seven-Day Meal Plan that ties together all of the advice and recommendations. *Ultimate Foods for Ultimate Health* tells you why, but, most importantly, it shows you how.

8 Provides Top Tips for Life in the Fast Lane

We live in a fast-paced, hectic world. Eating on the run, skipping meals, and frozen dinners are a way of life. No time to shop for food. No time to prepare food. We dine at our desks. We dine in our cars. The result is often a nutritional catastrophe—a diet of unhealthy fats, excess calories, and sodium, and not enough nutrition. A busy lifestyle is no excuse for a lousy diet, and neglecting our health, no matter how crazy life gets, is simply not an option. *Ultimate Foods for Ultimate Health* is geared for life in the fast lane. We provide fast food survival tips, like the two-slice pizza rule, and snacking on the run tips, such as the healthiest snacks to pack. There are also label reading tips, a frozen dinner checklist, and top tips for dining out. With *Ultimate Foods for Ultimate Health* your life can be healthy and high-speed.

9 Gets You Off the Couch

Our generation is the most sedentary in history. We've engineered activity out of our lives. We sit in cars. We stare at computer screens. We're glued to the tube. *Ultimate Foods for Ultimate Health* gives you 55 incredible reasons to move your body. Participation isn't optional. We provide 12 easy ways to build movement back into everyday life and 14 top tips for incorporating activity into your day. Recommended activities are provided, as well as tips for keeping your kids off the couch. *Ultimate Foods for Ultimate Health* is more than just an eating plan, it keeps you moving.

10 Still Leaves Room for Chocolate!

They say there's nothing better than a good friend . . . except a good friend with chocolate. It's true. Chocolate is calming, delectable, heavenly, intoxicating, irresistible, sexy, and sinful. The best news is that this mouth-watering food is actually good for you. *Ultimate Foods for Ultimate Health*

RESEARCH HIGHLIGHT
In an international study sponsored by the World Health Organization involving 34 countries around the world, the following countries were at the top of the list for having the most overweight children: Malta, the United States, England, and Canada.

RESEARCH HIGHLIGHT
People often have type 2 diabetes for several years before they're diagnosed. During this period, irreversible physical damage may occur. Diabetes is a particularly nasty disease that can cause serious complications such as blindness, kidney disease, greater risk for heart disease, strokes, amputations, and a host of other disorders. Children who develop type 2 diabetes face a much higher risk of kidney failure and death by middle age than people who develop type 2 diabetes as adults.

helps you choose the types of cocoa and chocolate with the highest amounts of disease-fighting anti-oxidants. It also provides chocolate recipes that are better for you than most, including the incredible Ultimate Healthy Chocolate Treat (page 308), the delicious Frozen Cocoa (page 270), and the truly divine Decadent Brownies (page 306). Let's face it, how could an eating plan be an Ultimate Eating Plan without chocolate?

The Bottom Line

Ultimate Foods for Ultimate Health is a super nutritious and incredibly delicious eating plan. It fights disease, whittles your waistline, gives great advice, and is designed for today's world. It's the best investment you can make in you. Here's to happy reading and tasting—and to being the healthiest you can be!

Have fun on your journey.
Sincerely,

Liz Pearson & Mairlyn Smith

P.S. Before starting any new eating plan or exercise program, be sure to check with your family doctor.

QUOTE OF THE DAY
It's estimated that one in two women and one in four men over the age of 50 in North America are at risk of an osteoporosis-related fracture. "Despite these staggering numbers, most people do not realize their personal risks of developing osteoporosis or suffering a related fracture. Osteoporosis may be a silent disease, but we cannot afford to be silent about it."
—Judith Cranford, Executive Director, National Osteoporosis Foundation

RESEARCH HIGHLIGHT
A sedentary lifestyle is a major cause of death, disease, and disability. Physical inactivity doubles the risk of cardiovascular disease, type 2 diabetes, and obesity. It also increases the risks of colon and breast cancer, high blood pressure, lipid disorders, osteoporosis, depression, and anxiety.

GOOD FATS, BAD FATS

FOR ULTIMATE HEALTH

» Optimize your intake of poly-unsaturated fats (including the omega-3 fats) and mono-unsaturated fats.

» Limit your intake of unhealthy saturated and trans fats.

THE RIGHT FAT

The traditional Japanese and Mediterranean diets of the 1960s are considered among the healthiest in the world. They're linked to remarkably low rates of disease, including heart disease and most cancers. However, these diets are surprisingly different from one another when it comes to their fat content. The traditional Japanese diet is very low in fat (less than 10% of the calories come from fat), whereas the Mediterranean diet is much higher in fat (as much as 40% of the calories come from fat). The types of fats used in both of these diets are primarily healthy or good fats. Olive oil is the mainstay of the Mediterranean diet, while fish provides a lot of omega-3 fats for the Japanese. The lesson: it's the type of fat you eat, not the quantity, that has the most significant impact on your health. Fat can definitely be a good thing, and choosing the right fats can slash your risk of many diseases. Polyunsaturated fats (especially the omega-3s) and monounsaturated fats are healthy. They're found in plant-based foods, including most vegetable oils (the omega-3 fats also come from fish). The fats you want to limit are the artery-clogging saturated fats (found in high-fat milk products and fatty meats) and trans fats (found in some processed and deep-fried foods).

Canola Oil: Omega-3 Fats & More

For ultimate health canola oil is recommended. Here are three reasons why canola oil gets my endorsement:

1 Omega-3 All-star

Omega-3 fats are nutritional heroes. There are two types of omega-3 fats: those that come from plants

RESEARCH HIGHLIGHT
Fat in our diet helps us absorb fat-soluble vitamins (A, E, D, and K). It also helps us absorb valuable plant carotenoids, like beta-carotene and lycopene, which are found in fruits and vegetables. In a study from Iowa State University, people who ate a salad with fat-free dressing didn't absorb any carotenoids, whereas a reduced-fat or full-fat dressing resulted in a substantially greater absorption of these important compounds.

QUESTION OF THE DAY
Should I buy low-fat products? It's important to focus on products that contain healthy fats. However, choosing lower fat products also makes sense, especially if you're watching your waistline. Fat is a concentrated source of calories (twice as many as the same amount of protein or carbohydrate). Less fat generally means less calories.

and those that come from fish (the benefits and recommendations for the omega-3 fats found in fish are detailed in the fish chapter). Very few foods are naturally rich in omega-3 fats, with the exception of foods like canola oil, flaxseeds, and walnuts. The greatest claim to fame for plant source omega-3 fat (also referred to as alpha-linolenic acid) is its ability to help the heart keep a strong and regular beat. A major cause of heart attacks is an irregular or chaotic heartbeat (also referred to as arrhythmia) that ultimately causes the heart to stop beating. These fats may also protect the endothelium (the cells that line blood vessel walls) as well as reduce inflammation (an inflammatory environment promotes the development of heart disease).

2 Lowers Your LDL Cholesterol

When we replace unhealthy saturated and trans fats in our diet with healthy polyunsaturated and monounsaturated fats—like those found in canola oil—we can lower our LDL cholesterol levels. LDL cholesterol is the "bad" or "artery-clogging" cholesterol that travels in our bloodstream and deposits cholesterol along artery walls. Canola oil contains polyunsaturated fats, including the omega-3 fats, but is also very high in healthy monounsaturated fats. In addition, canola oil has the lowest saturated fat content of most vegetable oils (all oils contain at least some saturated fat).

3 Balanced Ratio of Omega-6 to Omega-3 Fats

There are two types of polyunsaturated fats: omega-6 and omega-3 fats. Canola oil contains fairly equal amounts of these two fats (2:1 ratio). In contrast, corn, sunflower, safflower, and soybean oil (and products such as margarine or salad dressings made with these oils) contain significantly higher quantities of the omega-6 fats. Both omega-3 and omega-6 fats are considered healthy fats. However, research suggests a more balanced intake of these fats may provide optimal disease protection.

CLEAR THE CONFUSION
I don't like fish. Can I get my omega-3 fats from foods like canola oil, flaxseed, and walnuts instead? No. While both plant and marine sources of omega-3 fats protect our health, marine source omega-3 fats provide significantly greater protection. They're incorporated directly into cell membranes throughout the body, including tissues in the heart, brain, and eyes. Both sources of omega-3 fats should be included in the diet.

RESEARCH HIGHLIGHT
In the Lyon Heart Study, a healthy diet combined with a high intake of plant source omega-3 fats (much of which came from a canola-enriched margarine) was linked to a 70% reduction in fatal heart attacks.

RESEARCH HIGHLIGHT
In the Harvard Male Health Professionals Study involving over 47,000 men, the heart-protective effect achieved by consuming plant source omega-3 fats was even more significant than reducing saturated fat in the diet.

Olive Oil: Proven Track Record & Plenty of Antioxidants

For ultimate health extra virgin olive oil is recommended. Here are two reasons why extra virgin olive oil gets my endorsement:

1 Backbone of the Mediterranean Diet

You simply can't ignore that a hallmark of the Mediterranean diet, one of the healthiest diets in the world, is olive oil. While many foods contribute to the success of this diet, olive oil is an important part of the equation. People who regularly consume olive oil as part of a healthy diet live longer and have lower rates of heart disease and cancer.

2 Healthy Monounsaturated Fats & Beneficial Plant Compounds

Olive oil is very rich in healthy monounsaturated fats. When substituted for unhealthy trans and saturated fats, it helps lower LDL (bad) cholesterol. But that's not all. Olive oil contains a multitude of health-protective plant compounds, including phenols. Phenols have strong antioxidant and anti-inflammatory effects that promote heart health and help protect against cancer. Extra virgin olive oil is best because it's less processed and has higher quantities of these disease-fighting compounds.

Saturated Fats Are Bad, Trans Fats Are Nasty

For ultimate health limit your intake of saturated fats.

High intakes of saturated fats can cause the LDL (bad) cholesterol in your blood to increase. This causes plaque to build up on artery walls and ultimately increases your risk of a heart attack and stroke. Saturated fats may also increase your risk of type 2 diabetes, Alzheimer's, and some cancers. Saturated fat is found in high fat milk products (whole milk, cheese, butter, cream, ice cream) and fatty meats (hamburgers, hot dogs, sausages, salami, bologna, ribs, chicken wings). It's important to choose low-fat milk products and lean meats (more advice on this in the milk and meat chapters). Foods containing coconut oil, palm oil, palm kernel oil, or lard should be avoided because of their high saturated fat content.

For ultimate health limit your intake of trans fats.

Trans fats are nasty. Also referred to as hydrogenated fats, these man-made fats are used by food companies to increase the stability and shelf life of their products. Trans fats are considered as much as 10 times more harmful than saturated fats. In addition to increasing our LDL (bad) cholesterol levels, they may decrease our HDL (good) cholesterol. Our HDL cholesterol helps carry cholesterol

OLIVE OIL

RESEARCH HIGHLIGHT
The health-promoting properties of olive oil can be partly explained by the presence of beneficial plant compounds called phenols. In a study from the University of Cordoba in Spain, 21 people with high cholesterol levels consumed either phenol-rich olive oil or olive oil with most of the phenols removed.

Only the phenol-rich olive oil significantly increased levels of nitric oxide and reduced levels of oxidative stress in the blood. Nitric oxide is important for blood vessel health and dilation. Reducing oxidative stress helps prevent the damage to artery walls that leads to heart disease.

RESEARCH HIGHLIGHT
Some research suggests that olive oil may reduce the risk of rheumatoid arthritis. In a study from the University of Athens Medical School in Greece, people with the lowest lifetime consumption of extra virgin olive oil were over twice as likely to develop the disease compared to those with the highest intake.

out of our bloodstream to the liver for disposal. Trans fats also stiffen our arteries and increase our risk of type 2 diabetes as well as numerous other diseases.

How to reduce your trans fat intake:

» Trans fats can be found in some processed foods like cookies, crackers, microwave-popcorn, and hydrogenated margarine. Buy trans fat free versions of these products.

» Deep-fried foods, like french fries, donuts, and chicken nuggets can be a major source of trans fat. When dining out avoid deep-fried foods (best idea!) or ask if the oil they use is trans fat free.

» Milk and meat products naturally contain small amounts of trans fats. Buy low-fat or lean versions of these products.

For ultimate health a heart-healthy margarine instead of butter is recommended.

One headline screams "margarine: the healthy choice"; the next headline declares "butter is definitely best." What should we believe? A heart-healthy margarine gets my vote for two reasons.

1 The fat and calorie content of margarine and butter are the same. A good margarine, however, contains mostly healthy fats, including the much needed, omega-3 fats. Butter contains mostly unhealthy saturated fats. Two teaspoons of a good margarine (10 mL) contains only 1 gram of saturated fat. The same amount of butter contains 5 grams of saturated fat. To keep our blood cholesterol levels healthy, replacing unhealthy fats with healthy fats is key.

2 Vitamin E and vitamin D are both all-star disease fighting vitamins that most of us don't get enough of. A heart-healthy margarine is an excellent source of both of these vitamins (vitamin D is added to all margarine in Canada, but only to some in the United States). Butter isn't a source of these important nutrients.

Liz's definition of a heart-healthy margarine (many brands fit this profile):

» non-hydrogenated (trans fat free)

» low in saturated fat (2 g or less per serving)

» at least 0.4 grams of omega-3 fats per serving

Please Note

Don't be alarmed if you see ingredients like palm oil (high in saturated fat) on the ingredient list of some margarines. Small amounts are used to make margarine spreadable. As long as the margarine is still low in saturated fat (2 g or less per serving), it's still a healthy choice.

QUESTION OF THE DAY
What do you think of other oils like flaxseed, hemp, or grapeseed? I recommend ground flaxseed, instead of flaxseed oil, as it provides more benefits, including a greater ability to fight cancer (see flax chapter pages 86–89). Hemp oil is rich in omega-3 fats. However, both the canola oil and ground flaxseed recommended in this book meet that particular need. Grapeseed oil contains some beneficial plant compounds, but it's also high in omega-6 fats (research suggests we need less omega-6 fats and more omega-3s in our diet). I stand by my recommendation for the use of canola and extra virgin olive oil.

TRUE OR FALSE?
The amount of cholesterol in the food you eat is the major cause for the cholesterol in your blood to rise. False: For most people, it's the saturated and trans fats that are most harmful to blood cholesterol levels.

If you suffer from heart disease, consider using a margarine with added plant sterols, such as Smart Balance, Benecol, or Take Control (widely available in the United States). Plant sterols are compounds that help lower LDL (bad) cholesterol levels. These products are currently not available in Canada.

ONE FAT SERVING	
	1 tsp (5 mL) canola oil or extra virgin olive oil
	1 tsp (5 mL) heart-healthy margarine
	1 tsp (5 mL) full-fat mayonnaise or salad dressing
	1 Tbsp (15 mL) light or low-fat mayonnaise or salad dressing

Your Daily Fat Quota

For ultimate health consume 3 to 6 servings of healthy fats each day.

This includes the canola or extra virgin olive oil you use in cooking or baking, as well as margarine, salad dressing, mayonnaise, and other high-fat spreads. Most women (especially older women and anyone having trouble managing their weight) should choose the lower number of fat servings (3–4), while active men may enjoy the higher number of servings (5–6). Most other people fall somewhere in between (these guidelines apply to the rest of the book wherever there's a range of servings). Please note that other foods recommended in this book, like nuts and flaxseed, are also a source of dietary fat (guidelines for recommended quantities of these foods are included in subsequent chapters).

TRANS FATS

QUOTE OF THE DAY
Following a comprehensive research review the National Institute of Medicine concluded "there is no level of trans fatty acids that is safe to consume."

RESEARCH HIGHLIGHT
In the Harvard Nurses' Health Study involving over 80,000 women, those women who consumed the most trans fats were 50% more likely to develop heart disease and almost 40% more likely to develop type 2 diabetes.

GOOD ADVICE
Just because a product label screams "trans fat free," don't assume it's a healthy product. Many manufacturers are replacing artery-clogging trans fats with artery-clogging saturated fats. Look for products that are both "trans fat free" and "low in saturated fat" (2 g or less of saturated fat per serving).

» Look for salad dressings and mayonnaise made with extra virgin olive oil or canola oil.

» Don't buy fat-free salad dressings or mayonnaise. We need some healthy fats in our diet.

» Beware of salads served in restaurants. A large Caesar salad can contain more than 12 servings (12 teaspoons) of fat. Ask restaurants to go easy on the dressing or better yet, ask for your dressing on the side. Use low-fat or light dressing if available.

» Exception to the 3 to 6 servings rule: if you're trying to lose weight, consume 1 less serving of fats on the days you consume one full serving of nuts (¼ cup/60 mL), peanut butter (2 Tbsp/30 mL), avocado (2 Tbsp/30 mL), or olives (8 olives).

ULTIMATE FOODS FOR ULTIMATE HEALTH

Replace unhealthy saturated and trans fats with the healthy polyunsaturated and monounsaturated fats found in canola oil and extra virgin olive oil. Use a heart-healthy margarine instead of butter. Enjoy 3 to 6 servings of healthy fats each day.

MARGARINE

RESEARCH HIGHLIGHT
In a study from the Texas Southwestern Medical Center involving 46 families, switching from butter to soft-tub margarine caused LDL (bad) cholesterol levels to decrease an average of 11% for adults and 9% for children. Have you made the switch?

GOOD ADVICE
Instead of spreading your bread with butter or margarine, another option is to do as they do in the Mediterranean. Dip your bread into a small amount of spiced olive oil—delicious and good for you!

PHENOMENAL FRUITS & VEGETABLES

FOR ULTIMATE HEALTH

» Optimize your overall intake of whole fruits and vegetables.

» Optimize your intake of nutrient-rich, brightly-coloured fruits and vegetables.

» Optimize your intake of disease-fighting superstars: apples, berries, broccoli, pomegranate juice, spinach, and tomato-based foods.

ULTIMATE DISEASE PROTECTION

This is the part of the book where I want to jump up and down, scream and shout, do back flips, front flips, and other incredibly amazing feats. The reason for my theatrics is that I need you to pay attention to a message I know you've heard a million times before: eat your fruits and vegetables! Now, here's the problem. Even though you've heard this simple message over and over again, my guess is you still underestimate its value. Everyone's looking for a magic bullet when it comes to health. News flash: there is no magic bullet. Eating more fruits and vegetables is about as close as it gets.

Fruits and vegetables are disease-fighting power-houses. They contain a complex mix of health-protective vitamins, minerals, fibre, and literally hundreds of beneficial plant compounds. Name almost any disease, including heart disease, stroke, cancer, diabetes, Alzheimer's, obesity, and cataracts, and I guarantee that eating more fruits and vegetables will help reduce your risk. In the world of disease prevention, fruits and vegetables simply can't be beat.

How Do Fruits & Vegetables Protect Your Health?

Antioxidant Superheroes

Fruits and vegetables contain nutrients and plant compounds that act as antioxidant all-stars in the body. Antioxidants prevent nasty molecules called free radicals from damaging our cells. We all have free radicals in our body, created when our bodies use oxygen to produce energy. When we're exposed to things like cigarette smoke, ultraviolet light, radiation, or pollution, additional free radicals are created. Without antioxidants, free radicals can damage our cells, which ultimately leads to disease. Damage to our DNA—the blueprint our cells use to reproduce—can lead to cancer. When LDL (bad) cholesterol becomes damaged, it's able to penetrate and build up along artery walls, leading to a heart attack or stroke. Eye tissue damage can increase the risk of cataracts or macular degeneration (the leading cause of adult blindness), while injury to brain tissue can increase the risk of diseases such as Alzheimer's.

Beyond Antioxidants

Other ways that fruits and vegetables help protect against disease include:

» preventing the formation of blood clots that can cause a heart attack or stroke

» lowering LDL (bad) cholesterol levels

» maintaining the health of blood vessel walls, including a healthy blood pressure

» stimulating the immune system, which plays a central role in disease protection

» influencing important enzymes in the body that help prevent, block, and suppress the development of cancer and other diseases

» reducing inflammation—an inflammatory environment promotes the development of many diseases, including heart disease, cancer, and diabetes

» helping maintain a healthy body weight

Your Daily Produce Quota

For ultimate health enjoy 7 to 10 (ideally closer to 10) servings of fruits and vegetables each day.

To maximize your intake of health-enhancing nutrients like vitamin C, carotenoids (beta-carotene, lycopene, lutein, zeaxanthin), folate, potassium, fibre, and antioxidant-rich plant compounds like flavonoids, you need to reach for at least 7, ideally closer to 10, servings of fruits and vegetables each day. For those of you who think this sounds like a truckload of fruits and vegetables, let me assure you it's only a wheelbarrow full (just kidding!). It's easier than you think. See the table on the next page for what one serving looks like.

For ultimate health eat most of your fruits and vegetables whole. Limit your intake of fruit juice to no more than 1 cup (250 mL) daily.

My overall nutrition philosophy is that foods should be eaten as close to their natural state as possible. This means eating most of your fruits

FRUITS + VEGGIES

RESEARCH HIGHLIGHT

In the report "Food, Nutrition & the Prevention of Cancer," 15 of the world's leading researchers of diet and cancer reviewed over 4,500 studies. Fruits and vegetables came out on top as the food most likely to reduce cancer risk.

GOOD ADVICE

If you want your kids to love eating fruits and vegetables, be sure to do two things. First, serve fruits and vegetables over and over and over again. Children, especially when they're young, need to be exposed to a new fruit or vegetable as many as 10 times before they'll accept it (most parents give up after less than two tries). Second, be a great role model—eat and really enjoy fruits and vegetables yourself. One of the strongest predictors of what children eat is what their parents eat.

and vegetables whole. Although fruit juice can be a valuable source of nutrition, it's also a concentrated source of sugar and calories and doesn't contain the fibre found in whole produce. One cup (250 mL) of fruit juice contains anywhere from 5 to 9 teaspoons of naturally-occurring sugar and 120 to 160 calories. Limit your fruit juice to no more than 1 cup (250 mL) each day. Vegetable juice is much lower in sugar and calories, but can be high in sodium. Choose low-sodium varieties whenever you can.

Top 10 Tips for Meeting Your Fruit & Veggie Quota

1 Never miss a meal. Include at least 1 to 2 servings of fruits or veggies at every meal and at snack times. This is so important! Most people simply can't meet their daily quota any other way.

2 Don't leave home without them. Never (and I mean never!) leave home without packing some portable fruits or vegetables in your knapsack, purse, briefcase, or the glove compartment of your car. You'll get hungry, and rather than play vending-machine roulette or stopping at a convenience store (that only makes it convenient to eat poorly), reach for your personal stash of veggies or fruit. Easy-to-carry options include apples, pears, bananas, mandarin oranges or clementines, canned fruit cups, baby carrots, cherry or grape tomatoes,

ONE SERVING FRUITS & VEGETABLES	
	1 medium-sized fruit or vegetable (an apple, orange, carrot, or pear)
	½ cup (125 mL) raw, cooked, or frozen fruit or vegetable (a scoop of cooked peas or a small bowl of sliced peaches)
	½ cup (125 mL) juice (a small glass of orange or tomato juice)
	1 cup (250 mL) salad (a small side salad)
	¼ cup (60 mL) dried fruit (a medium-sized handful of raisins)

RESEARCH HIGHLIGHT
In the DASH study (Dietary Approach to Stop Hypertension), consuming 8 to 10 servings of vegetables and fruit each day—along with an overall healthy diet—was associated with a decrease in blood pressure normally only achieved with the use of medication. Potassium is just one of the nutrients found in fruits and vegetables that helps maintain blood pressure health.

QUESTION OF THE DAY
"I like fruit, but I'm not too keen on veggies. Can I get my 7 to 10 daily servings by eating just fruit?" Not a good idea for two reasons. First, because vegetables generally contain fewer calories than fruit, they should make up at least half of your daily produce intake. Second, because different kinds of vegetables and fruit contain different kinds of nutrients and beneficial plant compounds, eating a wide variety of both is your best bet for optimal disease protection.

GOOD ADVICE
Become famous for the wonderful fruit and veggie trays you bring to parties. Let everyone get healthy together!

dried fruits, and grapes. Carrying a small pack of wet wipes with you is also a good idea—it makes cleanup a breeze.

3 Eliminate the competition. The more cookies, chips, and candy you have in your cupboards or your desk at work, the less likely you are to reach for fruits or vegetables (sad, but true). Keep unhealthy but tempting goodies out of sight and out of reach (better yet, don't keep them around at all!). Then make the good stuff easy to see—and reach for. Keep a bowl filled with fruit on your kitchen counter at home and on your desk at work. Your family and co-workers will thank you for it. Always have baby carrots or cut-up veggies in your fridge. Make them the first thing you see when you (or your kids) open the fridge door.

4 Make room for frozen and canned. Who said canned or frozen fruits and vegetables aren't quality nutritional choices? On the contrary, these vegetables and fruits are harvested at their peak of ripeness and prepared for canning or freezing within hours of being picked. This guarantees great nutrition as well as great taste. In contrast, fresh produce—especially during the winter months—can lose valuable nutrients during travel and storage time. In one study, frozen spinach, after one year, was found to retain more than twice the vitamin C of fresh spinach from the same crop

that had been in the refrigerator for just seven days. Because most frozen vegetables are made with no added salt, they're a better choice than canned vegetables.

5 Put on your chef hat. Who likes soggy, overcooked, unseasoned vegetables? Yuck. So don't eat them that way. In the traditional Mediterranean diet, vegetables are considered tasty and delicious (even by children!). That's because they're served using herbs, spices, and other seasonings to create a variety of flavours and colours. Vegetables should look and taste great. Help your veggies come alive with garlic, ginger, or onions. Nutmeg or cinnamon compliment squash, carrots, and sweet potatoes. Best advice: try every vegetable recipe in this book (we'll make a veggie lover out of you yet!).

6 Order right when dining out. Research shows that people who dine out eat significantly less fruits and vegetables—especially at fast-food restaurants. To prevent this from happening:

» Order a salad as an appetizer or even as a main course. Ask for low-fat or light dressing on the side so you can control how much you consume.

» Ask whether the entrée comes with vegetables. If not, order extra veggies on the side (french fries don't count!).

QUESTION OF THE DAY
"Should I avoid avocados since they're so high in fat?" Absolutely not. Avocados contain important health-protective nutrients like potassium, folate, beta-carotene, lutein, vitamins K and E, as well as beneficial plant sterols. They're high in fat and calories (one whole avocado will set you back about 300 calories and 30 grams of fat). However, the type of fat they contain is primarily heart-healthy monounsaturated fat. My advice: enjoy avocados in small quantities as a replacement to other sources of fat in your diet. Have mashed avocado instead of butter or cream cheese on your bread or bagel. Instead of mayo, enjoy a few slices of avocado in your sandwich. When using a fat-free dressing on your salad, add some diced avocado.

GOOD ADVICE
Most people fail to meet potassium needs, an especially important nutrient for healthy blood pressure. Fruits and vegetables rich in potassium include bananas, potatoes, sweet potatoes, dried fruits, winter squash, cantaloupe, kiwi, orange juice, tomato juice, pomegranate juice, and prune juice.

» Supplement take-out dinners with vegetables and fruit from home. Microwaved veggies are fast and easy, and canned fruit like mandarin orange sections make a quick dessert.

7 Sensational smoothies. They're great for kids and adults alike. All you need is a blender and your imagination. Mix ½ cup (125 mL) of your favourite fresh or frozen fruits with 1 cup (250 mL) low-fat milk, soy milk, yogurt, or fruit juice. Use more fruit for a thicker smoothie. Give Mairlyn's sensational smoothie recipes on pages 266–68 a whirl. Beware of store-bought smoothies: they often contain only small amounts of real fruit and lots of added sugar.

8 Go for convenience. Pre-washed, pre-bagged salads make it easy to enjoy salad every single day of the year. Ready-to-serve veggie trays and fruit platters, as well as pre-chopped or pre-shredded veggies and fruits, are widely available at most supermarkets. Don't let cleaning and chopping come between you and your produce.

9 Double up. If you normally take one scoop of peas, take two. Instead of four spears of asparagus, have eight. It doesn't get any easier than this!

10 Dip and dunk. Raw veggies were born to be dipped (most kids would agree!). Go wild with carrot sticks, red pepper strips, and broccoli or cauliflower florets and serve them with a creamy light or low-fat salad dressing. Fresh fruit such as bananas, berries, or orange sections taste great dipped in low-fat, fruit-flavoured yogurt or low-fat chocolate pudding.

The Organic Debate

Should you buy organic produce? Let's look at both sides of the debate.

Why You May Not Need to Buy Organic:

» The American Cancer Society says, "At present there is no evidence that residues of pesticides at the low doses found in foods increase the risk of cancer."

» The American Institute for Cancer Research says, "Recent science indicates that the benefits of eating a wide variety of vegetables and fruits each day far outweigh any risks associated with pesticide residues."

» Simple household preparation, like rinsing and scrubbing, can remove anywhere from 30 to 100% of pesticide residues.

» Based on a report from the Environmental Working Group, the following fruits and vegetables are least likely to contain pesticide

QUESTION OF THE DAY

"What's the best type of fruit juice to drink?" That's a tough question. Orange juice gets top marks for its vitamin C, folate, and potassium content, plus the fact you can buy it calcium-enriched (most of us, including children and teens, are sorely lacking when it comes to calcium). Purple grape juice (made from concord grapes) is especially high in disease-fighting antioxidants, pomegranate juice even more so. My advice: enjoy ½ cup (125 mL) of orange juice in the morning and ½ cup (125 mL) of pomegranate juice later in the day. Mixing them together for an orange/pomegranate juice combo is also an option.

GOOD ADVICE

Frozen and canned veggies and fruit offer great nutrition and save you money and time. To limit sodium, buy frozen vegetables with no added salt instead of canned veggies. Avoid frozen veggies with high fat sauces. Buy canned fruit packed in its own juice or light syrup.

residues: asparagus, avocados, bananas, broccoli, cauliflower, corn, kiwi, mangos, onions, papaya, pineapples, and peas.

» Organic produce is more expensive and less widely available.

Why you may want to consider organic:

» Switching to organic produce can result in lower pesticide levels in the body.

» Exposure to pesticides poses a greater health risk to children and pregnant women.

» Organic produce may contain higher quantities of disease fighting, antioxidant-rich plant compounds such as flavonoids.

» Based on a report from the Environmental Working Group, the following fruits and vegetables are most likely to contain pesticide residues: apples, bell peppers, celery, cherries, imported grapes, nectarines, peaches, pears, potatoes, red raspberries, spinach, and strawberries.

Bottom line: for the most vulnerable groups, children and pregnant women, buying organic produce is a reasonable decision, especially when buying those fruits or vegetables that are more likely to contain pesticide residues. For the rest of us, if affordable, buying organic may be beneficial, and certainly can't hurt. Most important advice: don't stop eating your fruits and vegetables and be sure to thoroughly rinse and scrub them under running water before eating.

The Colour of Nutrition

For ultimate health eat a wide variety of dark green, orange, red, and purple/black fruits and vegetables.

When it comes to fruits and vegetables, colour is an excellent indication of nutritional content and disease-fighting potential. Brightly coloured fruits and veggies are generally higher in nutrients and beneficial plant compounds that fight disease. This is especially so when both the skin and flesh are bright in colour. Here's a list of produce that deserves to be featured on your daily menu:

Dark Green: asparagus, artichokes, broccoli, Brussels sprouts, green peppers, kiwis, and dark leafy greens like spinach, kale, and romaine

Orange: apricots, cantaloupes, carrots, oranges, mangos, papayas, pumpkins, squash, and sweet potatoes

Red: apples, cherries, cranberries, red or pink grapefruits, red cabbage, red peppers, strawberries, raspberries, tomatoes, and watermelon

Purple/Black: blackberries, dates, plums, and prunes

Disease-Fighting Superstars

For ultimate health enjoy each of the following foods at least three times per week: apples, berries, broccoli, pomegranate juice, spinach, and tomato-based foods.

An Apple a Day *Does* Keep the Doctor Away

Apples are available year-round. They're convenient, great for eating on the run, inexpensive, and children rank them as their favourite fruit. And that's not the best news. Apples are loaded with antioxidant-rich flavonoids. The antioxidant activity of one apple is equivalent to about 1,500 mg of vitamin C. Preliminary research—including human, animal, and test tube studies—has found that apples may:

» reduce the risk of heart disease or stroke by lowering and preventing damage to LDL (bad) cholesterol, as well as prevent the formation of harmful blood clots

» prevent the development and spread of numerous cancers, including cancers of the lung, prostate, and breast

» protect the health of the aging brain

» reduce inflammation

» reduce the risk of asthma and allergies

The key to healthy apple eating is to eat the skin. The skin contains five times more disease-fighting flavonoids. Red Delicious and Granny Smith apples are especially high in these antioxidants. Apple juice is not. For something different, try dusting apple slices with cinnamon (my kids love them this way) or serve them with thin slices of reduced-fat, aged cheddar cheese.

When in Doubt, Eat Broccoli

"Broccoli harbours what could be the most powerful anti-cancer compound ever detected." This was front page news of the *New York Times* in March, 1992. We've been on a broccoli feeding frenzy ever since—definitely a good thing. Broccoli is a member of the cruciferous family. Other cruciferous vegetables include Brussels sprouts, bok choy, cabbage, cauliflower, collards, kale, rutabaga, and turnips (enjoy them all!). Broccoli and kale rank highest in this group in terms of overall nutritional value; however, all cruciferous vegetables have one thing in common: they contain potent anti-cancer compounds called indoles and isothiocyanates (sulforaphane is one of the best-known isothiocyanates). These cancer-fighting compounds block the enzymes in the body involved in the initial stages of cancer development and help detoxify carcinogens (cancer-causing compounds) before they damage your cells. They also help stop cancer cells from

DRIED FRUITS

QUESTION OF THE DAY
"Are dried fruits good for you?" Yes, in small quantities. When the water is removed from fruit, the fruit generally becomes more concentrated in vitamins, minerals, and fibre. However, water-soluble nutrients like vitamin C are lost during processing. Dried fruits are a great eat-on-the-run snack and most are loaded with antioxidants. Dates and prunes (dried plums) rival berries in their ability to fight cell-damaging free radicals. The downside is that dried fruit is also concentrated in sugar and calories. Limit yourself to no more than one serving (¼ cup/60 mL) per day.

spreading and cause them to self-destruct (also referred to as cell suicide). Cruciferous vegetables are linked to a lower risk of many types of cancer, including lung, prostate, colon, stomach, ovarian, and breast. Encouraging girls to eat their broccoli during their teen years—the time when breast tissue is forming—may help reduce their breast cancer risk later in life. Lastly, a broccoli-rich diet may also lower the risk of heart disease and stroke, protect brain and eye health, and kill the type of bacteria that causes stomach ulcers.

Should you eat your broccoli raw or cooked? Research suggests the anti-cancer compounds in cruciferous vegetables are more available to your body when they're eaten raw or lightly steamed. Most important, don't boil them. The compounds are water-soluble and will be lost in the water. If you love cheese on your broccoli, don't despair. A small serving (1 Tbsp/15 mL) of a product like Cheez Whiz Light, contains about 30 calories and just over 1 gram of fat. I know with my kids, a lot more broccoli goes down when a bit of cheese sauce is along for the ride. Another great way to enjoy steamed broccoli is with a squeeze of lemon juice and a sprinkle of Parmesan cheese.

Popeye Was Right—Eat Your Spinach!

Popeye the sailorman had it right—spinach is good for you! Cornell University agrees. They put spinach at the top of the list as the vegetable we should eat more often based on its exceptional antioxidant profile and ability to suppress cancer. Here are four great reasons to make this nutritional powerhouse a regular part of your day:

1 Spinach is a cancer-fighting superstar. It's loaded with carotenoids like beta-carotene, the B vitamin folate, and a large supply of antioxidant-rich plant compounds.

2 A daily helping of spinach is what the eye doctor orders to reduce your risk of cataracts and macular degeneration. Spinach, along with other dark leafy greens, is rich in lutein and zeaxanthin. These nutrients absorb the sun's most damaging ultraviolet rays and stop nasty free radicals from damaging eye tissues.

3 The folate in spinach fights more than just cancer. It can slash your risk of heart disease and Alzheimer's as well as reduce your risk of having a baby with neural tube defects during pregnancy.

4 Vitamin K doesn't get the attention it deserves. It plays a crucial role in bone strength, blood clot-

APPLES

RESEARCH HIGHLIGHT
In a Harvard study involving over 38,000 women, those who consumed one or more apples per day were 28% less likely to develop type 2 diabetes.

RESEARCH HIGHLIGHT
In a study from Cornell University, rats were injected with a cancer-causing agent and fed the human diet equivalent of one, three, or six apples a day. The risk of breast cancer was reduced by 17%, 39%, and 44% respectively.

ting, and heart health by preventing hardening of the arteries. To maximize your intake of this often neglected nutrient, eat spinach.

Make it easy to eat spinach or other dark leafy greens more often. Always have pre-washed, pre-bagged spinach on hand, along with your favourite light or low-fat salad dressing. I make a big batch of Mairlyn's Unbelievably Delicious Raspberry Salad Dressing (page 144) and use it all week long. Don't forget to try Mairlyn's spinach recipes on pages 147–48.

Blueberries: Berry Good for the Brain

And the award for "the most delicious anti-oxidant-boosting food on the planet" goes to (drum roll please) . . . berries! I'm talking black-berries, raspberries, strawberries, cranberries, and of course, the antioxidant all-star, the blueberry. Berries are mega-stars in the antioxidant world. Perhaps the most exciting news, however, is the potential of berries to protect your brain. In animal studies from Tufts University, blueberries improved motor skills (balance and co-ordination) and reversed short-term memory loss that comes with aging. A blueberry-rich diet prevented symptoms of Alzheimer's in mice that were genetically programmed to develop the disease. And

in research from the University of South Florida, mice that were fed blueberries suffered 50% less stroke-induced brain damage. Berries appear to protect the brain through multiple mechanisms. They shield against free radical damage, reduce inflammation, enhance brain cell communication, increase the formation of new brain cells, and even result in new pathways within the brain. Pretty incredible if you ask me! Bottom line: if you're not a berry eater, I suggest you become one.

All types of berries can fit into a healthy diet. Fresh, dried, frozen, and cooked berries all demonstrate excellent antioxidant activity. I enjoy a large serving of blueberries on my cereal every morning (I buy frozen when fresh isn't available and let them thaw in a bowl overnight in the fridge). Frozen berries are also perfect for whipping up into tasty smoothies. For a treat, heat berries in the microwave and serve over low-fat frozen yogurt.

Pomegranate Juice: The Miracle Worker

A recent advertising campaign for pomegranate juice claims, "Not all miracle workers are people." I was a skeptic at first. Now I'm a believer. The research is simply too impressive to ignore. From heart disease, to cancer, to brain health, pomegranate juice is a truly exciting food. It contains more

RESEARCH HIGHLIGHT
Iceberg lettuce is a nutritional weakling. Romaine is better. Spinach is best. Darker greens mean more nutrition and better defense against disease. Spinach, for example, contains about 4 times more potassium, 7 times more folate, 8 times more vitamin E and vitamin C, 18 times more vitamin A, 20 times more vitamin K, and 44 times more lutein and zeaxanthin than iceberg lettuce.

Other great greens include kale, collards, swiss chard, turnip greens, mustard greens, and beet greens. Eat up.

RESEARCH HIGHLIGHT
Researchers from Johns Hopkins University School of Medicine have determined that broccoli sprouts contain about 20 times more cancer-fighting compounds than mature broccoli. As a result, they now grow and sell

these sprouts (www.brassica.com). Is there a downside? Raw sprouts of any kind can be a source of harmful bacteria and can cause food poisoning. People who are more vulnerable to infection, including young children and older adults, should avoid them.
P.S. Mature broccoli contains considerably more vitamin C, vitamin A, and fibre than broccoli sprouts.

polyphenols (plant compounds with exceptional antioxidant activity) than beverages like red wine, blueberry juice, cranberry juice, and green tea. Here's why I recommend you drink it:

» It's great for your heart. It helps prevent the type of damage to your LDL (bad) cholesterol that allows it to penetrate and build up on artery walls. It also helps maintain healthy blood pressure.

» It helps fight cancer by preventing the development and spread of cancerous cells.

» It boosts immunity and may stop you from getting sick through its ability to kill viruses.

» It provides excellent brain protection. When consumed by a mother during pregnancy, it may even protect her baby's brain.

» It may reduce your risk of inflammatory diseases like arthritis by protecting cartilage and other tissues.

While I generally recommend eating whole fruits rather than fruit juice, pomegranate juice is the exception to the rule. Because the entire fruit is crushed to make the juice, including the skin, the juice contains more antioxidants and beneficial plant compounds. Pomegranate juice, however, is a concentrated source of sugar and calories containing about 160 calories and 8½ teaspoons (45 mL) of naturally-occurring sugar per 1 cup (250 mL). Have no more than about ½ cup (125 mL) each day. If you suffer from heart disease, 1 cup (250 mL) daily is acceptable. And don't forget to try the Purple Pomegranate Smoothie on page 268.

Tomatoes' Secret Ingredient: Lycopene

There's one very good reason to enjoy processed tomato products like tomato sauce, tomato juice, and salsa: lycopene. Lycopene is a plant compound belonging to the carotenoid family (other famous carotenoids include beta-carotene and lutein). Lycopene demonstrates the highest antioxidant activity of all carotenoids. Its strongest claim to fame is its potential to reduce the risk of some cancers, especially prostate cancer. It's also good for the heart. In the Harvard Health Professionals Follow-up Study involving almost 47,000 men, having tomato products like tomato sauce and pizza four times a week was associated with a 34% lower risk of prostate cancer. In a similar study involving almost 40,000 women, a daily serving of tomato-based foods was linked to a 30% lower risk of heart disease.

The key to getting more lycopene in your diet is to increase your intake of processed tomato products. Although raw tomatoes, as well as watermelon, papaya, pink guava, and pink or red

BERRIES

RESEARCH HIGHLIGHT
Cranberries—including cranberry juice, dried cranberries, and even cranberry sauce—help prevent urinary tract infections by stopping bacteria from adhering to the bladder wall.

QUESTION OF THE DAY
"Are blueberries the best berry to eat?" All berries are antioxidant all-stars; however, blueberries, especially wild blueberries, are considered the leaders of the pack. However, some researchers predict that "purple" berries like elderberries, black currants, and chokeberries may soon start making headlines because they too are chock full of antioxidants.

grapefruit all provide lycopene, processed tomato products, like tomato sauce and tomato juice, contain the most. During processing, heat breaks down the cell walls of tomatoes, making the lycopene more available for your body to absorb. The easiest way to get more lycopene in your diet—even on the busiest days—is with a small glass or can of tomato juice. Remember, processed tomato products can be high in sodium, so go for low-sodium options when possible.

GOOD ADVICE

Don't drink tomato juice by itself. Have it with a meal or snack that contains some fat. That way your body can better absorb the health-protective lycopene that tomatoes are famous for. A small handful of nuts and a glass of tomato juice make an awesome snack combination. The same advice goes for other carotenoid-rich fruits and vegetables. For example, to get more beta-carotene from baby carrots enjoy them with a small amount of low-fat or light dip.

ULTIMATE FOODS FOR ULTIMATE HEALTH

Enjoy 7 to 10 servings of fruits and vegetables daily. Limit fruit juice to no more than 1 cup (250 mL) per day. Eat a wide variety of dark green, orange, red, and purple/black fruits and vegetables. For maximum disease protection, have each of the following at least three times per week: apples, berries, broccoli, pomegranate juice, spinach, and tomato-based foods.

POMEGRANATE JUICE

RESEARCH HIGHLIGHT

In a study from the Lipid Research Laboratory in Israel, 10 patients with heart disease consumed 1 cup (250 mL) of pomegranate juice daily for one year. Thickness of the artery wall was reduced by as much as 30% and systolic blood pressure by 21%.

Dr. Michael Aviram, one of the lead researchers, concluded, "The potential exists for high-risk patients to be spared bypass surgery simply by drinking pomegranate juice."

SPICE UP YOUR LIFE

FOR ULTIMATE HEALTH

» Optimizeyour intake of herbs,
  spices, onions, and garlic.

» Limityour intake of sodium (salt).

THREE REASONS TO SEASON

There are three excellent reasons to increase your intake of various herbs, spices, onions, and garlic. First, herbs and spices are an exceptional source of disease-fighting antioxidants. Second, these foods contain an assortment of beneficial plant compounds that protect against heart disease, cancer, diabetes, and more. Third, these foods add so much wonderful flavour to food that you can use less salt, thus lowering your risk of high blood pressure. There's never been a better time to spice up your life.

The Antioxidant Power of Herbs and Spices

For ultimate health increase your intake of a wide variety of herbs and spices.

Since ancient times, herbs and spices have been used to flavour food, but more importantly, they've been considered essential tools for fighting illness and disease. Herbs and spices are loaded with health-protective plant compounds called phenols and flavonoids. A recent study by the United States Department of Agriculture found that herbs and spices rival the antioxidant content of fruits and vegetables. Their plentiful supply of antioxidants enables them to wage war against cell-damaging free radicals before they cause disease. Herbs and spices also help boost our immunity by fending off viruses and bacteria. They can reduce our risk of cancer by impacting enzymes in the body involved in the development and spread of cancer. A wide variety of herbs and spices have beneficial effects, including allspice, basil, cumin, ginger, rosemary,

QUOTE OF THE DAY
"Adding a moderate amount of herbs may go a long way toward boosting the health value of a meal, especially as an alternative to salt and artificial additives."
—Shiow Wang, United States Department of Agriculture

QUOTE OF THE DAY
"The cancer-protective antioxidant power of herbs and spices is at least as great as that of fruits & vegetables."
—American Institute of Cancer Research

RESEARCH HIGHLIGHT
Flavonoids are health-protective plant compounds that fight disease. Herbs and spices commonly used in the traditional Mediterranean diet, although added in small quantities, significantly contribute to flavonoid intake due to their frequent consumption.

sage, thyme, bay leaf, dill, marjoram, tarragon, and peppermint. Certain herbs and spices, however, like cloves, cinnamon, oregano, and turmeric are gaining superstar status in the seasoning world.

The Seasoning Superstars

For ultimate health make cloves, cinnamon, oregano, and turmeric a regular part of your diet.

Cloves, cinnamon, oregano, and turmeric are at the top of the list of antioxidant-rich herbs and spices. They excel in their ability to prevent diseases caused by free radicals. They're exceptional at boosting immunity by killing a wide variety of bacteria and viruses. They're linked to an improvement in insulin sensitivity (less insulin is required to move sugar out of the blood and into the cells). This may help in the prevention and management of diabetes. Their strong anti-inflammatory action holds promise for reducing the risk of inflammatory disorders such as rheumatoid arthritis. Turmeric, in particular, appears to be a potent cancer fighter. It slows the spread of cancer, the growth of new cancer cells, and causes cancer cells to die. Diets rich in turmeric are linked to a lower risk of breast, prostate, lung, and colon cancer.

Spice Up Your Day

» Sprinkle ground cinnamon on apple slices or oatmeal.

» Add ¼ to ½ teaspoon (1 to 2 mL) of ground cinnamon or cloves to shakes or smoothies.

» Add whole cloves and cinnamon sticks to your pot of tea.

» Add a variety of herbs and spices to salad dressings and meat marinades.

» Use recipes that feature turmeric (most often found in curry powder), cinnamon, cloves, or oregano. Many of the baked goods in this book are chock full of cinnamon.

Please Note

Although fresh herbs are generally higher in antioxidants, dried herbs and spices still demonstrate excellent antioxidant potential. Dried herbs and spices should be used within six months of purchase. Buy the smallest quantities you can and store in airtight containers away from heat and light.

Health Promoting Onions & Garlic

For ultimate health make onions and garlic a regular part of your diet.

GOOD ADVICE
By adding herbs and spices to your salad dressing, you can increase the antioxidant power of your salad by as much as 200%.

RESEARCH HIGHLIGHT
Turmeric, a spice often found in curry powder, has been called the "wonder spice." In a review of 300 papers by a researcher from the University College of London, turmeric was linked to a lower risk of many diseases including heart disease, cancer, diabetes, Parkinson's, and cataracts. The study concluded there's ample evidence that the consumption of turmeric both prevents and treats disease.

RESEARCH HIGHLIGHT
In a study from the Beltsville Human Nutrition Research Center, 60 people with type 2 diabetes consumed either ½, 1, or 2½ teaspoons (2, 5, or 12 mL) of cinnamon daily. After 40 days, all levels of cinnamon intake resulted in significant decreases in blood sugar levels, triglycerides, and LDL (bad) cholesterol. Dr. Richard Anderson, the lead researcher, called it one of the most significant nutritional discoveries he had seen in 25 years.

Garlic may stink and onions may make you cry, but they're well worth adding to your diet. Onions and garlic, as well as leeks and chives, are all members of the allium family. They contain important sulfur compounds linked to a lower risk of cancer and heart disease. These compounds help activate enzymes in the body that help detoxify cancer-causing compounds before they damage cells. They also help prevent cancer through their effects on cell growth and reproduction. By reducing the "stickiness" of the blood, they lower the risk of potentially deadly blood clots that lead to heart attack or stroke. Both raw and cooked onions and garlic appear to provide health benefits and are used in many of the recipes in this book. Onions are also an important source of health-protective flavonoids in the diet.

Sodium: Enough Already

For ultimate health lower your sodium intake by adding less salt to foods, but more importantly, by reducing your intake of high sodium processed, packaged, and fast foods.

Salt has been called one of the deadliest ingredients in the food supply. It leads to stroke, heart attack, heart failure, and kidney disease. In excess, it's also linked to a higher risk of stomach cancer and may be detrimental to bone health. Here's the problem: time-crunched families that rely on packaged or processed foods, and make fast food a regular part of their lifestyle, are eating sodium by the truck-load (slight exaggeration). In fact, over 75% of consumed sodium comes from processed or packaged foods, as well as food from restaurants. The other 25% comes from salt added during cooking or at the table, as well as the sodium that's naturally present in food.

So, how much sodium should you be eating? Most people should aim for less than 2,300 mg of sodium each day (about 1 teaspoon/5 mL of salt) and ideally closer to 1,500 mg. Because some people are more sensitive to the blood pressure-raising effects of sodium than others—including older adults, African Americans, and those who already suffer from high blood pressure, diabetes, or kidney disease—they should limit their daily sodium intake to 1,500 mg or less.

Sodium Shakedown

The vast majority of people in North America are eating way too much sodium. Here are 15 tips to help you slash the salt from your diet:

1 Become an avid label reader. Sodium is a hidden ingredient in many processed or packaged foods, even those that don't taste salty. Use your daily sodium limit of 2,300 mg as your benchmark.

RESEARCH HIGHLIGHT
Curcumin is the active ingredient in turmeric and is responsible for its yellow colour. Researchers from UCLA and the Department of Veterans Affairs concluded that curcumin may be a powerful weapon against Alzheimer's disease. Curcumin slowed the accumulation of plaque and broke up existing plaque in the brains of mice (the type of destructive plaque associated with Alzheimer's).

GOOD ADVICE
When you eat meat cooked at high temperatures, it can cause your cells to produce an enzyme that causes cancer. Garlic can help prevent this enzyme from forming. Add garlic to your homemade hamburger patties and steak marinades.

RESEARCH HIGHLIGHT
Researchers from Cornell University found pungent onion varieties like New York Bold, Western Yellow, and shallots have the highest antioxidant activity and are the best for inhibiting the growth of cancer cells. The sweetest tasting onions, including the beloved Vidalia, showed little cancer-fighting ability.

2 Look for soups or frozen dinners that contain less than 500 to 600 mg per serving (this is still not low-sodium, but is about as good as it gets). Choose snack foods like crackers, popcorn, or nuts that are unsalted or low in sodium (120 mg per serving or less).

3 Compare brands. Sodium content can vary tremendously for the same food from one brand to another.

4 Add little or no salt to meals or in cooking.

5 Buy "no added salt," "reduced-sodium," or "low-sodium" packaged foods.

6 Limit intake of ham, bacon, sausage, hot dogs, and most deli or processed meats.

7 Look for low-sodium salad dressings, or try the salad dressings in this book.

8 Limit cured, smoked, and pickled foods.

9 Buy lower-sodium processed tomato products, including tomato sauce, tomato juice, and salsa.

10 Drain and rinse canned beans.

11 Use nutrition information available from fast food restaurants to choose lower-sodium options. At restaurants where this information isn't available, ask your server if menu items can be prepared without salt and for sauces and dressings to be served on the side.

12 Rice and pasta are naturally low in sodium, but those sold in boxes with added ingredients are often salt landmines.

13 Eat higher sodium foods, like cheese, in small quantities.

14 Eat more fresh foods like whole fruits, vegetables, meat, poultry, and fish.

15 Last, but certainly not least, don't forget to season your foods with lemon or lime juice, vinegars, garlic, onions, herbs, and spices. Consider ready-made herb and spice mixtures, like Mrs. Dash.

HEALTHY BLOOD PRESSURE

QUOTE OF THE DAY
"There is clear evidence that salt intake is linked to high blood pressure—one of the main risk factors for heart disease. It remains important for people to reduce levels of salt in food preparation and at the table."
—Peter Hollins, Director General of the British Heart Foundation

GOOD ADVICE
If you want healthy blood pressure, slashing sodium isn't enough. You also need to maintain a healthy weight and exercise regularly. If you consume alcohol, do so in moderation (one to two drinks daily). Make sure your diet is rich in foods containing calcium, magnesium, and especially potassium—three nutrients that play an important role in blood pressure health.

SODIUM INTAKE

GOOD ADVICE

If your diet is loaded with salt, the best way to cut back is slowly but surely. Studies show that a gradual reduction in sodium intake over 8 to 12 weeks decreases the desire for salty foods.

RESEARCH HIGHLIGHT

The DASH-Sodium trial (Dietary Approach to Stop Hypertension) looked at the effect of a high, medium, and low-sodium intake (3,300 mg, 2,400 mg, and 1,500 mg per day) on blood pressure. Results were consistent: the greater the reduction in sodium, the greater the reduction in blood pressure.

RESEARCH HIGHLIGHT

In the Northern Manhattan Study, consuming more than 4,000 mg of sodium daily—a typical intake for many North Americans—was linked to a 90% higher risk of stroke. The risk was consistent regardless of whether or not the person had high blood pressure.

A "WHOLE" LOT MORE
WITH WHOLE GRAINS

FOR ULTIMATE HEALTH

» Optimize your intake of whole grain foods.

» Optimize your intake of whole grain
  cereals.

» Limit your intake of refined grains.

THE "WHOLE" FOOD

Thousands of years ago in ancient Rome bread was made using only part of the grain (white bread) rather than the whole grain (whole grain bread). Wealthy Romans preferred this more expensive and exclusive white bread. Darker breads were considered food for the poor. The Romans had it wrong. They were unaware of what I refer to as one of the golden rules of nutrition—for better health you've got to eat the "whole" food. Whole grains fight heart disease, stroke, cancer, and diabetes as well as help you maintain a healthy body weight. In contrast, refined grains like white bread are tied to a higher risk of disease.

The Whole Grain Story

All grains, whether from wheat, oats, rice, barley, or other sources, are made up of three parts: the bran, the endosperm, and the germ. Each part contributes something special. When grains are refined to make foods like white bread or white rice, the bran and germ are discarded. Here's the problem. When you throw away the bran and the germ, you throw away a whole lot of the good stuff. For example, over 80% of the health-protective plant compounds (many which demonstrate potent antioxidant activity) are found in the bran and germ. Many nutrients are found there as well. We can see this by comparing the nutritional value of white flour to whole wheat flour. Whole wheat flour contains:

» 2 times more calcium and selenium

» 3 times more copper and phosphorus

» 4 times more potassium, zinc, and fibre

RESEARCH HIGHLIGHT
In the Iowa Women's Health Study involving over 11,000 postmenopausal women, the risk of dying from any cause—including heart disease and cancer—was found to be significantly lower in women who ate more whole grains than refined grains.

QUESTION OF THE DAY
"I've heard it's not good to eat foods that are high on the glycemic index. What types of foods should I avoid?" The glycemic index is a measure of how fast a particular food is likely to raise your blood sugar. Some studies suggest that people who eat a lot of foods with a high glycemic index may increase their risk of heart disease, diabetes, some cancers, and even obesity. Generally, less refined whole grain products, especially barley and oats, have a lower glycemic index. Most important advice? Enjoy a wide variety of whole grains, whole fruits and vegetables, and beans (all healthy sources of carbohydrates). Eat smaller, more frequent meals. Limit the amount of highly processed, refined grains you eat. Maintain a healthy weight and exercise regularly.

» 6 times more magnesium

» 12 times more lutein and zeaxanthin

» 14 times more vitamin E

The Bottom Line
With whole grains you get a whole lot more.

Please Note
Whole grains are also naturally higher in iron and B vitamins, including folate. These nutrients, however, are added back to white flour. That's why we say white flour is "enriched."

Health Protection and Whole Grains
How do whole grains reduce your risk of heart disease, cancer, diabetes, and more? Like fruits and vegetables, whole grains contain a complex mix of disease-fighting vitamins, minerals, fibre, and beneficial plant compounds. Here are just some of the ways they protect your health.

Creates a Healthy Gut Environment
Whole grains are rich sources of fermentable carbohydrates, including fibre, resistant starch, and oligosaccharides. A fermentable carbohydrate is one that resists digestion until it reaches your colon, where it serves as food for the bacteria there.

During this fermentation process, health-protective substances (short chain fatty acids) are produced, which provide numerous benefits. For example, they inhibit the growth of cancerous tumors in the gut.

Keeps Things Moving Along
People who eat a lot of whole grains are much less likely to suffer from constipation. The fibre in whole grains increases stool bulk. This promotes quicker elimination of body wastes, reducing the amount of time the colon is exposed to potential cancer-causing substances. Whole grains also reduce hemorrhoids and diverticular disease (pouches or pockets that form in the wall of the colon). It's been said that we spend about three years of our life in the bathroom. Shouldn't those years be as enjoyable as possible?

Lowers Cholesterol
Whole grains decrease LDL (bad) cholesterol levels, thereby reducing the buildup of plaque on artery walls. Oats, rye, barley, and psyllium are highest in the type of fibre (soluble fibre) linked to cholesterol lowering. Whole grains also help maintain a healthy blood pressure and reduce injury to blood vessel walls.

Contains Health-Protective Nutrients & Plant Compounds
Whole grains are an important source of disease

WHOLE GRAINS

RESEARCH HIGHLIGHT
In the Harvard Male Health Professionals Study involving over 42,000 men, those who consumed the most whole grains were 18% less likely to suffer from heart disease. Men with the highest intake of added bran slashed their risk of heart disease risk by 30%.

RESEARCH HIGHLIGHT
In the Harvard Nurses' Health Study involving about 75,000 women, those who ate the most whole grains reduced their risk of heart disease by 25%, stroke by over 30%, and diabetes by almost 40%. In addition, women who ate the most high-fibre whole grains

were almost 50% less likely to experience major weight gain over a 12-year period. In contrast, diets heavy in refined grains and low in whole grains were linked to an expanding waistline as well as an almost 60% greater diabetes risk.

fighting nutrients (vitamin E and selenium) and plant compounds (phenols, flavonoids, lignans, phytates), which act as potent antioxidants. Vitamin E and selenium are found in highest concentration in the germ, while many of the health-protective plant compounds are in the bran (the antioxidant power of wheat bran is 20 times greater than white flour). Antioxidants protect against cancer, heart disease, and even aging by reducing cell damage caused by free radicals.

Good for Blood Sugar

Whole grains contain a variety of substances—fibre, magnesium, and various plant compounds—that reduce the risk of diabetes. They improve insulin sensitivity (less insulin is required to move sugar out of the blood), enhance insulin secretion, and result in a slower, more sustained release of sugar into the blood.

Minimizes Your Waistline

Many studies link a smaller waistline to high fibre and whole grain foods. Whole grains are generally more slowly digested and absorbed. They fill you up and delay the return of hunger. In contrast, refined grains like white bread are linked to an expanding waistline, especially fat stored around the belly (the most dangerous type of body fat for your health).

ONE SERVING GRAINS	
	1 slice of bread
	½ hamburger bun, English muffin, small bagel
	half of a 6-inch (15-cm) pita bread
	one 6-inch (15-cm) tortilla
	½ cup (125 mL) cooked brown rice, barley, bulgur, or quinoa
	½ cup (125 mL) cooked pasta
	5 crackers
	one 4-inch (10-cm) pancake
	1 small muffin
	¾ cup (175 mL) cooked cereal
	1 oz (30 g) ready-to-eat cereal, equal to about ¾ to 1 cup (175 to 250 mL) of most cereals
	Be sure to look for 100% whole wheat or whole grain options.

Going for Grains

For ultimate health enjoy 5 to 8 servings of grain products each day. Ideally all the servings should be whole grain.

RESEARCH HIGHLIGHT
In a study from The National Institute of Environmental Medicine in Sweden involving over 60,000 women, those who ate 5 or more servings of whole grains a day were 33% less likely to develop cancer of the colon.

RESEARCH HIGHLIGHT
Metabolic syndrome has been called a cardiovascular disease time bomb. A person with metabolic syndrome has a cluster of the most dangerous heart attack risk factors, including abdominal obesity, high blood triglycerides, low HDL cholesterol, high blood pressure, and insulin resistance.

Several studies, including the Framingham Offspring Cohort Study involving almost 3,000 men and women, conclude that whole grain eaters have a significantly lower risk of metabolic syndrome. Refined grain eaters, on the other hand, have an increased risk.

But, Is It Really Whole Grain?

Choosing whole grain foods can be tricky. Food companies excel at making foods that aren't whole grain appear to be whole grain. Here are some tips to help you become a whole grain detective:

» Don't be fooled by beautiful pictures of whole grains on package labels or labels that say "multi-grain," "made with whole wheat," "whole grain blend," "source of whole grains," or "contains whole wheat." Numerous products, including many multi-grain or seven-grain breads, as well as many crackers, tortillas, pita breads, and bagels, are made with a mix of white flour and whole grains, often with white flour as the dominant ingredient. Look for labels that say "made with 100% whole grains."

» Read the list of ingredients. Avoid products that contain "wheat flour," "enriched flour," "unbleached flour," or "untreated flour." This is just another way for food companies to say "white flour." Look for products that say "whole wheat flour." Rolled, instant, quick, or steel-cut oats all qualify as whole grain. Degerminated or degermed corn or cornmeal aren't a whole grain. Neither is pearled barley.

» The Whole Grains Council (www.wholegrains council.org) considers the following foods and flours as whole grain: amaranth, barley, brown rice, buckwheat, bulgur, corn and whole corn- meal, emmer, farro, Kamut grain, millet, oat- meal and whole oats, popcorn, quinoa, sor- ghum, spelt, teff, triticale, whole rye, whole wheat, wheat berries, and wild rice.

» Choose whole grain products, but don't forget fibre. Look for products that contain a mini- mum of 2 grams of fibre per serving and ideally 4 to 6 grams of fibre or more.

Cereal: The Best Breakfast Choice

For ultimate health start most days with a bowl of high fibre, whole grain cereal. Here's why:

» People who eat cereal regularly are more likely to meet their daily nutrient requirements.

» The right cereal significantly boosts your fibre intake for the day.

» The average antioxidant activity of many whole grain cereals is equal to, or exceeds, many fruits and vegetables.

» People who eat cereal for breakfast are more likely to have a healthy body weight.

» Cereal served with milk helps contribute to your daily requirement of calcium and vitamin D— two nutrients most people don't get enough of.

BREADS + PASTA

QUESTION OF THE DAY
"Are rye or pumpernickel breads considered whole grain?" Many people mistakenly believe that if the bread is dark in colour it must be whole grain. Although some whole grain rye breads are available, many pumpernickel and rye products are made mostly with white flour and caramel, or another added colouring.

QUESTION OF THE DAY
"Is it better to buy breads that have been stone-ground?" Stone-ground refers to a technique for grinding grains. It usually means that the grain is coarser. Some research indicates that grains with a larger particle size are better for your health. If you buy stone-ground bread, make sure it's whole grain or whole wheat.

QUESTION OF THE DAY
"Is coloured pasta better for you than plain pasta?" No. When bits of spinach, tomatoes, or other vegetables are added to plain pasta dough to colour it, the amount used per serving is usually equivalent to about 1 teaspoon (5 mL). This amount has no significant nutritional value. The healthiest pasta you can eat is 100% whole grain or whole wheat.

» Whole grain cereal is linked to a significantly lower risk of death from heart disease and other causes. Cereal fibre has consistently been associated with a reduced risk of type 2 diabetes.

» Cereal is quick and fits easily into life in the fast lane.

Ten Terrific Tips for Building a Beautiful Bowl of Cereal

Consider these 10 essential steps before sitting down to your next bowl of cereal:

1 Choose a cereal that's made with 100% whole grains or a very high fibre bran cereal. Most bran cereals are technically not whole grain (they're made primarily with the bran portion of the grain), but they're still an excellent choice. Remember, when you eat the bran, which protects the grain from disease, insects, ultraviolet light, and harsh weather, it's also the part of the plant most protective of our health. That's why eating the skin on fruits and vegetables also makes such good sense.

2 Go for fibre. Most women need 25 grams of fibre per day, while most men need 38 grams. That's a challenging goal to reach, especially when you consider that most people average about 15 grams of fibre each day. Meeting your daily fibre quota is far more achievable when you start the day with a cereal that's fibre-rich. Cereals like All-Bran, All-Bran Buds, or Fibre 1 contribute as much as 12 grams of fibre per ½ cup (125 mL) serving. If you don't like these cereals on their own, consider mixing them with a whole grain cereal that you do like. I often mix All-Bran with Cheerios.

3 Hot cereals like oatmeal aren't as high in fibre as bran cereals. One serving (¾ cup/175 mL) contains 3 grams of fibre. Oatmeal is still a good choice since the type of fibre it contains helps lower blood cholesterol levels. To boost the fibre content, try sprinkling a tablespoon or two of wheat bran on your oatmeal.

4 Women, especially prior to menopause, may want to choose a cereal that's iron-enriched (iron will appear on the list of ingredients). Most cereals have added iron, with the exception of a few, like regular oatmeal (not instant oatmeal) and Shredded Wheat.

5 For extra disease-protection, as well as additional fibre, sprinkle 1 to 2 tablespoons (15 to 30 mL) of ground flaxseed on your cereal (more details about flax in the Fabulous Flax chapter).

6 Enjoy ½ to 1 cup (125 to 250 mL) of fresh fruit, such as blueberries, on your cereal. I use frozen wild blueberries, available all year round (I thaw them in the fridge overnight or microwave them

CONSUMING CARBS

QUESTION OF THE DAY
"I thought high carbohydrate diets were bad because they cause trigylcerides in your blood to go up—a risk factor for heart disease. Is this true?" Studies suggest that a diet high in refined carbohydrates (cakes, cookies, baked goods, and breads made with white flour) can increase blood triglyceride levels. However, a high carbohydrate diet that emphasizes whole grains, beans, and whole fruits and vegetables has a beneficial effect on triglyceride levels.

GOOD ADVICE
Looking for a whole grain snack? Popcorn and most low-fat baked tortilla chips are whole grain. Go easy on the toppings when it comes to popcorn. Enjoy baked tortilla chips with generous amounts of tomato-rich salsa.

briefly in the morning). A sliced banana or quarter cup of dried fruit like raisins are other great cereal additions.

7 Have skim or 1% milk with your cereal. With 2% or homogenized milk, too much artery-clogging saturated fat comes along for the ride.

8 What about sugar? The World Health Organization recommends no more than 10% of the calories we eat daily should come from "free sugars"—sugar added to foods and those naturally present in honey, syrups, and fruit juices. For most of us this means limiting sugar to about 10 teaspoons per day. Because sugar is added to so many foods, sticking to this daily quota can be a challenge. To determine the sugar content of any food, including cereal, divide the grams of sugar on the label by four to reach the amount of teaspoons (for example, a cereal with 16 grams of sugar per serving contains 4 teaspoons). Aim for cereals that contain two teaspoons or less per serving. If the cereal you buy is unsweetened, it's okay to add a teaspoon or two of sugar to your bowl. Sugar substitutes, like Splenda, are also an option.

9 Enjoy your cereal with a small glass of fruit juice—the vitamin C it contains will help you absorb more iron from the cereal.

10 Cereal isn't just a breakfast food. It makes a great after-school snack for kids and can even serve as supper on those days when you're just too exhausted to cook.

Five More Great Ways to Add Whole Grains to Your Day

Here are five more tips to assist you in your quest for whole grains:

1 It's challenging to find a muffin that's 100% whole grain at restaurants or grocery stores. Most restaurant or fast food muffins will also set you back about 400 calories and 30 grams of fat. Your best bet is to make your own muffins. To save time, make a double batch on weekends and pop them in the freezer in individual baggies. They thaw in no time. Be sure to try the muffin recipes in this book—they're loaded with good stuff and taste truly outstanding!

2 Why make a small batch of brown rice when you can make a bigger batch and enjoy it all week long? Cooked rice stores for up to five days in the fridge. Mairlyn has put together an incredible variety of quick and simple recipes for leftover brown rice. The Sensationally Simple Stir-Fried Rice on page 183 is one of my favourites.

BREAKFAST

QUESTION OF THE DAY
"How much oatmeal do I need to eat each day to lower the amount of cholesterol in my blood?" A review of 10 studies concluded that the daily consumption of 3 grams of soluble fibre from oat products results in lower blood cholesterol levels. To get that amount of soluble fibre you'd need to eat ½ cup (125 mL) of hot oat bran cereal, 1½ cups (375 mL) cooked oatmeal, three packets instant oatmeal, or 3 cups (750 mL) of Cheerios.

GOOD ADVICE
The best way to enjoy sugar is in small amounts to make healthy foods taste better. For example, have jam on your whole wheat toast, sugar on your whole grain cereal, or maple syrup on your whole grain pancakes. Avoid sugar-rich foods that are nutrient poor, like soft drinks, cakes, pies, cookies, and candy.

3 If you haven't switched to 100% whole wheat or whole grain pasta, what are you waiting for? They taste great and are significantly higher in fibre than regular pasta. I especially like the whole wheat spaghettini—the long and thin pasta. Serve it with a tomato-based sauce. Look for brands that are lower in sodium or try Mairlyn's Kid Friendly Spaghetti Sauce on page 197 (it's made with plum tomatoes and grape juice—it's amazing!). Stay away from artery-clogging alfredo or cream sauces. Pesto sauces made with olive oil are acceptable, but watch your serving size since they're a concentrated source of fat and calories.

4 A delicious way to start your Sunday morning is with a batch of whole grain pancakes (pages 287–91) or French toast (page 294). Serve them for dinner when you don't have time to prepare a more elaborate meal (my kids love whole grain pancakes—especially when I throw in a few chocolate chips). Try the "light" syrups, which contain about half the calories of regular syrup and still taste great.

5 Try new recipes that feature less familiar whole grains. Quinoa, for example, has a chewy texture and a nutty taste—a great alternative to brown rice. It's so rich in nutrients that some food experts refer to it as a super-grain. Mairlyn's Quinoa Pilaf on page 190 is quick, easy, and delicious. Wheat berries are whole kernels of wheat. They're fibre-rich and a great addition to soups and salads. The Blueberry Wheat Berry Salad on page 192 is super nutritious and has a wonderful crunchy texture. Barley, a great source of cholesterol-lowering soluble fibre, is another grain that can easily be added to soups or stews. The Barley Risotto on page 191 gets rave reviews every time it's made.

Pass On the White Bread

For ultimate health limit your intake of refined grains to no more than 1 to 2 servings daily. However, all your choices should ideally be whole grain.

While whole grains protect our health, research suggests that refined grains may be harmful to health—especially for people who are overweight or inactive. Refined grains lack many of the health-protective nutrients and plant compounds found in whole grains and may result in higher spikes in blood sugar levels. People who eat a lot of refined grains are more likely to suffer from diabetes, heart disease, and some cancers. They're also more likely to be overweight and to store fat around the belly. More fat around the waist indicates a significantly higher risk of many diseases.

How do you avoid refined grains? Read labels and limit your intake of breads, rolls, buns, English muffins, tortillas, and bagels made with white

RESEARCH HIGHLIGHT
Breakfast really may be the most important meal of the day. Researchers from the University of Florida reviewed 47 nutrition studies and concluded that children and teens who eat breakfast have superior overall diet quality, are less likely to be overweight, and have better mental function and school attendance records than those who skip the morning meal.

QUESTION OF THE DAY
"What is psyllium?" It's found in Kellogg's All-Bran Buds cereal, as well as laxatives such as Metamucil. People with high blood cholesterol levels or problems with regularity should consider making it a regular part of their diet.

flour. Many of the pancakes, waffles, muffins, crackers, cookies, cakes, and other baked goods found in restaurants and grocery stores are made with refined grains. The list of breakfast cereals that contain refined grains is very long and includes popular brands like Special K, Corn Flakes, and Rice Krispies. White rice, couscous, and basmati rice are all generally considered refined grains. However, whole wheat couscous and whole grain brown basmati are available in some stores.

Limiting your intake of refined grains can be particularly difficult if you dine out frequently. Many restaurants still serve primarily white bread or rolls, and whole wheat pasta is still nonexistent at most. Do your best by limiting your portion sizes and ask for whole grain options where possible.

Whole Grain, White Bread?

Are the new whole wheat white breads good for you? Relatively new to the market are breads made with white wheat rather than the traditional red wheat used to make most whole wheat products. White whole wheat has the same amount of fibre, vitamins, and minerals as red whole wheat, but its bran layer is lower in beneficial plant compounds like tannins and phenols. Studies from the University of Minnesota have shown that animals eating red wheat develop substantially fewer of the changes in cells lining the colon that precede colon cancer than animals consuming white wheat. In addition, many of the products made with white wheat (may be listed as ultragrain flour on the label) contain refined grains as well. Also new to the market are white breads made with refined white flour plus added fibre. Bottom line: these new products are certainly better than traditional white bread, but they're not as good as true whole grain and whole wheat products made with red wheat.

ULTIMATE FOODS FOR ULTIMATE HEALTH

Enjoy 5 to 8 servings of grain products each day. Ideally all the servings should be whole grain. A great way to start most days is with a bowl of high fibre whole grain cereal. If you have refined grains, limit your intake to no more than 1 to 2 servings daily.

GOOD ADVICE
Unless you want to watch your waistline expand, limit your intake of baked goods like muffins and scones from your local gourmet coffee shop. Here's just a sampling of items from Starbucks:

	Calories	Fat
Buttermilk Blueberry Muffin	460	21 g
Lemon Cranberry Scone	470	21 g
Butter Croissant	440	26 g
Sticky Bun	470	32 g
Breakfast Cookie	510	27 g
Marble Loaf	640	37 g

LOW-FAT MILK MAKES SENSE

FOR ULTIMATE HEALTH

» Optimize your intake of low-fat milk products.

» Optimize your intake of calcium and vitamin D.

NUTRITION & BETTER BONES

There are many logical and scientifically supported reasons to make milk products a regular part of your diet. The first and most obvious reason is your bones. Milk is your best dietary source of calcium and vitamin D—two absolutely essential nutrients for bone health. Another often overlooked reason is the concentrated hit of vitamins and minerals milk products provide. A diet devoid of dairy is often a poor diet, not just in respect to calcium and vitamin D, but for many other nutrients as well. Milk products may also slash your risk of high blood pressure, colon cancer, and even assist in your quest for a healthy body weight.

Building Better Bones

Imagine picking up a bag of groceries and breaking your wrist, getting a hug from your spouse and breaking your ribs, or losing 4 inches (10 cm) in height because the bones in your spine are so weak they start to collapse. This is osteoporosis—the disease of fragile or brittle bones. While many people have heard of it, most don't realize how devastating and debilitating it can be. It often leads to chronic disabling pain (especially fractures of the spine) and has a profound impact on quality of life. Fear, anxiety, depression, and loss of mobility are frequently reported in people who suffer from this disease.

The good news? Calcium and vitamin D make a difference. Your lifelong intake of these nutrients plays a major role in building and preserving bone mass as well as decreasing your risk of an osteoporotic fracture. Your best daily source of calcium and vitamin D is milk. In fact, milk has been called "the complete tool kit for healthy bones." In addition to calcium and vitamin D, it provides a variety

BONE HEALTH

QUOTE OF THE DAY
"Prevention of bone disease begins at birth and is a lifelong challenge. Physical activity and adequate calcium and vitamin D intake are now known to be major contributors to bone health for individuals of all ages."
—U.S. Surgeon General, Report on Bone Health and Osteoporosis

RESEARCH HIGHLIGHT
Japanese women have lower rates of osteoporosis even though they generally don't consume high amounts of calcium. Why? Fish, especially higher fat fish, is rich in vitamin D. Japanese women have high intakes of vitamin D because they eat fish so frequently— usually four or more times per week. Some researchers believe that a high intake of vitamin D may protect against osteoporosis, even when calcium intake is lower. Best advice: give your bones the best chance possible by staying active and getting plenty of calcium and vitamin D each and every day.

of nutrients that help build strong bones, including magnesium, protein, and phosphorus.

Here's what you should know about bone health & children:

» The majority of children and teens, including most teenage boys and almost all teenage girls, don't meet recommended intakes for calcium and vitamin D.

» Calcium and vitamin D intake during childhood and adolescence, along with physical activity, help build the strongest bones possible. Strong bones are better equipped to handle the bone loss that occurs later in life.

» Approximately 90 to 95% of bone mineral or bone mass is achieved by age 20, and the final 5 to 10% is added over the next 10 years.

» During puberty, there's a "bone growth spurt" and more than 25% of bone mass is accumulated at this time. This occurs at age 11 to 14 for girls and age 13 to 17 for boys.

» A 10% increase in peak bone mass (peak mineral content of bones) can result in a 50% reduction in fracture risk.

» During recent decades, children's intake of milk has declined, while their consumption of soft drinks has tripled. Most kids start drinking significantly more soft drinks beginning around age eight.

» Children and teens who see their parents drink milk with meals are much more likely to choose milk as well.

Here's what you should know about bone health beyond childhood:

» The majority of adults, especially older adults, don't meet recommended intakes for calcium and vitamin D.

» By age 30, we start to lose bone. Calcium and vitamin D help us maintain and preserve the bone we have.

RESEARCH HIGHLIGHT
Research suggests that the diet of early humans—from which our genetic make-up was programmed—was high in both calcium and vitamin D (much of the vitamin D came from daily exposure to the sun).

RESEARCH HIGHLIGHT
Do your kids drink milk at lunch? A study of children and teens aged 5 to 17 found that only those who drank milk at the noon meal met or exceeded the recommended daily calcium intake. In contrast, children who drank soft drinks, juice, or fruit drinks at lunch didn't meet daily calcium recommendations.

RESEARCH HIGHLIGHT
It's okay to give your kids chocolate milk. It's chock full of good nutrition and kids like it better than plain milk. In a study from the University of Vermont involving almost 4,000 children ages 5 to 17, those who consumed flavoured milk were found to drink fewer soft drinks and fruit drinks and had higher calcium intakes than those who didn't consume flavoured milk.

» Pregnancy and lactation increase requirements for calcium and vitamin D.

» Menopause is associated with rapid bone loss.

» By age 80, many women have lost an average of 30% of their peak bone mass.

» Even older individuals with poor bone health can improve their bone status with calcium and vitamin D.

» Osteoporosis isn't just a woman's disease. Men suffer from it too, just not as often.

» Other factors impact bone health. Genetics play a role. Smoking is bad for bones. Crucial for strong bones is physical activity. Resistance exercise, like lifting weights, and weight-bearing or high-impact activity are the best activities for bone health.

Milk: A Powerful Cocktail of Nutrition

Milk is a nutrient-rich food that's hard to replace. When you drink a glass of milk, you get so much more than calcium and vitamin D. You get a "package" of nutrients that includes generous quantities of phosphorus, riboflavin, vitamin A, vitamin B12, protein, potassium, zinc, and magnesium. That's why a diet without milk products compromises your intake of so many vitamins and minerals.

Replacing milk with soft drinks, fruit drinks, or even fruit juices, causes the nutritional quality of your diet to go down. It's important, however, to choose low-fat or fat-free milk products. High fat dairy, especially cheese, is a major source of artery-clogging saturated fat. Bottom line: for a whole lot of nutrition, make low-fat milk products a regular part of each day.

Beyond Bone Health

Although milk products have long been associated with the prevention of osteoporosis, here are other ways they can protect health.

The Blood Pressure Diet

The DASH study (Dietary Approach to Stop Hypertension) looked at the effects of diet on blood pressure. The greatest reductions in blood pressure were seen with a diet rich in fruits and vegetables (8 to 10 servings per day) and low-fat milk products (3 servings per day). The reduction in blood pressure was far greater than observed in any prior nutritional study of blood pressure regulation. Most important was the combination of vegetables, fruit, and milk products (fruits and vegetables alone lowered blood pressure but not by nearly as much as when combined with milk products). Calcium and potassium are two nutrients in milk that are important for blood vessel health

CHILD DEVELOPMENT

RESEARCH HIGHLIGHT
In a study from the University of Otago in New Zealand, the bone health of children who didn't regularly drink milk was compared to that of children who were regular milk drinkers. Kids who didn't drink milk were shorter, had smaller skeletons, and lower bone mineral density. They were also almost three times more likely to fracture a

bone, often through minimal impact or trauma.

RESEARCH HIGHLIGHT
Researchers from the Mayo Clinic have reported a significant increase in forearm fractures in children and teens. Compared to about 30 years ago, fracture rates have

increased 32% in males and 56% in females. Researchers speculate a major long-term health crisis surfacing in our youth due to lack of calcium and physical activity. The cast wearers of today may be the wheel chair users of the future due to osteoporosis-related hip fractures.

and dilation. Specific compounds, called peptides, found in milk proteins may also inhibit an enzyme that causes blood vessels to constrict.

Less Colon Cancer

People with high intakes of calcium and vitamin D may be less likely to develop cancer of the colon. Calcium binds to fatty acids and bile salts, which are potentially toxic to the colon, and also helps regulate the growth of the cells that line the colon wall. At least 1,000 milligrams of calcium each day from food or supplements (each serving of milk products provides about 300 mg) appears necessary to produce a beneficial effect. Vitamin D is also a powerful inhibitor of abnormal or cancerous cell growth. Your body makes vitamin D when sunlight strikes your skin, so those people who have limited exposure to sunlight are more likely to develop cancer of the colon.

Weight Control Assistance

Cutting calories, but still including low-fat dairy in your diet, may protect your waistline from expanding. Some evidence from human and animal studies has shown that high calcium diets inhibit the storage of body fat as well as enhance fat breakdown. Dairy food sources of calcium appear to have a significantly greater effect than calcium taken as a supplement.

ONE SERVING OF MILK PRODUCTS	1 cup (250 mL) milk
	1 cup (250 mL) buttermilk
	½ cup (125 mL) evaporated milk
	¾ cup (175 mL) yogurt
	2 slices (1½ oz or 45 g) hard cheese
	⅓ cup (75 mL) shredded cheese
	½ cup (125 mL) ricotta cheese
	2 oz (55 g) processed cheese
	4 Tbsp (60 mL) grated Parmesan cheese
ONE HALF SERVING OF MILK PRODUCTS	¾ cup (175 mL) ice cream
	½ cup (125 mL) frozen yogurt
	1 cup (250 mL) cottage cheese

CALCIUM

RESEARCH HIGHLIGHT
It's never too late to get more calcium and vitamin D in your diet. In a three-year French study involving over 3,000 older women living in nursing homes (many over 80 years of age), increasing the daily intake of calcium by 1,200 mg and vitamin D by 800 IU reduced hip fractures by 43%.

RESEARCH HIGHLIGHT
In the Continuing Survey of Food Intakes by Individuals involving almost 18,000 children, teenagers, and adults, higher milk product intake resulted in statistically significant and often large increases in the intake of essential nutrients, including magnesium, potassium, zinc, vitamin A, riboflavin, and especially calcium. The results reinforce the importance of milk products as a key calcium source, but also as a food associated with a whole "package" of nutrients.

Your Daily Milk Quota

For ultimate health enjoy 3 to 4 servings of low-fat milk products each day. Fortified soy milk can be used as an alternative to cow's milk.

To limit your intake of saturated fat, it's important to choose low-fat milk products.

Please Note

In addition to consuming milk products, some people may require a calcium supplement. A vitamin D supplement is recommended for most people (see supplement chapter, page 111, for more details).

Choose Milk & Yogurt More

For ultimate health choose milk and yogurt, especially a "probiotic" yogurt, more often than cheese. Here are 3 reasons why:

1 One serving of milk or yogurt contains about 10 times more potassium than a serving of cheese. This is because when cheese is made, potassium is lost in the liquid whey. Potassium is critical for healthy blood pressure and is also a nutrient that's extremely challenging to get enough of.

2 All milk is fortified with vitamin D. It's also added to some yogurt, but generally at lower levels. Cheese doesn't contain added vitamin D. Like potassium, the diets of most people are sorely lacking in this all-star, disease-fighting nutrient.

3 Yogurt can be a valuable source of "good-for-you-bacteria," also referred to as probiotics (read on to learn more).

Probiotic Yogurt: Healthy Food for Your Gut

When most people think of bacteria they think of something bad or dirty—something to be avoided. And yet more than 1,500 kinds of bacteria live along your gastrointestinal tract. Many of these bacteria are considered "good" or "friendly." That's because they help you combat the "bad" bacteria that may come your way, and may also help maintain the health of cells that line your gastrointestinal tract. While all yogurts are made with active bacterial cultures (yogurt is basically milk fermented by the addition of bacteria), some yogurts also contain added "good" bacteria, referred to as probiotics. Probiotics are defined as living organisms that can potentially promote health when consumed in sufficient quantities. The two most common bacterial cultures are lactobacillus acidophilus and bifidobacteria (or bifidus). If these bacteria are added to yogurt, their presence is generally identified on the product label or list of ingredients. Many of the recipes in this book use the probiotic yogurt Activia made by Danone.

Preliminary research suggests that consuming probiotics may:

PREVENTION

RESEARCH HIGHLIGHT
Women in an osteoporosis prevention study were given 1,000 mg of calcium daily either as a supplement (pill) or directly from milk products. The women getting their calcium from milk products improved their intake of calcium as well as 11 other nutrients. Bottom line: for more nutrition, milk products make sense.

RESEARCH HIGHLIGHT
A study from the University of New York involving more than 2,500 postmenopausal women found that women with low bone density (which may lead to osteoporosis) were 86% more likely to suffer from gum disease, which is the major cause of tooth loss in those over the age of 35. Calcium is thought to contribute to healthier gums by keeping the underlying bone strong.

RESEARCH HIGHLIGHT
When people at high risk for colon cancer increased their intake of low-fat milk products by 1,200 milligrams per day, the precancerous cells in the lining of their colon started acting like healthy cells.

» boost the immune system by defending against harmful viruses and bacteria

» reduce intolerance to lactose

» help with diarrhea that results from taking antibiotics (antibiotics kill both good and bad bacteria) or diarrhea caused by infection or virus

» protect against vaginal and bladder infections

» help prevent allergies and asthma in children (especially if consumed in early childhood and by the mother during pregnancy)

» ease symptoms of irritable bowel syndrome, Crohn's disease, and ulcerative colitis

» help fight cavities

» suppress the bacteria that cause stomach ulcers and stomach cancer

» protect cells of the colon and reduce colon cancer risk

» relieve constipation

Your Best Dairy Options

When shopping for milk products, keep the following tips in mind:

» Both skim and 1% milk are considered low in fat. Whole (homogenized) and 2% milk are high fat and should be avoided (children under the age of two can enjoy higher fat milk products and gradually make the shift to a lower fat diet). Breast milk is the best food for infants.

» Chocolate milk is a delicious way for kids and adults to get more milk in their diet. For fewer calories and less sugar, make your own. For example, adding two teaspoons of chocolate syrup to a glass of low-fat milk adds about 30 calories and 1½ teaspoons (7.5 mL) of sugar. In contrast, most store-bought ready-made chocolate milk contains an extra 60 to 80 calories and 4 to 5 teaspoons (20 to 25 mL) of sugar per 1 cup (250 mL) serving.

» Look for yogurt that is low-fat (no more than 3 grams of fat per serving), contains the highest amounts of calcium and vitamin D, and is a source of probiotics (good-for-you bacteria).

» Cheese is a major source of saturated fat in the North American diet. If you don't like the taste and texture of low-fat cheese, choose reduced-fat or "light" cheeses instead. Also, consider strong-flavoured cheeses like extra sharp cheddar. You tend to be satisfied with less.

» Most soft cheeses like Brie, Camembert, feta and goat's cheese are significantly lower in calcium than hard cheeses like cheddar, Swiss, mozzarella, and Parmesan.

LOW-FAT CHOICES

GOOD ADVICE
At your local coffee shop, stay away from specialty coffees made with added syrups, whole milk, and whipped cream. Some large sizes contain more than 500 calories and 16 grams of fat (including the artery-clogging, saturated fat). Your best bet at the coffee counter? A latte or cappuccino made with skim or 1% milk.

GOOD ADVICE
Just one scoop or ½ cup (125 mL) of Häagen-Dazs Extras Triple Chocolate Ice Cream will set you back 360 calories and a whopping 22 grams of fat (much of which is the artery-clogging, saturated kind). Be good to your heart and your waistline. Stick with low-fat frozen yogurt or "light" ice cream that contains no more than 120 calories per serving and 2 grams of saturated fat or less.

To get the same amount of calcium as one glass of milk you'd have to eat:	
Almonds	1 cup (250 mL)
Bok choy	1 cup (250 mL)
Broccoli	2¼ cups (550 mL)
Kale	1½ cups (375 mL)
Pinto beans	4 cups (1 L)
Spinach	8 cups (2 L)
Tofu (made with calcium)	½ cup (125 mL)

Please Note

You need to replace the calcium found in not 1 but 3 to 4 servings of milk products each day.

» Ricotta cheese contains about five times more calcium and three times less salt than cottage cheese.

» Cream cheese isn't a good source of calcium. You need to eat about 25 tablespoons (375 mL) to get the same amount of calcium as one glass of milk.

» Most processed cheeses, including processed cheese slices, are a source of calcium, but also contain at least twice as much salt. Use them less often, and when you do buy processed products, look for brands that are low in fat and contain the highest amount of calcium per serving.

» A serving of most store-bought puddings contains only one-third the calcium found in a glass of milk.

Calcium from Other Sources

If you don't like milk, can you get all the calcium you need from other foods like broccoli or almonds? Sure, if you're willing to eat almost 7 cups (1.75 L) of broccoli or 3 cups (750 mL) of almonds every single day. For most people, that's not likely to happen. What about calcium-fortified orange juice? One glass of juice can provide as much calcium as a glass of milk. However, fruit juice—because it's so high in sugar and calories—should be limited to no more than 1 cup each day. The only good

PROBIOTICS

RESEARCH HIGHLIGHT

Why has there been such a major increase in allergies and asthma in recent years? Some researchers believe that unhealthy diets, high in processed foods, are to blame. A poor diet is thought to be detrimental to our gut microflora (the good bacteria that live along our gastrointestinal tract). This alters our immune response so the body is no longer able to protect against allergens. The best advice for a healthy gut: eat a healthy diet (like the one outlined in this book!) and consider a probiotic yogurt (a yogurt containing "good-for-you" bacteria).

QUOTE OF THE DAY

Yogurt can be an important source of probiotics (good-for-you bacteria). Jeffrey Gordon, professor and researcher from Washington University said, "The trillions of microbes living in the human digestive system outnumber actual human cells 10-to-1. To ignore our microbial side would be to ignore an important contributor to our health and our biology."

alternative to cow's milk is fortified soy milk, which, like milk, also contains other bone-building nutrients like protein, vitamin D, and magnesium. With any calcium-fortified beverage, it's important to shake the container before pouring, because the calcium tends to separate out.

Avoiding Milk: Is It Necessary?

Do you avoid milk because of lactose intolerance? You may not need to. Several well-controlled studies have found that even people who suffer from lactose intolerance (also referred to as "lactose maldigestion") can consume ½ to 1 cup (125 to 250 mL) of milk without symptoms of intolerance as long as they consume it with meals. Solid food slows the digestive process and gives the body more time to digest the lactose. A study of African-American girls suffering from lactose intolerance also found that the colon adapts to milk products when they're consumed on a regular basis. Most yogurts and hard cheeses contain very little lactose and are well tolerated. Lastly, you can purchase milk, like Lactaid, that has the enzyme lactase added to break down the lactose.

MEETING CALCIUM NEEDS

GOOD ADVICE
The more often you dine away from home, the less likely you are to meet your recommended intake of milk products. Make milk products a part of your life at home and on the road.

RESEARCH HIGHLIGHT
In addition to consuming at least 3 servings of milk products daily, enjoying ½ to 1 cup (125 to 250 mL) of calcium-fortified orange juice each day can help ensure your calcium needs are met. The type of calcium found in Tropicana orange juice—calcium citrate malate—is better absorbed by the body than brands of orange juice that use tricalcium phosphate or calcium lactate.

MORE BEANS, PLEASE!

FOR ULTIMATE HEALTH

» Optimize your overall intake of
beans.

» Optimize your intake of soy and
soy products.

BEANS ARE THE BEST

Beans or legumes are an incredible food. They've earned a first-class reputation for their exceptional nutritional content, as well as their ability to fight heart disease, cancer, diabetes, obesity, and more. Researchers and health experts have referred to them as:

» the best human plant food there is

» a near-perfect food

» among the most nutritious foods on the planet

» one of the greatest foods you can eat to protect against disease

The Bottom Line

There's never *bean* a better time to make beans a regular part of your diet.

Ten Reasons to Be a Bean Eater

1 Beans contain a whole lot of nutrition in one little package. People who eat beans get more vitamins and minerals than people who don't.

2 Beans are the best source of plant protein, especially soybeans. Protein builds skin, muscle, bones, and hair. In fact, every cell in our body is constructed from the protein we get from foods. A protein-rich meal also helps keep hunger at bay. For those who suffer from diabetes or kidney disease, protein from plants is easier on the kidneys too.

3 Beans are rich in B vitamins, especially folate, which has been called "the nutrient that does almost everything." It helps prevent serious birth defects during pregnancy and may significantly lower your risk of heart disease and cancer, especially colon cancer. It may help ward off Alzheimer's disease, as well as reduce your risk of depression. It's a nutrient most of us simply don't get enough of.

LEGUMES

QUESTION OF THE DAY
"Is 'legume' just another word for beans?" When I talk about beans, I'm really referring to the legume family. Legumes, often referred to as dried beans and peas, are edible seeds from the pods of certain plants. The legume family includes peas (such as split peas, chickpeas, and black-eyed peas), beans (such as lima, navy, kidney, pinto, black, and soybeans) and lentils (such as red, brown, and green lentils). Green peas and green beans are considered vegetables.

RESEARCH HIGHLIGHT
The Food Habits in Later Life Study examined the eating habits of people over the age of 70 in four different countries: Japan, Sweden, Australia, and Greece. Beans (or legumes) came out as the food most linked to a longer life. In fact, beans were the only food consistently and significantly linked to survival across all populations.

4 Beans are an important source of magnesium, a mineral that helps build strong bones and reduces your risk of diabetes by enhancing the action of insulin.

5 Beans boost your intake of potassium, another nutrient sorely lacking in most people's diets. Potassium is essential for healthy blood pressure, can slash your risk of stroke, and reduces your risk of kidney stones.

6 Beans contribute significant amounts of other nutrients too, including calcium, iron, copper, zinc, phosphorus, and manganese—all essential nutrients for good health.

7 Beans are disease-fighting, antioxidant all-stars, especially those that are black or red in colour, like black beans and red kidney beans. Their antioxidant action comes from the health-protective plant compounds they contain, including flavonoids and phenols.

8 Beans are rich in carbohydrates, but they have a low glycemic index. This means the carbohydrates they contain are slowly released into the bloodstream and don't cause a quick or steep rise in blood sugar. This is important in the management and prevention of type 2 diabetes.

9 Beans are loaded with fibre—most contain a whopping 15 grams per cup. Eating more beans makes it possible to reach your recommended fibre target of 25 to 38 grams of fibre each day. Fibre is a health-protective superstar. It helps you maintain healthy blood sugar levels, lowers LDL (bad) cholesterol, makes you feel full longer so you eat less, and prevents constipation.

10 Beans are one of the best food sources of "resistant starch," a type of fibre that resists digestion and results in the production of a cancer-fighting compound in the colon called butyrate. Resistant starch is also considered a prebiotic—it encourages the growth of health-promoting good bacteria along your gastrointestinal tract.

Sensational Soy

Is soy a magic bullet? No. Is soy a sensational food? Yes. All beans are jam-packed with nutrition. The soybean, however, rises above all others. The protein quality of soybeans rivals foods like meat, milk, and eggs. Soy contains significantly more calcium, iron, magnesium, potassium, zinc, copper, and manganese than other beans. It's truly a superstar of nutritional value. Unlike other beans, soy isn't low in fat. However, the fat it contains is primarily the healthy-for-your-heart kind. Soy is

BEAN HEALTH

RESEARCH HIGHLIGHT
A review of more than 25 years of research by nutrition experts from Michigan State University concluded that eating 2 to 4 cups of beans each week can help reduce the risk of developing many of the deadliest diseases, including heart disease, diabetes, and cancers of the breast, colon, and prostate.

RESEARCH HIGHLIGHT
Data from the National Health and Nutrition Examination Survey found that people who included beans in their diets weighed an average of 7 pounds (3 kg) less and were 22% less likely to be obese than people who didn't eat beans. The bean eaters' diets were more nutrient-rich, containing more protein, fibre, potassium, niacin, folate, iron, zinc, copper, and magnesium. Their diets also included less fat and sugar.

also unique in that it contains a specific type of flavonoid called isoflavones. These isoflavones are referred to as phytoestrogens because they demonstrate estrogen-like or hormone-like activity in the body. The daily consumption of soy is a defining characteristic of the traditional Japanese diet, which is considered one of the healthiest diets in the world. Soy has been linked to a lower risk of heart disease and prostate cancer. Soy may reduce breast cancer risk, especially if consumed over the entire lifespan, and may also be good for bones.

Is It Safe to Eat Soy?

Some research—mostly animal studies using soy in very high doses—has linked soy to everything from reproductive problems, to impaired thyroid function, to increased breast cancer risk. Is it safe to eat? Overwhelming evidence shows soy isn't detrimental to health when consumed as part of a healthy diet in its naturally occurring food form (not from pills or supplements).

Here's what you need to know about soy:

» Soy provides the greatest health benefits when it replaces less healthy foods in the diet like meat, which is high in saturated fat.

» Soy should be enjoyed in quantities similar to Asian countries—about 1 to 2 servings daily. Remember, Asian countries have been con-suming soy safely for hundreds and hundreds of years.

» Eat whole soy foods. In research from the University of Illinois, mice with cancer were fed minimally processed soy (soy flour) or more highly processed forms of soy such as soy extracts and soy isoflavones. In the mice fed soy flour, tumors remained the same and didn't grow. In mice fed the more processed soy extracts and isoflavones, tumors increased in size. Researchers believe that eating highly refined components of soy, like those found in soy pills or supplements, have very different effects in the body than eating whole soy foods.

» How does soy impact breast cancer risk? A review of 18 studies by researchers from Johns Hopkins School of Medicine concludes that among healthy women, soy consumption reduces breast cancer risk by 14%. Soy consumed over the lifespan, especially during puberty when breast tissue is forming, may be most protective. Research based primarily on animal studies, however, questions whether soy's hormone-like effects can fuel cancer growth in women with high risk of breast cancer or who already suffer from the disease. Until further research gives a clear answer to this question, high risk women may want to limit soy foods

RESEARCH HIGHLIGHT
Researchers from the University of Guelph tested the antioxidant activity of plant compounds called flavonoids from the skin of 12 common bean varieties. Black beans came out on top, followed by red, brown, yellow, and white. In general, darker coloured beans were associated with higher levels of flavonoids, therefore higher antioxidant activity.

RESEARCH HIGHLIGHT
The glycemic index ranks carbohydrate-containing foods based on their effect on blood sugar levels. In a study from the University of Göttingen in Germany, people with type 2 diabetes consumed either a low glycemic index meal (legumes) or a high glycemic index meal (potatoes). Increases in blood sugar and insulin were delayed and much lower after eating the legume meal. Researchers concluded that people with type 2 diabetes may not need to count the carbohydrates in dried peas, the type of legume used in this study, because the carbohydrates are released so slowly into the bloodstream. This is a remarkable finding when you consider about 70% of the calories in most beans come from carbohydrates.

to a few servings a week and, most importantly, avoid soy in pill or supplement form. Soy may also interfere with tamoxifen, a breast cancer treatment drug.

» A review of 14 studies found little evidence that soy adversely affects thyroid function in healthy people. Soy foods, however, may interfere with the absorption of synthetic thyroid hormones. If you take these hormones because you have an under-active thyroid, you can still enjoy soy, but your dose of medication may need to be increased.

» Can the hormone-like effects of soy affect reproduction or development? A review by 14 independent scientists for The Center for the Evaluation of Risks to Human Reproduction, concludes that there is "negligible" concern about possible reproductive or developmental harm from plant estrogens found in soy products or soy baby formula. Having said that, experts are also quick to point out that when it comes to babies, breast milk is by far the best food option.

The Bottom Line
Soy is a nutrition packed food that, in moderation, deserves a regular place in most diets.

Bring on the Beans!

For ultimate health enjoy 1 to 2 servings of beans, which includes soy, at least four days a week. Beans are considered a replacement to meat. Fortified soy milk can also be used as an alternative to cow's milk.

Ten Great Ways to Say Hello to Beans (including soy)

1 Bean Dips—Like Hummus (Chickpea Spread)
Bean dips are great with cut-up veggies like carrot sticks, or wedges of whole wheat pita bread. They also make great sandwich fillings (try our Hummus Peanut Butter Sandwich Filling on page 220).

2 Have Them Roasted
This is a must-try recipe! Simply drain and rinse a can of chickpeas. Toss with about 1 Tablespoon (15 mL) olive oil and a few shakes of dried rosemary. Add a bit of salt and pepper to taste. Spread on a baking sheet. Bake at 350°F (180°C) for about 45 minutes. Let them cool for five minutes and serve warm. Great for snacking, and kids love them! Roasted soy nuts, now widely available in most supermarkets and health food stores, also make for a tasty on-the-run snack.

3 Super Soup
From minestrone, to black bean, to lentil soup—the options are endless. Research also suggests soup is

SOY

RESEARCH HIGHLIGHT
Okinawa is an island off the coast of Japan. More people live to the age of 100 here than anywhere else in the world. A typical Okinawan diet is low in fat, contains plenty of vegetables, and includes about 2 servings of soy each day.

QUESTION OF THE DAY
"Will eating soy help reduce menopausal hot flashes?" While some research suggests that soy may reduce the number or severity of hot flashes, most research suggests soy has minimal impact, if any.

RESEARCH HIGHLIGHT
In the Shanghai Women's Health Study, involving almost 75,000 women, those consuming about 2 to 3 servings of soy daily were 75% less likely to develop heart disease, almost 40% less likely to fracture a bone, and had significantly lower blood pressure than women who didn't regularly eat soy.

a super way to fill yourself up with fewer calories. Look for lower-sodium options.

4 So-Good Salads

Toss a handful of beans—chickpeas, kidney beans, or roasted soybeans—on top of your favourite green salad. If you live life in the fast lane, ready-made marinated bean salads are an absolute must. They're also a great alternative to a meat-filled sandwich in your brown bag lunch. Also, be sure to try Mairlyn's Amazing Artichoke and Chickpea Salad on page 223.

5 Chili: Not Just for Super Bowl Parties

I love chili. The spicier the better! Make a big batch and freeze it for those days when you don't feel like cooking. Try our Blazin' Black Bean Chili (page 207). Beans served with whole wheat tortillas, like bean burritos, or our Amazing Black Bean Quesadillas (recipe on page 217), are also superb.

6 Baked Beans

Canned baked beans make for a quick and tasty meal. Kids love them too—especially the after-effects! Jazz up your baked beans with the incredibly easy recipe ideas on pages 213–15.

7 Beans 'n' Rice

Beans and rice are a staple meal in many countries. Make them a staple in your house too. Be sure to

ONE SERVING OF BEANS	
	½ cup (125 mL) beans (any type)
	4 Tbsp (60 mL) hummus
	1 cup (250 mL) fortified soy milk
	3 Tbsp (45 mL) roasted soy nuts
	½ cup (125 mL) tofu or tempeh
	½ cup (125 mL) soy meat alternative
	3 Tbsp (45 mL) miso
	1 veggie burger

RESEARCH HIGHLIGHT
A Harvard study involving over 4,000 men and women from Costa Rica linked a daily serving of beans to a 38% lower risk of heart attack. The bad news is that many Latin American countries are shifting to a more Westernized diet and eating less nutrient-rich, disease-fighting beans.

QUESTION OF THE DAY
"Is it safe to eat soy that has been genetically modified?" Overall, I believe genetically-modified foods are safe. Biotechnology helps increase food production, reduce the use of pesticides, and benefits farmers and the environment.

RESEARCH HIGHLIGHT
Timing of soy intake was found to be important in a study from Vanderbilt University School of Medicine involving 3,000 Chinese women. Women who consumed the most soy between the ages of 13 and 15 were 50% less likely to develop breast cancer later in life. Researchers believe that eating soy during puberty may affect maturation of the mammary gland in such a way as to make breast tissue more resistant to the development of cancer.

make them with whole-grain rice. Try the Awesome Lentil and Rice Salad recipe on page 182.

8 Soy Smoothie

While it's fine to drink soy milk on its own, soy smoothies are perhaps the most delicious way to enjoy soy. Strawberry soy milk mixed with frozen berries is a great combo, and chocolate soy mixed with a frozen banana simply can't be beat. Try the Super Banana Chocolate Shake recipe on page 266.

9 Edamame: Green & Sweet

Edamame are soybeans that are harvested when the soybeans are still green and sweet-tasting. Edamame can be purchased pre-cooked from most sushi counters at your local supermarket. Simply squeeze the seeds from the pods directly into your mouth with your fingers. Edamame is also widely available frozen—simply boil for four to five minutes. Enjoy them as a snack, or add to foods like soups, salads, or rice. Try the Japanese-Style Edamame and Corn Salad on page 204.

10 Meatless Meals

Ground beef is a major source of artery-clogging saturated fat in the North American diet. Use soy meat alternatives, like Yves Veggie Ground Round, as a replacement to ground beef in foods like spaghetti sauce, lasagna, or shepherd's pie. Use tofu instead of meat in your favourite stir-fry. Have a veggie burger instead of a hamburger.

ULTIMATE FOODS FOR ULTIMATE HEALTH

Enjoy 1 to 2 servings of beans, which includes soy, at least four days of the week. Beans are considered a replacement to meat. Fortified soy milk can also be used as an alternative to cow's milk.

RESEARCH HIGHLIGHT

Researchers from the VA Medical Center and the University of Kentucky reviewed 11 studies to determine the effects of beans on heart health. Beans were linked to lower LDL (bad) cholesterol, triglycerides, and body weight—important factors in slashing the risk of heart disease.

RESEARCH HIGHLIGHT

In the Harvard Nurses Health Study II involving over 90,000 women, those who ate beans and lentils at least twice a week had a 24% lower risk of developing breast cancer than those who ate them less than once a month.

BEANS

GOOD ADVICE

Canned beans are a nutritious and time-saving alternative to cooking beans from scratch. The downside? They're loaded with salt. Most canned beans contain about 400 mg of sodium per ½ cup (125 mL) serving. By draining the canning liquid and rinsing, you'll cut the sodium by almost half.

GOOD ADVICE

Fact: beans give you gas (technical term: flatulence). If it's a problem for you, there are two options. Option one: try Beano, a product available at most supermarkets and drugstores. It contains the enzyme that helps break down the hard-to-digest sugars in beans that cause gas. It works! Option two: enjoy beans with those who know and love you (definitely the most fun option).

FATTY FISH IS FABULOUS

FOR ULTIMATE HEALTH

» Optimize your intake of omega-3 fats found in higher fat fish.

» Mnimize your intake of contaminants like mercury.

AN INCREDIBLE FAT

Slash your risk of heart disease and stroke. Chase away the blues. Protect your brain from the ravages of aging and diseases like Alzheimer's. Cut your risk of the most common cancers—breast, prostate, and colon. Reduce symptoms of inflammatory disorders like rheumatoid arthritis, inflammatory bowel disease, asthma, and allergies. Guard against eye diseases like macular degeneration and cataracts. Is it possible that the omega-3 fats found in higher fat fish like salmon, mackerel, herring, and rainbow trout can do all this and more? Accumulating research says yes. The omega-3 fats from fish are health protection all-stars. They're a must-have in any diet designed to prevent disease.

Outstanding Protection for Your Heart

The omega-3 fats in fish have been called as potentially potent as any high-tech heart drug, and one of the most overlooked defenses against heart disease. Some researchers consider these fats the most important nutritional factor for reducing the risk of heart disease. Scientists first suspected their importance back in the 1970s, after observing rock bottom rates of heart disease among natives of Greenland and the Japanese islanders on Okinawa, who both consume high amounts of seafood. Since then a large body of evidence has accumulated to support the heart-healthy benefits of higher fat fish. Not only are regular fish eaters less likely to have a heart attack or stroke, but if one does occur, it's much less likely to be fatal. In addition, damage to the heart muscle is greatly reduced.

Your heart loves the omega-3 fats from fish because they:

QUESTION OF THE DAY

"I don't like fish. Can I get my omega-3 fats from foods like flax, walnuts, and canola oil instead?" Both plant and marine (fish) source omega-3 fats are good for your heart. However, the marine omega-3 fats (also referred to as EPA and DHA) provide significantly greater protection from a long list of diseases as they're incorporated directly into cell membranes throughout the body, including tissues in the heart, brain, and eyes. Bottom line: both plant and marine sources of omega-3 fats should be included in the diet, but for best overall disease protection, the omega-3 fats from fish are a must!

RESEARCH HIGHLIGHT

In the Harvard Nurses Health Study involving over 80,000 females, it was found that those who ate fish at least two times a week were over 30% less likely to suffer from heart disease. They were also significantly less likely to die of a heart attack or suffer from a stroke.

» decrease the stickiness of your blood (this means blood clots are less likely to form, which are often the first step in a heart attack)

» stabilize the electrical activity of the heart so that it keeps a strong and regular beat (irregular heart beats are another leading cause of heart attacks)

» keep artery walls relaxed and dilated

» lower triglycerides in your blood—another type of blood fat linked to heart disease

» reduce inflammation of the artery wall, which in turn reduces the buildup of plaque (fatty deposits)

RESEARCH HIGHLIGHT
In the Lugawala Study involving two African village populations with similar genetics and lifestyles, the risk of heart disease was found to be significantly lower in the fish-eating village than in the vegetarian-eating village.

Brain Food

Some researchers believe that humans evolved in coastal areas because the omega-3 fats from fish are so critical for healthy brain development. The brain is an astonishing 60% fat and it needs the omega-3 fats from fish for optimal function. These fats are incorporated directly into the cell walls of your brain. They boost levels of the brain chemical serotonin and increase the number of connections between brain cells. In fact, the omega-3 fats from fish are concentrated in the brain right where the brain cells communicate with each other and all the signals pass back and forth. They help preserve thinking skills as we get older, especially memory, and are linked to better intelligence and school performance in children. Low blood levels of omega-3 fats are also associated with attention deficit hyperactivity disorder, Alzheimer's, bipolar disorders (also known as manic depression), schizophrenia, and depression. Is it any wonder the omega-3 fats from fish are called "fertilizer for the brain"?

RESEARCH HIGHLIGHT
Medical doctors at two Copenhagen hospitals confirmed that eating fish regularly helps prevent the buildup of plaque (fatty deposits) that narrows the arteries. The doctors performed 40 autopsies and determined that the degree of plaque present in the coronary arteries was inversely proportional to the amount of omega-3 fat from fish in the fatty tissue.

RESEARCH HIGHLIGHT
Smog isn't good for your heart, but omega-3 fats from fish can help. Elderly nursing home residents in heavily polluted Mexico City who took daily fish-oil supplements were significantly less likely to experience the type of abnormal heart rhythms caused by pollution that lead to heart attacks.

RESEARCH HIGHLIGHT
If two people have the same amount of plaque (fatty deposits) on their artery wall, why is one person more likely to have a heart attack? Plaque stability may be the reason. Plaque that's more stable is less likely to rupture and cause a heart attack or stroke. Fish oil promotes plaque stability. It gets incorporated directly into the plaque, reduces inflammation, and makes the plaque less likely to burst.

RESEARCH HIGHLIGHT
Animal research from Louisiana State University suggests that mothers who eat fish rich in omega-3 fats during pregnancy and while nursing, and who continue to feed their babies such a diet after weaning, may dramatically reduce their daughters' risk of developing breast cancer later in life.

RESEARCH HIGHLIGHT
Eat fish for better bones. Research from Purdue University has found that the omega-3 fats from fish stimulate the bone-building cells in the membrane that covers the long bones in your body. These bone-building cells lay down the protein matrix on which calcium and other minerals are deposited.

QUESTION OF THE DAY
"Is it okay to eat shellfish, like shrimp?" Shellfish, including shrimp, crab, clams, oysters, lobster, mussels, and scallops are low in fat, including unhealthy saturated fats, and rich in nutrients like protein, iron, copper, zinc, and selenium. Although shrimp, lobster, and crab contain moderate amounts of cholesterol, they can easily fit into a healthy diet—especially when you avoid other high cholesterol foods, like eggs, on the same day.

RESEARCH HIGHLIGHT
In a 30-year study from the Karolinska Institute involving more than 6,000 Swedish men, those who didn't eat fish had a two- to three-fold higher risk of prostate cancer than those who ate moderate or high amounts.

Cancer Fighting Omega-3s

Evidence suggests that the diet of early humans, which our genetic makeup was programmed for, contained equal amounts of omega-3 fats and omega-6 fats. Some researchers believe that an imbalance of these fats may fuel cancer growth, especially when the diet is very rich in the omega-6 fats and lacking in the omega-3 fats. A more balanced intake of these fats appears to reduce both the development and the spread of cancerous cells. Omega-6 fats are found in safflower oil, sunflower oil, corn oil, soybean oil, and products such as salad dressing or mayonnaise made with these oils. Meat can also contribute significant amounts of these fats, since many animals, such as beef cattle, are fed a diet rich in omega-6 fats. Fish, as well as other foods recommended in this book like canola oil and flaxseed, help increase the omega-3 content of your diet. Optimizing your intake of the omega-3 fats, especially from fish, appears most beneficial for decreasing your risk of breast, prostate, and colon cancer.

The Anti-Inflammatory Diet

Chronic or excessive inflammation has been referred to as the fire within or a body at war with itself. Omega-3 fats decrease inflammation by increasing the production of anti-inflammatory hormone-like substances called eicosanoids.

RESEARCH HIGHLIGHT
In a study of almost 3,000 Finnish, Italian, and Dutch men, those who regularly ate fatty fish were 34% less likely to die from heart disease. No association was found between eating lean fish and heart disease. Moral of the story: while lean fish is still a healthy choice, it's the fatty fish that you need to put on your plate more often.

RESEARCH HIGHLIGHT
The omega-3 fats from fish have been called "the happy fats" and "Prozac from the Sea." Dr. Joseph Hibbeln, from the National Institute of Health, found that countries with the highest fish consumption—Japan, Taiwan, and Korea—have the lowest rates of depression. Countries with the lowest fish consumption—New Zealand, Canada, West Germany, France, and the United States—have the highest rates of depression.

Rates of postpartum depression are 50 times higher in countries where women don't eat fish. Even homicide, murder, and suicide rates are linked to a low intake of fish.

QUOTE OF THE DAY
"Omega-3 fats have immense public health significance for the control of the current epidemic of heart disease."
—Dr. William Connor, Oregon Health & Science University

They may provide benefits for inflammatory disorders like rheumatoid arthritis, multiple sclerosis, lupus, asthma, allergies, psoriasis, and inflammatory bowel disorders like ulcerative colitis. Eating higher fat fish regularly is recommended, but for many inflammatory disorders, fish oil supplements are necessary for maximum effectiveness. Here are some examples of how the omega-3 fats can help:

» Women who eat fatty fish or take fish oil during pregnancy may reduce allergy and asthma risk in their children.

» Fish oil capsules can reduce the throbbing and stiffness associated with arthritis.

» For people with asthma, the temporary narrowing of the airways triggered by vigorous exercise may be prevented.

» For inflammatory diseases of the bowel, fish oil may reduce pain and result in longer remission times. Preliminary research suggests that combining fish oil with a diet high in flavonoids (found in foods like berries, apples, cinnamon, and tea) may provide even more protection against inflammation.

Omega-3s for Healthy Eyes

It's been said that "sick eyes occur in a sick body." If you want healthy eyes, take care of your body. Part of taking care of your body is eating a diet that contains omega-3 fats from fish. These fats are especially important for eye health as they're a major structural component of eye tissue, particularly in the retina. They promote the survival of photo receptor cells (cells that detect light and allow us to see), enhance cell communication, and decrease inflammation. An omega-3 rich diet is linked to a lower risk of cataracts (clouding of the lens of the eye), age-related macular degeneration (distorted central vision and the leading cause of blindness in older adults), and dry eye syndrome (tear glands produce fewer tears). Perhaps seafood should be called *see*-food (chuckle, chuckle).

RESEARCH HIGHLIGHT
A study from the Australian National University involving more than 3,500 older adults, found that eating fish just once per week cut the risk of macular degeneration (leading cause of adult blindness) in half compared to eating fish less than once per month.

QUESTION OF THE DAY
"Is smoked salmon a good source of omega-3 fats?" Unfortunately, no. Smoked salmon contains less than one-quarter of the omega-3 fats found in fresh salmon. Much of the beneficial fats are lost during the smoking process.

GOOD ADVICE
Do you suffer from diabetes? If so, eat your fish! People with diabetes are much more likely to develop heart disease and die from it. They need the protection that fish oils provide. In research involving 5,000 women with type 2 diabetes who were part of the Harvard Nurses Health Study, those who consumed at least two fish meals per week were over 35% less likely to suffer from heart disease.

RESEARCH HIGHLIGHT
Can eating fish turn back the clock? In a study from Rush University Medical Center involving almost 4,000 people over the age of 65, those who ate fish two or more times per week had the mental function of a person four years younger.

RESEARCH HIGHLIGHT
In research from Sheffield University, 70 depressed patients who hadn't been helped by drugs such as Prozac were given a supplement containing omega-3 fats from fish. After 12 weeks, 69% of the patients showed marked improvement, compared with 25% given a placebo (dummy pill).

Your Weekly Fish Quota

For ultimate health enjoy 2 servings of higher fat fish each week.

ONE SERVING OF HIGHER FAT FISH	3 oz (85 g) fish (about the size of a deck of cards) ¾ cup (175 mL) flaked or canned fish

GOOD ADVICE

If you don't want dry, tough fish, don't overcook it! Most fish requires just 10 minutes of cooking time for each inch (1 inch/2.5 cm) of thickness. Properly cooked fish will flake easily with a fork.

QUESTION OF THE DAY

"Should I buy foods that contain added omega-3 fats?" There has been an explosion of products on the market fortified with omega-3 fats. Most contain relatively small amounts of these added fats, and the omega-3 fats they do contain often come from plant sources such as flaxseed or canola oil rather than from fish and algae (EPA and DHA), which are the most beneficial to your health. My advice: if you buy products with added omega-3 fats, look for EPA or DHA on the label. Most important, to make sure you optimize your intake of omega-3 fats, don't stop eating your fish or taking a fish oil supplement.

Higher fat fish include salmon, herring, mackerel, sardines, and rainbow trout. Anchovies and pickled herring are also high in omega-3 fats; however, they're also very high in salt. Enjoy them on occasion. Most tuna is low in omega-3 fats; however, bluefin tuna (often available at higher end restaurants) and white or albacore canned tuna are better sources of these fats. Unfortunately, these tuna choices are also often higher in mercury and should be avoided most of the time (see safe fish guidelines below). Most frozen fish sticks and fast-food fish sandwiches are a poor source of omega-3 fats (not to mention that some of these products are loaded with nasty trans fats).

But Is It Safe?

When you look at the powerful impact fish can have on our health, it's tempting to call it a wonder food. But is it safe to eat? What about contaminants like mercury, dioxin, or polychlorinated biphenyls (also known as PCBs)? Fish eating is generally safe and provides far more benefits than potential harm; however, it's best to limit our overall intake of seafood and avoid certain kinds of fish.

Here are some fish guidelines to help you get maximum benefits with minimum risks:

» It's prudent to limit your intake of all types of seafood to no more than 2 to 4 servings per week (serving size of 3 oz/85 g).

GOOD ADVICE

Pregnant and nursing women: eat your fish. The omega-3 fats in fish are essential for the healthy development of your baby's brain and eyes. This development takes place in the womb and throughout the first year of your baby's life. But avoid shark, swordfish, king mackerel, tilefish, and tuna as they may contain unsafe amounts of mercury.

RESEARCH HIGHLIGHT

The Children of the '90s Study involves 14,000 British children who have been followed from development in the womb through their early teens. Results so far indicate that eating higher fat fish during pregnancy leads to better language and communication skills.

RESEARCH HIGHLIGHT

In a study from the University of Southern California involving almost 700 mothers with asthma, those mothers who regularly ate higher fat fish while pregnant were 70% less likely to have children that developed asthma. Researchers believe the omega-3 fats in fish dampen the type of inflammation involved in asthma. Other research suggests that fish consumption by pregnant women also reduces allergy risk in their children.

» Women who may become pregnant, pregnant women, nursing mothers, and young children need to be especially careful about making safe fish choices.

» Limiting your intake of mercury is particularly important. It's a contaminant that accumulates in the body and can cause substantial damage to the kidneys, heart, brain, and central nervous system. It's also linked to a significantly higher risk of heart disease.

» Fish that contain the highest amounts of mercury should be avoided. These include shark, swordfish, king mackerel, and tilefish (also called golden bass or golden snapper). Limit your intake of Chilean sea bass, lobster, Spanish mackerel, orange roughy, grouper, red snapper, and halibut.

» Tuna may also contain significant amounts of mercury, especially tuna steaks and white or albacore canned tuna. The tuna used in sushi may also be high in mercury (sushi made with salmon is a better choice). Canned light tuna (made with skipjack, not yellowfin) is generally low in mercury and is your safest tuna option. My overall recommendation, however, is to choose fish like salmon most often, in order to benefit from the omega-3 fats they provide.

» Salmon is low in mercury and one of the most delicious ways to get your omega-3 fats. Farmed salmon has been found to contain more contaminants, like PCBs and dioxin, than wild salmon. Both Health Canada and the FDA in the United States state that the levels of contaminants in both farmed and wild salmon don't pose a risk to human health when consumed in moderate amounts. My recommendation is to choose wild salmon if available but that enjoying farmed salmon a few times per week can also be a safe and healthy choice.

» Check local advisories about the safety of fish caught by family and friends in your local lakes, rivers, and coastal areas.

» Lastly, never eat undercooked clams, mussels, or oysters as they may contain harmful bacteria and viruses.

Fish Oil Capsules Instead?

For ultimate health people suffering from heart disease, high triglycerides, depression, and inflammatory disorders should consider a fish oil supplement.

Numerous studies, including a study from Harvard Medical School, have found fish oil capsules are safe and don't contain detectable levels of contaminants such as mercury, PCBs, and dioxin. In

RESEARCH HIGHLIGHT
In the Cardiovascular Health Cognition Study involving over 3,500 elderly men and women, eating fatty fish more than twice a week was associated with 28% lower risk of dementia and 41% lower risk of Alzheimer's. However, the protective effect was only present for those who didn't have a genetic predisposition for Alzheimer's.

RESEARCH HIGHLIGHT
Research from the University of Toyama in Japan shows that the anti-inflammatory effects of omega-3 fats help prevent periodontitis (gum disease). Periodontitis is responsible for most tooth loss in adults.

GOOD ADVICE
Short on time? Frozen fish (not breaded) is a tasty and convenient alternative to fresh fish. I always have frozen salmon fillets in my freezer for quick and easy dinners.

QUESTION OF THE DAY
"What should I look for when buying a fish oil supplement?" Consumer Reports tested 16 major brands of fish oil supplements. All supplements were in good shape, contained the amounts of omega-3 fats advertised, and didn't contain significant levels of contaminants. Conclusion: look for supplements that contain the amount of fish oil you want (most people want 1 gram of fish oil, EPA and DHA combined), and are least expensive.

addition, with certain diseases or conditions, such as heart disease, it's almost impossible to meet recommended intakes for omega-3 fats by eating fish alone.

Here's what you need to know about popping a fish oil pill instead of eating fish:

» If you're generally healthy, your goal should be to eat fatty fish twice a week. In addition to omega-3 fats, higher fat fish like salmon is very rich in protein, vitamin D, vitamin B12, and selenium, and contains significant amounts of niacin, vitamin B6, and potassium. If you rely on supplements, you miss out on the long list of nutrients that fish provides. If you really don't like fish (and have tried each and every incredible salmon recipe in this book!) or if you don't always manage to put two fatty fish meals on your menu each week, take a fish oil supplement to make up the shortfall (two fatty fish meals or two fish oil supplements per week). Each fish oil capsule should contain 1 gram of fish oil.

» If you're diagnosed with heart disease, you should take 1 gram of fish oil supplements daily (except on those days that you eat fatty fish). People at high risk for developing heart disease, such as people who suffer from diabetes, should also consider a daily fish oil capsule.

» If you have been diagnosed with high blood triglycerides, you should take 2 to 4 grams of fish oil from supplements per day.

» If you suffer from depression, at least 1 gram of fish oil from supplements per day may be helpful.

» If you suffer from inflammatory disorders like rheumatoid arthritis, psoriasis, or inflammatory bowel diseases you may need to take at least 3 grams of fish oil from supplements each day.

» All fish oil supplements should be a combination of EPA and DHA (the two types of omega-3 fats found in fish).

Please Note

Before taking fish oil supplements, always discuss with your doctor. This is especially important if taking 3 grams of fish oil or more per day as it may interfere with some medications, such as anticoagulant drugs.

QUOTE OF THE DAY

"Fish is likely the single most important food to eat for health, based on the evidence."
—Dr. Darivsh Mozaffarian, Harvard School of Public Health

RESEARCH HIGHLIGHT

In a report in the *American Journal of Preventive Medicine*, eight leading experts concluded the following: the benefits of eating salmon are at least 100-fold greater than the estimates of harm, which may not exist at all.

RESEARCH HIGHLIGHT

The GISSI trial is one of the largest population studies to look at the benefits of taking fish oil capsules on the risk of heart disease. In this study, involving over 11,000 Italian men and women with pre-existing heart disease, those who took 1 gram of fish oil daily slashed their risk of dying from a heart attack by 45%.

QUESTION OF THE DAY

"I take cod liver oil everyday. Do you recommend this?" If you take fish oil, I recommend oil from a fatty fish like salmon. I don't recommend cod liver oil. Cod liver oil isn't a rich source of omega-3 fats. It's significantly more likely to contain contaminants and it's also too high in vitamin A. Too much vitamin A can interfere with bone growth and may promote fractures.

Omega-3 Content of Seafood
(per 3 oz/85 g portion)

High Source

Salmon, Atlantic	1.8 g
Anchovy, canned	1.7 g
Herring, Atlantic	1.7 g
Mackerel, Pacific and Jack	1.6 g
Salmon, Chinook	1.5 g
Salmon, pink, canned	1.4 g
Herring, Atlantic, pickled	1.2 g
Sardines, Pacific, canned	1.2 g
Tuna, bluefin	1.2 g
Salmon, coho	1.1 g
Salmon, sockeye, canned	1.0 g
Trout, rainbow	1.0 g
Mackerel, Atlantic	1.0 g

Moderate Source

Bluefish	0.9 g
Sardines, Atlantic, canned	0.8 g
Smelt, rainbow	0.8 g
Tuna, white, canned	0.7 g
Bass, freshwater	0.7 g
Sea bass	0.7 g
Swordfish	0.7 g
Mussels	0.7 g
Pollock, Atlantic	0.5 g

Low Source

Flatfish (flounder/sole)	0.4 g
Crab, Alaska king	0.4 g
Halibut, Atlantic and Pacific	0.4 g
Oysters	0.4 g
Sea trout	0.4 g
Smoked salmon	0.4 g
Whiting	0.4 g
Scallops	0.3 g
Shrimp	0.3 g
Snapper	0.3 g
Perch	0.3 g
Catfish	0.2 g
Fish sticks	0.2 g
Grouper	0.2 g
Haddock	0.2 g
Tuna, light, canned	0.2 g
Tuna, yellowfin	0.2 g
Cod, Atlantic	0.1 g
Lobster	0.1 g
Mahi mahi	0.1 g
Pike, northern	0.1 g
Orange roughy	0.0 g

Source: USDA Nutrient Database

ULTIMATE FOODS FOR ULTIMATE HEALTH

Enjoy two servings of higher fat fish, like salmon, each week. People suffering from heart disease, high triglycerides, depression, and inflammatory disorders should consider a fish oil supplement in consultation with their doctor.

MORE CHICKEN, LESS BEEF, & EGGS ARE OKAY

FOR ULTIMATE HEALTH

» Moderate your intake of poultry (skin removed).

» Limit your intake of red meat and processed meats.

» Minimize your intake of the harmful compounds formed when meat is cooked.

» Moderate your intake of eggs.

WHERE'S THE BEEF?

Is it okay to eat red meat like beef, veal, lamb, and pork? Compared to other sources, meat (especially beef) provides substantial amounts of highly available (easily absorbed) iron and zinc. Many people—especially females—fail to get enough of these two nutrients. Even mild deficiencies of iron and zinc are linked to poor growth, impaired learning ability, reduced work performance, and lower resistance to infections. Meat also contributes significant amounts of protein, vitamin B12, selenium, phosphorus, niacin, vitamin B6, and riboflavin. There is, however, a dark side to the meat story. High intakes of red meat and processed meats in particular can cause cell damage and may increase the risk of some cancers and possibly type 2 diabetes. Eating too many fatty meats can also cause arteries to clog, leading to a heart attack or stroke. My advice: don't stop eating meat, but be sure to follow my five rules for healthy meat eating.

The Five Rules for Healthy Meat Eating

Rule #1: Minimize Your Portion Size

For ultimate health a "deck of cards" serving size is recommended for meat.

ONE SERVING OF MEAT	2 to 3 oz (55 to 85 g) lean meat or poultry 2 slices lean cold cuts (2 oz/55 g)

RESEARCH HIGHLIGHT
In research from the Karolinska Institute in Sweden involving over 60,000 women, high intakes of red or processed meats (like bacon, sausage, hot dogs, ham, and salami) were linked to a 66% higher risk of stomach cancer, a 73% higher risk of pancreatic cancer, and more than double the risk of distal colon cancer (cancer near the end of the colon).

RESEARCH HIGHLIGHT
In the Harvard Nurses Health Study involving almost 70,000 women, every one-serving increase in red meat increased the risk of type 2 diabetes by 26%. For processed meats, like bacon and hot dogs, the risk was increased by as much as 73%.

RESEARCH HIGHLIGHT
For a smaller waistline, eat less meat. In research from Tufts University involving 55,000 women, 40% of meat eaters were overweight compared to 29% of vegans (who eat no animal foods) and semi-vegetarians (who eat milk and fish).

Vegetarians generally have lower rates of disease than meat-eaters. Countries that have the lowest rates of disease, like the Mediterranean and Japan, eat meat, but not in large quantities. For example, Japan eats about one-third as much meat as the United States. How much meat should you eat? You need two to three servings of meat, poultry, fish, or alternatives like eggs, beans, or nuts each day. Each serving of meat, poultry, or fish should be about the size of a "deck of cards" (3oz/85g). This means meat shouldn't be the main focus of your meal. Enjoy meat in stir-fries, stews, kabobs, and fajitas where other foods like veggies and whole grains take center stage.

Rule #2: It's Gotta Be Lean

For ultimate health eat only lean meat and poultry.

Evidence suggests that the diet upon which humans evolved included meat. However, the meat consumed was primarily wild game, which is extremely lean. Today, meat is a major source of artery-clogging saturated fat in the North American diet—primarily due to our consumption of ground beef like hamburgers and fatty processed meats like salami, bacon, sausages, and hot dogs. If you're going to eat meat, it's got to be lean. Here are my tips for a lean meat diet:

1 For beef or pork, round and loin cuts are generally the leanest. Sirloin steak, pork tenderloin, and pork center loin chops are good examples of lower fat loin cuts. Eye of round, top round, and bottom round are good examples of lower fat round cuts (round cuts are tougher and need to be cooked by moist heat methods like stewing or braising). Stay away from ribs. Just six pork side ribs can set you back a whopping 55 grams of fat and 750 calories. All cuts of veal are lean except veal cutlets (ground and cubed) and breast.

2 If you buy ground meat, choose "extra lean." Brown the meat and drain off the fat before adding to foods like chili, spaghetti sauce, or shepherd's pie. Be wary of pre-made frozen burgers that can ring in at more than 30 grams of fat for just one burger. Compare labels and opt for lean or fat-reduced burgers instead.

3 For chicken or turkey, breast meat is the leanest. However, all cuts can be enjoyed as long as the skin is removed (dark meat is higher in iron and zinc). About 50 to 80% of the fat is in the skin, and it's the not-so-healthy saturated kind. Chicken wings are particularly lethal. Just six wings can boost your fat intake by almost 50 grams and your calorie intake by close to 800 (now that's scary!).

4 Choose low-fat luncheon meats such as lean roast beef, turkey, chicken, and ham, rather than salami or bologna, which contain as much as 10

QUOTE OF THE DAY
"A meal that's both tasty and cancer protective should contain a high proportion of foods like fruits, vegetables, and grains that are rich in cancer-fighting substances and a much smaller proportion of meat."
—Dr. Ritva Butrum, American Institute for Cancer Research

GOOD ADVICE
Dining out at a steakhouse? Avoid the prime rib—it's highest in fat. Go for a sirloin steak or filet mignon. Trim any visible fat and choose the smallest serving size available. Most restaurants serve steaks that are at least two to three times larger than the "deck of cards" serving size that's recommended (taking some home in a doggy bag is always a good idea). Some restaurants boldly serve a 72-oz (2,040-g) steak. That's 24 times more meat than you need in one sitting!

RESEARCH HIGHLIGHT
In the CARDIA study involving over 4,300 men and women, higher intakes of red meat and processed meat were linked to a significantly higher risk of high blood pressure.

times more fat. Stay away from high fat bacon, sausages, and hot dogs.

5 The leanest lamb cuts are leg, arm, and loin.

Rule #3: Cook Safely

For ultimate health cook meat to minimize the formation of cancer-causing compounds.

When you cook meat, poultry, or fish by high-heat methods such as pan frying, broiling, or grilling, potent cancer-causing compounds called heterocyclic amines (HCAs) can form on the surface of the meat. The longer the food is cooked, and the higher the temperature, the greater the number of HCAs. These cancer-causing compounds appear to preferentially target cells in our colon, prostate (in men), and breast (in women). They can cause genetic mutations that may ultimately lead to cancer. In addition, when the fat from meat, poultry, or fish drips onto hot coals or the burner when grilling, another type of cancer-causing compound called polycyclic aromatic hydrocarbons (PAHs) form. These PAHs are deposited onto the food when the smoke rises. Does this mean you should never eat foods cooked on the barbecue or by other high-heat methods? No, but it does mean that you need to take some precautions.

Cooking Tips for Healthy Meat Eating (When Pan Frying, Broiling, or Grilling)

1 Marinate your meat before cooking it. A marinade that contains beneficial plant compounds, including antioxidants, can reduce the formation of cancer-causing compounds from 40 to 90%. Effective marinade ingredients include extra virgin olive oil, green or black tea, garlic, lemon juice, and most herbs and spices including turmeric, oregano, and rosemary.

2 Choose lean, well-trimmed meats to grill. They have less fat to drip onto the flames. Remove the skin from poultry.

3 For faster cooking times, keep meat portions small. Skewered kebobs cook the fastest on the grill. Stir-frying small strips of meat is your best option when pan-frying.

4 Consider precooking meats in the oven or microwave and then grilling them briefly for flavour. In one study, meat that was microwaved for 2 minutes before cooking formed 90% less cancer-causing compounds.

5 Keep flipping and lower the temperature. Research has found that cooking hamburger patties at a lower temperature and turning them frequently

CANCER RISKS

RESEARCH HIGHLIGHT
Based on research from the University of Guelph, breast-feeding mothers who consume charred meats are passing potentially cancer-causing compounds on to their babies.

RSEARCH HIGHLIGHT
In a study from the National Cancer Institute involving over 29,000 men, eating very well done meat regularly was associated with a 40% higher risk of prostate cancer.

RESEARCH HIGHLIGHT
In the Iowa Women's Health Study involving over 42,000 women, consistently eating very well-done steak, bacon, and hamburgers was linked to an almost five times greater risk of breast cancer.

accelerates the cooking process and helps prevent the formation of cancer-causing compounds.

6 Remove all charred or burned portions of food before eating.

7 Stewing, simmering, and braising are all considered safer cooking methods for meat. Baking or roasting meat is also safer, especially if the oven temperature is kept below 325°F (160°C).

8 Don't worry about grilling your veggies, fruit, or soy burgers. Only meat, fish, and poultry form cancer-causing compounds during cooking.

Rule #4: Beware of Processed Meats

For ultimate health choose fresh meat over processed meats whenever possible.

Meat is considered processed if it contains added preservatives like salt, nitrites, or nitrates. Cold cuts, bacon, sausages, hot dogs, and most pre-made hamburgers fall into this category. The sodium content of most processed meats is alarming. Too much salt can increase blood pressure and the risk of a heart attack or stroke. A salty diet also boosts the risk for stomach cancer. Preservatives added to processed meats, like nitrites and nitrates, can be converted to compounds called nitrosamines during cooking and in the body. Nitrosamines are linked to a higher cancer risk, especially for cancer of the colon. Although some food manufacturers are making an effort to add less sodium and preservatives to their products, eating fresh meat whenever possible is the healthier choice. For example, putting leftover fresh cooked chicken from last nights dinner in your sandwich is better than chicken from the deli counter that contains added salt and preservatives. If you do eat processed meats, be sure to look for brands that are lower in fat and sodium.

Rule #5: Limit Red Meat

For ultimate health enjoy red meat no more than two to three times per week. Choose chicken, fish, or meatless meals, like beans, more often.

Red meat is linked to a higher overall risk of disease than chicken or fish. Why? At least part of the reason may be due to the iron. Red meat, chicken, and fish all contain a type of iron called heme iron. Beef, however, contains twice as much heme iron as chicken or fish. Getting enough iron in our diets is absolutely essential, but getting too much may actually be harmful to health. Heme iron is considered cytotoxic, which means in excess it can be toxic or damaging to cells. For example, research has shown it can damage the lining of the colon and cause the type of abnormal cell growth that leads to colon cancer. Excess iron also increases the production of free radicals in the body, which causes additional injury to body cells.

RESEARCH HIGHLIGHT
In a study from the Dunn Human Nutrition Unit in England, researchers examined cells from the lining of the colon from people who consumed a red meat, vegetarian, or high fibre diet for 15 days. They discovered that red meat raises the level of nitroso-compounds in the large bowel that can alter DNA (the blueprint our cells use to reproduce), which increases the likelihood of cancer.

QUESTION OF THE DAY
"If I don't eat a lot of red meat, how can I meet my needs for iron?" Good animal sources include chicken, seafood, and eggs. Fortified breakfast cereals are one of your best plant sources, as well as whole grains, beans, dried fruit, nuts, and seeds. Boost the absorption of the iron found in eggs and plant foods by enjoying foods rich in vitamin C at the same meal (like orange juice, red pepper, kiwi, strawberries, or broccoli).

In the Harvard Nurses' Health Study, the risk of developing type 2 diabetes climbed in tandem with heme iron consumption. In another study from the Netherlands, high heme intake was associated with a 65% greater risk of heart disease. This doesn't mean you should stop eating red meat. Red meat helps many women meet their iron needs. Simply limit your intake of red meat to two to three servings weekly. In most studies, the harmful effects of eating meat were seen in people eating one to two servings of red meat every day. Eat chicken, fish, or alternatives to meat, like beans, more often. I also recommend including plenty of plant-based foods like whole grains, fruits, and vegetables along with your meat as these foods help protect your cells from damage.

Have Eggs Instead?

For ultimate health omega-3 eggs are recommended. Have no more than one egg each day and about 3 to 4 eggs each week.

If you like eggs, put up your hand. My hand is definitely up. Eggs are low in fat and contain a whole lot of nutrition in one neat, little package. They contain more than 15 nutrients that are essential to good health—all for only 70 calories. Nearly all of the nutrition is found in the yolk, with the exception of protein, which is why I recommend eating the whole egg, not just egg whites as some people do. Eggs are a good source of lutein and zeaxanthin—nutrients also found in dark leafy greens and linked to a reduced risk of cataracts and age-related macular degeneration (a leading cause of blindness in older adults). They're also rich in choline—a nutrient required for the normal function of all cells. Research suggests that choline may be particularly important for early brain development and may help prevent neural tube defects (birth defects involving the brain or spine). Pregnant women should definitely enjoy eggs. Lastly, eggs are easy on the pocketbook and make for fast, easy meals. They're especially great for dinners on the fly when you don't have the time or energy for a more elaborate meal. But what about the cholesterol?

Here are my guidelines for healthy egg eating:

» Saturated fats and trans fats in food, not cholesterol, are the main factors that cause the cholesterol in your blood to increase. Research demonstrates that about 70% of the population can safely consume eggs in moderation (one egg per day). However, some people are more sensitive to cholesterol in food than others. These people, called cholesterol-responders or hyper-responders, experience a significant increase in blood cholesterol levels when they regularly eat cholesterol-rich foods like eggs. People with

RESEARCH HIGHLIGHT
In a study by the American Cancer Society involving almost 150,000 men and women, high intakes of red or processed meat (about 2 to 3 oz/55 to 85 g daily) was linked to a 50% higher risk of distal colon cancer (cancer near the end of the colon) and a 70% higher risk of rectal cancer. Long term consumption of poultry and fish was associated with a lower risk of colon cancer.

RESEARCH HIGHLIGHT
In the EPIC study involving 10 European countries and over 500,000 men and women, high intakes of red and processed meat (about 5.5 oz/160 g daily) was linked to a 35% higher risk of colon cancer. Low fibre diets also increased colon cancer risk. Fish was linked to a 31% lower colon cancer risk. Those who ate the most red meat and the least fish were 63% more likely to develop cancer of the colon.

QUESTION OF THE DAY
"Are brown eggs more nutritious than white eggs?" The breed of hen determines the colour of the eggshell. White hens lay white eggs and dark hens lay brown eggs. Shell colour has nothing to do with egg quality, flavour, or nutritional value.

diabetes, especially if they're overweight, appear to be more likely to fall into this category. They should consider limiting egg consumption to just a few times per week.

» The American Heart Association recommends that cholesterol be limited to less than 300 mg daily. One egg contains about 215 mg of cholesterol. Have no more than one egg each day and ideally no more than about 3 to 4 eggs per week (a healthy diet contains a wide variety of foods). On the days you do have an egg, avoid other high cholesterol foods, like shrimp and lobster. You can also limit your intake of cholesterol by choosing lean meats and low-fat milk products.

» Buy omega-3 eggs instead of regular eggs. These designer eggs are produced by chickens fed a special diet, which can include foods like flaxseed and algae. These eggs are significantly higher in omega-3 fats and vitamin E. Some chickens are fed marigolds to produce eggs that are higher in lutein. Omega-3 eggs contain both plant source omega-3 fats, as well and some EPA and DHA (the more beneficial type of omega-3 fats found in fish). But you still need to eat your fatty fish. One omega-3 egg contains very small amounts of EPA and only 90 mg of DHA. In comparison, a serving of salmon (3 oz/85 g) contains 587 mg of EPA and 1,240 mg of DHA. We need two servings of fatty fish each week to meet recommended intakes for EPA and DHA.

ULTIMATE FOODS FOR ULTIMATE HEALTH

You need 2 to 3 servings of meat, poultry, fish, or alternatives like eggs, beans, or nuts each day. Enjoy a "deck of cards" serving size for lean meat and poultry (skin removed). Cook using methods to minimize the formation of cancer-causing compounds. Choose fresh meat over processed meat whenever possible. Limit red meat to 2 to 3 servings per week. Choose chicken, fish, or meatless meals, like beans, more often. Buy omega-3 eggs and have no more than one egg daily and about 3 to 4 eggs each week.

RESEARCH HIGHLIGHT
Researchers from the University of Arizona reviewed 224 studies that covered more than 30 years. They concluded that dietary cholesterol (the cholesterol found in food) has only a limited effect on blood cholesterol (the amount of cholesterol in your blood). Saturated fats (found in higher fat meat and dairy products) and trans fats (found in deep-fried foods and some processed foods) are much more likely to cause an increase in blood cholesterol levels. Foods like beans, whole grains, nuts, fruits, and vegetables can help lower blood cholesterol levels.

RESEARCH HIGHLIGHT
Based on the Harvard Nurses' Health Study and the Health Professionals Follow-Up Study involving over 115,000 women and men, no evidence was found of a significant overall link between egg consumption and the risk of heart disease or stroke. Higher egg consumption was linked, however, to a higher risk of heart disease in people with diabetes.

GO NUTS!

FOR ULTIMATE HEALTH

» Optimize your intake of nuts
   and seeds.

NUTS: HEROES NOT VILLAINS

In the early 1990s fat was considered the villain. People stopped eating nuts. Nut consumption dropped by a whopping 40%. Then came the science—study after study demonstrated that nuts deserve a prominent place in a healthy diet. Yes, nuts contain fat, but it's mostly the healthy-for-your-heart kind. They also contain an impressive mix of protein, fibre, vitamins, minerals, and beneficial plant compounds that amplify their disease fighting potential. Plus, they easily fit into a busy lifestyle and they taste great. Most people (myself included) love nuts. Bottom line: with nuts you get outstanding nutrition, exceptional portability, and terrific taste combined with a top-notch ability to protect your health. Go nuts!

Health Protection at Its Best

Nuts most deserving reputation comes from their ability to protect your heart. Five large-scale, population studies—Adventist Health Study, Iowa Women's Health Study, Nurses' Health Study, Physician's Health Study, and the CARE study—link eating nuts to significantly lower rates of heart disease. The relationship is remarkably strong and consistent. People who eat nuts regularly are much less likely to have a heart attack and far less likely to die of one. Eating nuts is also linked to a lower risk of diabetes, some cancers, and macular degeneration. Not surprisingly, people who eat nuts live longer too!

How do nuts protect your health? Similar to other health-protective foods, nuts contain a complex mix of nutrients and plant compounds. Nuts are generally rich in:

» **monounsaturated and polyunsaturated fats**— the heart-healthy fats that help lower LDL (bad) cholesterol in your blood

PREVENTION

GOOD ADVICE
Want more nutrition in your diet? Eat nuts. People who add nuts to their diet significantly boost their intake of beneficial nutrients like protein, vitamin E, folate, calcium, magnesium, copper, zinc, iron, and fibre. At the same time they decrease their intake of unhealthy saturated fats and trans fats. Have you had your nuts today?

RESEARCH HIGHLIGHT
Why do most vegetarians have lower rates of heart disease? Is it because they don't eat meat? Some researchers believe it's because vegetarians are regular nut eaters. Making nuts a daily part of your diet can be as powerful as taking medications to lower blood cholesterol. Just one handful daily can slash your risk of a fatal heart attack by as much as 45%.

RESEARCH HIGHLIGHT
In the Harvard Nurses Health Study involving over 80,000 females, eating nuts five or more times per week was associated with a 27% lower risk of type 2 diabetes. Having peanut butter five or more times per week slashed risk by 21%.

» **vitamin E**—an antioxidant that helps prevent free radical damage and may reduce the risk of heart disease, stroke, Alzheimer's, and some cancers (including prostate)

» **folate**—a B vitamin that helps prevent DNA changes that may lead to cancer. Lowers blood levels of homocysteine (an amino acid that may cause blood vessel wall damage)

» **selenium**—enhances immunity, helps protect against cancer, and reduces inflammation

» **potassium**—essential for healthy blood pressure and may reduce the risk of stroke

» **magnesium**—important for bone and blood vessel health. May reduce the risk of diabetes and some cancers (including colon)

» **zinc**—essential for healthy immune function. May lower the risk of macular degeneration and some cancers (including prostate)

» **arginine**—a building block of protein and precursor to nitric oxide, which is a potent dilator of blood vessel walls

» **fibre**—helps lower blood cholesterol and manage blood sugar levels

» **flavonoids**—plant compounds with potent antioxidant activity that protect against heart disease, cancer, and Alzheimer's

» **sterols**—plant compounds that bind with cholesterol and lower blood cholesterol levels

The Nut Plan

For ultimate health enjoy ½ to 1 serving of nuts or seeds five or more days per week.

GALLSTONES

RESEARCH HIGHLIGHT
Nuts are rich in several nutrients that may protect against gallstones, such as healthy fats, fibre, magnesium, and vitamin E. Gallstones are hard stone-like structures formed within the gall bladder. They can be very painful and cause infections or damage to the gallbladder, liver, or pancreas. In the Harvard Health Professionals Follow-up Study and the Nurses' Health Study, men and women who ate nuts five or more times per week reduced their risk of gallstones by 25 to 30%.

ONE SERVING OF NUTS	1 oz (30 g) nuts—a small handful or about ¼ cup (60 mL)
	1 oz (30 g) seeds—about 2 to 3 Tbsp (30 to 45 mL)
	2 Tbsp (30 mL) peanut butter—about the size of a ping-pong ball
	To be even more specific,
ONE SERVING OF NUTS IS ABOUT	6–8 Brazil nuts
	10–12 macadamia nuts
	14 walnut halves
	18 cashews
	20 pecan halves
	21 hazelnuts
	23 almonds
	28 peanuts
	49 pistachio nuts
	167 pine nuts
	3½ Tbsp sunflower seeds
	3½ Tbsp sesame seeds
	2 Tbsp pumpkin seeds

Good, Better, Best

Are some nuts or seeds healthier than other nuts? Here are the facts:

» Overall, most nuts and seeds are nutrient dense and contain a nutful (or seedful) of great nutrition.

» Almonds are one of the most nutrient-rich nuts, especially high in calcium, magnesium, potassium, and vitamin E.

» Walnuts are the best source of the omega-3 fats and are rich in antioxidants.

» Peanuts are higher in protein and niacin than most other nuts, and especially rich in folate.

» Hazelnuts are high in potassium, vitamin E, and antioxidants.

» Pecans demonstrate the highest antioxidant activity of all nuts.

» Cashews contain high amounts of magnesium, potassium, and zinc.

» Pine nuts are highest in vitamin K and are rich in zinc, manganese, and magnesium.

» Pistachios contain the most potassium and vitamin B6 and are rich in plant sterols.

» Brazil nuts are highest in magnesium, are rich in potassium, and are absolutely loaded with sele-

NUTRIENTS + MINERALS

RESEARCH HIGHLIGHT
In a study by the USDA involving almost 10,000 adults who participated in the Continuing Survey of Food Intakes by Individuals, only 8% of men and 2% of women met recommended intakes for vitamin E. Eating more nuts and seeds, especially almonds, sunflower seeds, and hazelnuts, can help boost your intake of this important nutrient. Nuts are also an important source of magnesium and fibre—two other nutrients that most people fall short of.

GOOD ADVICE
Want some selenium? Eat a Brazil nut. Studies suggest that selenium is a mineral with strong anti-cancer potential. It's recommended that we get at least 55 mcg of selenium daily. Brazil nuts are the best source of this nutrient. Just one Brazil nut (not one serving, just one nut!) contains about 80 mcg.

nium. They're also higher in unhealthy saturated fat than most other nuts.

» The least nutritious nut is the macadamia nut. It's also higher in unhealthy saturated fat than other nuts.

» Sunflower seeds are nutrient-dense like almonds. They're high in potassium, selenium, folate, vitamin E, and plant sterols.

» Pumpkin seeds are rich in protein, magnesium, and iron.

» Sesame seeds are the best for zinc, fibre, and plant sterols and are also high in iron and magnesium.

Moral of the Story
Eating a variety of nuts and seeds makes the most sense.

Important Advice for Nut Lovers

To keep your nut eating as healthy as possible, keep in mind the following advice:

» Don't consume more than 1 serving of nuts or seeds daily (½ serving if you're trying to lose weight or having trouble maintaining a healthy weight). The fat and calories add up quickly. For example, 1 serving of most nuts is about 175 calories and 16 grams of fat. Make that 3 or 4 servings and you'll be wolfing back closer to 700 calories and over 60 grams of fat.

» Coconuts should not be on your eat-more-often list. Almost 90% of the fats they contain are the artery-clogging saturated kind.

» There's little nutritional difference between raw, dry-roasted, and oil-roasted nuts (because nuts are already high in fat they don't absorb much oil during roasting), but be sure to avoid nuts that have been oil-roasted in hydrogenated or trans fats.

» Whenever possible, choose nuts and seeds with no added salt.

» Buy peanut butter or other nut butters that are low in saturated fat (2 grams or less per serving) and trans fat free. If you see "hydrogenated oil" on the ingredient list, don't be alarmed. Some manufacturers add small amounts of hydrogenated or trans fats to prevent the fat from separating out.

» Don't buy light or fat-reduced peanut butter. You get less of the healthy fats, more sugar, and save few, if any, calories.

» If you buy natural peanut butter (made with just peanuts), keep it in the fridge so the fat doesn't separate from the peanut mixture.

HEART HEALTH

GOOD ADVICE
Eat almonds with the skin on. The brown skin on almonds is an important source of flavonoids (plant compounds with potent antioxidant activity). In research from Tufts University, it was found that flavonoids in almond skins work in synergy with the vitamin E in almonds to protect artery walls from damage and reduce the risk of heart disease.

RESEARCH HIGHLIGHT
In the Adventist Health Study involving over 31,000 men and women, researchers looked at 65 different food items to see which foods were most beneficial for heart health. Nuts came out at the top of the list. In addition to slashing the risk of heart disease by 40% or more (even in men and women over 80 years of age), regular nut eaters experienced an extra 5.6 years of life expectancy—free from heart disease.

» Last, but not least, remember that a peanut butter sandwich is a great fast food alternative on those nights when you don't feel like cooking. Peanut butter and banana is definitely one of my favourites.

Sometimes I Feel Like a Nut

Six Easy Ways to Enjoy Nuts

1 Sprinkle on cereal.

2 Sprinkle on salads.

3 Enjoy with cooked veggies, rice, or pasta.

4 Use in stir-fries.

5 Snack on them (portable and great for hectic days).

6 Eat a peanut butter sandwich (try with either apple slices, lettuce, raisins, banana, or even kiwi for something different).

SNACKING

GOOD ADVICE
Skip the pretzels and enjoy a handful of nuts instead. Nuts produce more eating satisfaction and feelings of fullness than carbohydrate-rich snacks like pretzels (not to mention loads more nutrition). The crunchy texture, along with the protein, fibre, and fat, make nuts a more satisfying snack. Just be sure to stop at a handful.

FANTASTIC FLAX

FOR ULTIMATE HEALTH

» Optimize your intake of ground flaxseed.

THE POWER OF FLAX

Humans have consumed flaxseed since the beginning of civilization. One of the greatest of all the medieval kings, King Charlemagne, considered the seeds of the flax plant so healthy he wrote a series of laws requiring his subjects to consume a certain amount each year. More recently, researchers have referred to flax as one of the most promising foods of the 21st century and a treasure trove of nutrients. These tasty, tiny, reddish-brown seeds contain a unique mix of beneficial plant compounds, healthy fats, and fibre. Flax's greatest claim to fame is its ability to fight cancer, especially cancers of the breast and prostate. It's also good for your heart.

Cancer Fighting Lignans, Healthy Fats, & Fabulous Fibre

Here are three first-rate reasons to make flax a regular part of your diet:

The Lignans

Lignans are beneficial plant compounds that demonstrate potent anti-cancer activity. Flax is by far the richest food source of lignans, containing over 100 times more than other lignan-containing foods like broccoli, berries, and whole grains. Some seeds, such as pumpkin and sesame seeds, are also a source of this plant compound. Lignans act as both antioxidants and phytoestrogens in the body. As antioxidants they prevent the type of damage caused by free radicals that can lead to heart disease or cancer. As phytoestrogens—plant compounds with estrogen-like activity—lignans appear to provide powerful protection against hormone-sensitive cancers, like breast and prostate cancer. They decrease cancer risk by influencing the production, availability, and action of hormones.

QUESTION OF THE DAY

"Where do I buy flax?" As the awareness of the health benefits of flax increase, so does its availability. If you can't find it at your local supermarket (be sure to ask), it's widely available at health food stores and most bulk food stores.

QUESTION OF THE DAY

"Which is better, brown flaxseed or golden flaxseed?" Some distributors of golden flaxseed claim it's nutritionally superior to brown flaxseed. Research from the Flax Council of Canada, however, indicates that both types are good choices and very similar in composition.

RESEARCH HIGHLIGHT

In a study from the University of Medicine and Pharmacy of Iasi in Romania involving 40 patients with high blood cholesterol levels, those consuming 2½ tablespoons (45 mL) of ground flaxseed daily, combined with a healthy diet, saw significant reductions in total cholesterol, LDL (bad) cholesterol, and triglyceride levels—all risk factors for heart disease.

For example, by reducing the availability of estrogen, they help block both the development and spread of cancer cells (high blood levels of estrogen can stimulate tumor growth). In animal research, mice or rats injected with cancer cells and then fed flaxseed are less likely to develop tumors. If tumors do form, there are fewer of them and they're much smaller in size. Human studies—particularly with breast cancer—confirm flax's potential as a valuable tool for both cancer prevention and treatment. Flaxseed has also been found to enhance the anticancer effects of tamoxifen, a drug used to treat women who have breast cancer.

The Omega-3s

In addition to lignans, flax is also the best plant source of omega-3 fats, also referred to as alpha-linolenic acid or ALA (this fat was also discussed in the Good Fats, Bad Fats chapter). The Institute of Medicine recommends a daily intake of 1.1 grams of ALA for women and 1.6 grams for men. One tablespoon of ground flaxseed contains 1.8 grams of ALA. Results from the Health Professionals Follow-Up Study, the Lyon Diet Health Study, the Multiple Risk Factor Intervention Trial, and the Nurses' Health Study indicate that people who consume more ALA are less likely to have a heart attack. If they do have a heart attack, they're less likely to die from it. That's because ALA helps your heart keep a strong and regular beat. Irregular heart beats (called arrhythmias) are a leading cause of heart attacks. Substituting unhealthy trans fats or saturated fats with unsaturated fats, like ALA, can reduce blood cholesterol levels. Lastly, small amounts of ALA are converted in the body to EPA and DHA (the type of omega-3s found in fish that provide additional health benefits).

The Fibre

Flaxseeds are a rich source of fibre. A mere ¼ cup (60 mL) of ground flax contains 9 grams of fibre. The same amount of wheat bran, often touted as the fibre all-star, contains about 6 grams of fibre. Flax contains both soluble and insoluble fibre.

BREAST CANCER

RESEARCH HIGHLIGHT
In a study from the University of Toronto involving 32 postmenopausal patients with newly diagnosed breast cancer, those who consumed a muffin containing 3 tablespoons of ground flaxseed daily saw significant reductions in tumor cell growth and increases in tumor cell death.

RESEARCH HIGHLIGHT
In a study from the University of Toronto, rats were fed flaxseed while nursing their young. The young rats were later injected with a carcinogen that would cause breast cancer to develop. Rats from the mothers who had been fed flaxseed were significantly less likely to develop tumors and the tumors that did develop were much smaller in size. Researchers concluded that exposure to lignans when breast tissue is forming may reduce the risk of breast cancer later in life.

ONE FLAX SERVING	1 tablespoon (15 mL) of ground flaxseed

While both types of fibre play a role in protecting your heart, soluble fibre is especially important for lowering blood cholesterol levels. Several studies have reported lower levels of total cholesterol and LDL cholesterol (the artery-clogging kind) in people who consume flax regularly. Soluble fibre also helps manage and prevent diabetes by keeping blood sugar levels in check. For gastrointestinal tract health, studies in older adults show that eating flax helps increase the frequency of bowel movements (frequent movements make for happier people!). It's the insoluble fibre in flax that has the capacity to hold water, which helps soften the stool and allows it to move through the colon more quickly (in case you wanted to know).

Flax Facts and Recommended Intake

For ultimate health consume 1 to 2 servings of ground flaxseed each day.

One to two tablespoons of flax daily appears to be a safe and reasonable amount—optimizing your intake of plant source omega-3 fats and providing lignans and some fibre. Don't have more than three tablespoons (45 mL) of flax on any given day. Flax is a food we're still learning about and the research is still in the early stages. Most foods are best consumed in moderate amounts and as part of a well-balanced diet.

MENSTRUAL PAIN REDUCTION

RESEARCH HIGHLIGHT

In a study from the University of Toronto, pre-menopausal women with menstrual cycle-associated breast pain (cyclical mastalgia), experienced significant pain reduction after consuming 3 tablespoons (45 mL) of ground flax in muffins every day for four months. Some studies also suggest flaxseed may ease symptoms of menopause.

Seven Need-To-Know Flax Facts & Tips

1 Eat ground flax. Whole flaxseeds often pass through the gastrointestinal tract undigested. You can buy flax pre-ground or grind it up yourself with a coffee grinder.

2 Whole flaxseed can be stored at room temperature for up to one year. Ground flaxseed can be stored in an airtight, opaque container for up to 90 days in the refrigerator.

3 The easiest way to enjoy flax is to sprinkle it on your cereal each morning. You can also add it to yogurt or blend it into smoothies. Another tasty option is to mix ground flax with a bit of honey or peanut butter and spread it on whole wheat toast.

4 In this book there are numerous recipes for muffins containing flax. Each muffin contains one tablespoon (15 mL) of ground flax. Try them— they're outstanding!

5 The flax content of store-bought flax breads or muffins varies widely. If you do buy them, choose products that contain ground flax combined with 100% whole grains such as whole wheat flour (many products contain whole flaxseeds combined mostly with white flour).

6 I don't recommend flaxseed oil. The oil contains omega-3 fats, but it doesn't contain the cancer-fighting lignans or fibre found in ground flax.

7 For more information on flax, including recipes, visit www.flaxcouncil.ca.

ULTIMATE FOODS FOR ULTIMATE HEALTH

Enjoy 1 to 2 servings of ground flaxseed each day.

CANCER-FIGHTING LIGNANS

RESEARCH HIGHLIGHT
Flax is the best food source of plant compounds called lignans. Research from the Technical University of Munich in Germany involving over 450 pre-menopausal women linked a high intake of lignans to an almost 60% lower risk of breast cancer.

RESEARCH HIGHLIGHT
In a study from Duke University Medical Center, 25 men with prostate cancer who ate 3 tablespoons (45 mL) of ground flaxseed daily, as part of a low-fat diet, were able to slow the progress of their cancers between the time they were diagnosed and the time of surgery.

GOOD ADVICE
Eat ground flaxseed. Unless chewed very well, whole flaxseeds pass through the body undigested. In a study from Wageningen University in the Netherlands, 12 healthy people ate either whole or ground flaxseed for 10 days. People who ate ground flaxseed absorbed almost twice as many cancer-fighting lignans.

DITCH THE SOFT DRINKS, DRINK WATER, & TAKE TIME FOR TEA

FOR ULTIMATE HEALTH

» Optimize your intake of green or black tea.

» Optimize your overall intake of fluids, including water.

» Limit your intake of soft drinks.

THE BEVERAGE QUESTION

What combination of beverages best contributes to long-term health? This is an interesting and important question. We know water is absolutely essential to good health. Name almost any major function of the human body and water plays a starring role. In fact, every living cell in our bodies depends on water to carry out their essential functions. We need milk for healthy bones. Fruit juice is nutritious, but we need to limit our intake to one cup daily. Vegetable juice is also healthy (low-sodium varieties are best). An occasional diet soft drink is okay, but they tend to crowd out healthier beverages. Regular sugar-sweetened soft drinks are all-round bad news (more on this later). What about coffee versus tea? Coffee doesn't appear to be a major risk factor for heart disease or cancer and has been linked to a lower risk of type 2 diabetes and Parkinson's disease. In moderate amounts (about two to three cups daily and no more than about 300 to 400 mg of caffeine per day), coffee can fit into a healthy diet. However, if you want the ultimate disease-fighting diet, I believe tea, especially green tea, is a better choice than coffee.

Drink Your Flavonoids

If you'd like to sip on a cup full of antioxidants, look no further than a cup of green or black tea. Both types of tea come from the same plant (the *Camellia sinensis* bush) and are loaded with plant compounds called flavonoids. Because green and black tea are processed differently (black tea is fermented, green tea isn't), the type of flavonoids they contain are different. Green tea contains generous quantities of a flavonoid called

QUOTE OF THE DAY
"Tea cannot replace the nutritional value of fruits and vegetables, but it is a good complimentary source of antioxidants."
—Dr. John Weisburger, Chair of the 2nd International Symposium on Tea and Human Health

RESEARCH HIGHLIGHT
Does tea reduce the risk of breast cancer? Based on a research review by the University of Minnesota, drinking five cups of green tea daily is linked to a 22% lower risk of breast cancer. Some studies also link green tea to a lower risk of prostate, colon, lung, and ovarian cancer.

RESEARCH HIGHLIGHT
Based on a review of 17 studies by the University of North Carolina School of Public Health, drinking three cups of tea per day may reduce your risk of a heart attack by 11%.

epigallocatechin gallate (more frequently referred to as EGCG). Black tea contains mostly thearubigens and theaflavins. The good news: both types of tea display antioxidant activity and both demonstrate the ability to fight disease. Is green tea better? Green tea has stronger antioxidant activity and appears to protect health better than black tea, especially when it comes to cancer, but both are good choices.

Here are some ways tea may act as a bodyguard for your health:

» Reduces cancer risk by preventing free radical damage and by influencing enzymes in the body that reduce the development and spread of cancer cells.

» Promotes heart health by reducing free radical damage and protecting the health of the artery wall.

» Protects against age-related diseases, including Alzheimer's, by protecting brain cells from damage.

» Boosts immune system and fights off bacteria and viruses, including the flu.

» Protects against arthritis by reducing cartilage damage caused by inflammation.

» Reduces symptoms of asthma by blocking the release of histamine.

» Fights cavities by preventing bacteria in the mouth from forming plaque on the teeth.

» Reduces diabetes risk by having an insulin-like effect on blood sugars.

Please Note

As with most foods, tea provides the best health protection when consumed on a daily basis over much of the lifespan and as part of a healthy diet.

Cup of Tea, Mate?

For ultimate health drink 3 to 6 cups of green or black tea each day. Choose green tea more often than black as it appears to provide better health protection.

Three things you should know about tea:

» Skip the decaf and drink regular. Decaffeinated black or green tea contains about 50% less flavonoids than regular tea. If you're concerned about the caffeine content, don't be. Black tea contains about 45 mg of caffeine per cup, while green tea contains about 30 mg. That's three to four times less than the amount found in a cup of coffee (coffee contains about 130 mg of caffeine per cup). Having 300 to 400 mg of caffeine daily is considered a safe and moderate amount. Even at six cups of tea daily (as long as you're not getting caffeine from many other

QUESTION OF THE DAY
"Does adding milk to tea reduce its antioxidant activity?" No. Based on research from the National Institute of Nutrition, milk doesn't appear to interfere with the body's ability to absorb or use the health-promoting antioxidants found in tea.

QUESTION OF THE DAY
"Is it true that drinking green tea will help me lose weight?" Some research suggests that green tea may boost metabolism and lower body fat. More research is needed, however, to determine if green tea can actually help you lose weight and by how much. Your best weight control strategy: eat less, move more.

GOOD ADVICE
Don't drink your tea scalding hot! While tea is generally linked to lower rates of disease, drinking your tea when it's very hot may increase your risk of cancer of the esophagus.

sources), you're within the recommended limit for caffeine. Consider drinking your tea earlier in the day rather than late in the afternoon or evening so the caffeine doesn't interfere with a good nights sleep.

» Tea bags and loose-leaf tea are both good sources of antioxidants.

» If you're having trouble meeting your needs for iron as many women do—especially pre-menopausal women—consider drinking tea between meals or at least one hour after meals. Tea decreases the absorption of non-heme iron. This is the type of iron found in plant foods, like cereal or bread. Black tea may reduce non-heme iron absorption by 70 to 80%. Green tea reduces iron absorption about half as much as black tea.

» Both oolong and white tea come from the same plant as black and green tea. They're also good choices, especially white tea. White tea is made from tea leaves not yet fully open, the buds still covered with a fine white hair. Preliminary research suggests that white tea may have even stronger antioxidant and disease fighting potential than green tea.

QUESTION OF THE DAY
"Do herbal teas provide the same health benefits as green or black tea?" Many herbal teas, including rooibos, peppermint, and chamomile, contain antioxidant-rich plant compounds like phenols and flavonoids that may benefit your health. At this time, however, there's more research supporting the benefits of drinking green or black tea. My advice: enjoy your regular green or black tea throughout the day. Later in the afternoon or evening, sit back and relax with a caffeine-free herbal tea, such as one of those listed above.

RESEARCH HIGHLIGHT
In a study from Case Western Reserve University, mice were injected with a substance that causes a condition similar to rheumatoid arthritis in people. They were then given either water or green tea (equivalent to a human drinking about 4 cups daily) as a regular part of their diet. In the green-tea group, less than half the mice developed arthritis, while in the water group, over 90% did.

GOOD ADVICE
For a more powerful mix of antioxidants, spice up your tea. Chai tea is usually brewed with milk and a mixture of spices. Whether or not you brew your tea with milk, make it a habit to add spices like cinnamon sticks and cloves to your teapot. Be wary of Chai tea that comes from your local coffee house: depending on the size and whether it's made with whole milk, these drinks can contain 8 to 14 teaspoons (40 to 70 mL) of added sugar and nearly 200 to 400 calories per serving.

QUESTION OF THE DAY
"How long should I brew my tea to get the most antioxidants?" 85% of the antioxidants are released in about three to five minutes. Don't reuse your tea bag.

RESEARCH HIGHLIGHT
Based on research from the University of Florida, flavonoids in green tea may help maintain our thinking skills as we age by reducing nerve damage to our brain. In a study with mice, green tea flavonoids reduced the build-up of a type of plaque associated with Alzheimer's by as much as 54%.

GOOD ADVICE
If you love iced tea, make your own. Because of the processing and time spent sitting on the shelf, most ready-made and powdered iced teas contain little or no flavonoids. For an antioxidant-rich iced tea beverage, try one of the recipes on pages 273–74.

Water—The Forgotten Nutrient

For ultimate health drink at least 4 to 6 cups (1 to 1.5 L) of water each day.

The importance of water is best illustrated by the fact that we can live for several weeks without food, but only a few days without water. Water makes up more than 70% of the body's tissues and plays a role in nearly every body function. A few of water's many tasks are to regulate temperature, cushion joints, bring oxygen and nutrients to the cells, and remove waste from the body. Drinking lots of water or other fluids also helps prevent constipation and reduces the risk of kidney stones.

Why 4 to 6 cups (1 to 1.5 L)? We actually need about 10 to 12 cups (2.5 to 3 L) of fluids daily to replace the water we lose all day long through breathing, perspiring, and trips to the toilet. All types of fluids, with the exception of alcoholic beverages, can help us meet this need. Most of us consume at least half of our daily fluid needs from beverages other than water. For example, on a typical day following the eating plan recommended in this book, you might consume 2 cups (500 mL) of milk, 1 cup (250 mL) of fruit or vegetable juice, and 3 cups (750 mL) of tea. If you add 4 to 6 cups (1 to 1.5 L) of water to your day, your daily fluid quota has been met.

Six Water Drinking Tips

1 Make it a habit to carry water with you at all times.

2 Keep a bottle or pitcher of water with you at work to enjoy throughout the day. If it's there, you'll drink it! If it isn't, you won't!

3 Every time you brush your teeth, drink a glass of water.

4 When dining out, always ask for water with your meal.

5 Drink extra water before, during, and after physical activity.

6 Both tap and bottled water are considered safe and healthy choices, although not all bottled water contains fluoride, which is important for dental health.

Soft Drinks: Liquid Candy

For ultimate health avoid regular, sugar-sweetened soft drinks and limit the consumption of diet soft drinks to no more than 1 to 2 servings daily, if at all.

Some researchers feel that sugar-sweetened soft drinks are so detrimental to health they should

SOFT DRINKS

QUOTE OF THE DAY
"Soft drinks such as soda and so-called 'sports drinks' are the biggest single source of kids' calories. Any serious plan to make a dent in childhood obesity would put curbing soda consumption at the top of the list."
—Michael Jacobson, Center for Science in the Public Interest

RESEARCH HIGHLIGHT
In the Nurses Health Study II involving over 90,000 women, drinking one or more regular soft drinks per day was linked to an 83% higher risk of type 2 diabetes. Increasing soft drink consumption was also linked to an increase in body weight.

QUOTE OF THE DAY
"Parents and health officials need to recognize soft drinks for what they are—liquid candy—and do everything they can to return those beverages to their former role as an occasional treat."
—Michael Jacobson, Center for Science in the Public Interest

carry a warning on their labels similar to those on cigarette packages. Here are six reasons to take regular soft drinks off your shopping list:

1 Soft drinks are called liquid candy for good reason. One can of pop (12 oz/375 mL) contains about 10 teaspoons (50 mL) of sugar and nothing in the way of vitamins, minerals, or other nutrients that are good for your health. The jumbo-sized soft drinks that are sold in some convenience stores and movie theatres contain more than 30 teaspoons of sugar per serving.

2 Soft drinks are considered a leading cause of obesity. They provide a concentrated liquid hit of calories yet do little to actually make you feel less hungry. In a study from the Children's Hospital in Boston, each additional soft drink serving was linked to a 60% increased risk of obesity.

3 Soft drinks may increase your risk of type 2 diabetes. In a study from the University of California, children with a high intake of sugar from soft drinks showed signs of poor beta cell function (a measure of the pancreas' ability to produce insulin) and a lower insulin response (less insulin was produced by the cells).

4 Soft drinks crowd out healthier beverages. It's no surprise that as people drink more pop, they also decrease their intake of healthy beverages, like milk, which is so important for strong bones.

5 Soft drinks can lead to a mouthful of cavities. The sugar and acid content of soft drinks is a lethal combination for dental health. The acid in soft drinks (even diet soft drinks) breaks down the enamel that guards your teeth. The sugar in soft drinks can cause plaque to build up on teeth and cavities to form.

Diet soft drinks are a healthier choice than regular sugar-sweetened soft drinks. But what about the safety of sugar substitutes like aspartame? Although entire websites are devoted to the dangers of aspartame (also known as NutraSweet or Equal), the majority of research suggests it's safe to consume in moderation. Because there have been fewer safety concerns with sucralose (also known as Splenda), it's the sugar substitute I most often recommend. The long-term risk of consuming any sugar substitute is unknown (most have only been on the market for the last 10 to 20 years), so using them in small amounts makes the most sense. If you enjoy diet soft drinks, limit your intake to no more than one to two servings daily.

GOOD ADVICE

No slurping! Slurpees are partially frozen beverages that come in various fruit and soda flavours. Like soft drinks, they're loaded with sugar. A small slurpee (16 oz/454 mL) contains 13 teaspoons of sugar, a medium slurpee (29 oz/828 mL) about 24 teaspoons, and a large slurpee (41 oz/1.18 L) a whopping 34 teaspoons of sugar.

QUESTION OF THE DAY

"Are sports drinks a healthier choice than soft drinks?" Many experts feel that drinking sports drinks instead of soft drinks is simply substituting one bad product for another. Although most sports drinks contain fewer calories than regular soft drinks, their primary ingredients are the same—sugar and water. As for the additional electrolytes found in some sports drinks, like sodium and potassium, unless you're involved in endurance sports like long distance running, most people can get all the electrolytes they need simply by eating a healthy diet and meeting their fluid needs by drinking water.

ULTIMATE FOODS FOR ULTIMATE HEALTH

Enjoy 3 to 6 cups (750 to 1.5 mL) of green or black tea each day. For better health protection, choose green tea more often. Make it a habit to drink at least 4 to 6 cups (1 to 2.5 L) of water daily. Avoid regular sugar-sweetened soft drinks and have no more than 1 to 2 servings of diet soft drinks daily, if at all.

RED WINE FOR GOOD HEALTH?

FOR ULTIMATE HEALTH

» Moderate your alcohol intake (wine,
beer, liquor), if you choose to drink.

A LITTLE IS GOOD

Alcohol has been called the Dr. Jekyll and Mr. Hyde of preventive medicine. If you drink a little, it's good for you. If you drink a lot, it's bad for you. Alcohol in moderation (one to two drinks daily) can reduce your risk of heart disease, stroke, type 2 diabetes, and more. Drinking beyond moderation is linked to a higher risk of stroke, heart failure, liver damage, many types of cancer, as well as a higher risk of accident or injury. Bottom line: moderation is the only way alcohol fits into a healthy diet.

Heart Health & More

How does alcohol, when consumed in moderation, protect health? Understand first that all alcohol—wine, beer, and liquor—can protect health, not just red wine, as commonly believed. It's the actual alcohol, also referred to as ethanol, in these beverages that's responsible for most of the health benefits. These health benefits include the following:

» Heart-health. Alcohol increases levels of HDL (good) cholesterol in the blood—the type of cholesterol that carries cholesterol out of the bloodstream and to the liver for disposal. Alcohol also reduces the formation of potentially harmful blood clots. Many heart attacks and strokes are caused by blood clots forming in a partially blocked artery. By reducing inflammation, alcohol may also reduce plaque build-up on artery walls.

» Protect against type 2 diabetes. Moderate alcohol consumption can decrease resistance to

RESEARCH HIGHLIGHT
According to the Center for Disease Control and Prevention, excessive alcohol consumption or alcohol abuse shortens lives an average of 30 years.

QUOTE OF THE DAY
"An individual's risk for developing alcoholism is difficult, if not impossible, to determine."
—American Heart Association Science Advisory

QUOTE OF THE DAY
"A large number of recent studies have consistently demonstrated a reduction in coronary heart disease with moderate consumption of alcohol. Any prohibition of alcohol would then deny such persons a potentially sizable health benefit."
—Dr. Thomas Pearson, Nutrition Committee, American Heart Association

RESEARCH HIGHLIGHT
In a review of 32 studies, drinking alcohol in moderation was linked to a 33 to 56% lower risk of type 2 diabetes. Heavy drinkers, or those who consumed more than three drinks per day, increased their risk of diabetes by as much as 43%.

insulin. This means less insulin is required to maintain healthy blood sugar levels.

» Preserve your thinking skills. Alcohol may protect against age-related declines in our cognitive function (our ability to think, learn, and remember).

Please Note

Alcohol provides the greatest benefit to people who are middle-aged and older—the time when the risk of heart disease or type 2 diabetes is greatest. For many young adults, the risks of consuming alcohol outweigh the benefits. Mounting evidence shows that the still-maturing teenage brain is particularly susceptible to damage from heavy drinking. Breast tissue in teenage girls and women before the birth of their first child may also be more susceptible to damage from alcohol.

Alcohol & Cancer

Alcohol is a significant cause of cancer worldwide. It's most often linked to cancers of the mouth, throat, esophagus, breast, and colon. One of the ways alcohol is believed to increase cancer risk is by damaging our DNA—the blueprint our cells use to reproduce. Cancer risk is greatest in people who consume three or more drinks daily. Even in moderate amounts (one drink per day), alcohol may increase the risk of breast cancer in women. This risk appears to be significantly higher in women who don't get enough folate in their diet. Folate is a B vitamin found in foods like asparagus, spinach, broccoli, orange juice, beans, fortified cereals, and peanuts. Post-menopausal women who take hormones and drink alcohol appear to have an especially high breast cancer risk.

The Red Wine Debate

In 1991, the television show 60 Minutes aired a segment about the "French Paradox" and the possible benefits of drinking red wine. The following month, sales of red wine surged by 44% in the United States! If you choose to drink alcohol, should red wine be your beverage of choice? It's probably your best option. Red wine is as beneficial as other forms of alcohol and may provide additional health benefits. It contains plant compounds called flavonoids, which are also found in tea, cocoa, grape, and pomegranate juice, and various fruits and vegetables. Other alcoholic beverages, such as dark beer, also contain flavonoids. These plant compounds, which act as antioxidants in the body, may provide additional health benefits for the heart. For example, they may help prevent damage to artery walls and help keep blood vessels relaxed or dilated. Some experts question whether the flavonoid content of red wine is enough to provide significant health protection. However, there

RESEARCH HIGHLIGHT
Almost 100 studies link moderate alcohol consumption to a healthier heart, including a 20 to 40% lower risk of ischemic stroke or heart attack. According to Harvard researchers, the lowest risk of heart attack is seen among women and men who drink moderately three to four days per week.

RESEARCH HIGHLIGHT
In a review of 35 studies by Tulane University School of Public Health, having five or more drinks daily increases the risk of ischemic stroke (blood clot blocks blood flow to the brain) by 69% and doubles the risk of hemorrhagic stroke (blood vessel bursts in the brain). Compared to non-drinkers, light to moderate drinkers (one to two drinks daily) lowered stroke risk by 17 to 28%.

RESEARCH HIGHLIGHT
In the Cardiovascular Health Study involving almost 6,000 men and women 65 years and older, having one to six drinks per week was linked to a 54% lower risk of dementia (loss of memory and ability to think logically). Heavier alcohol consumption (two or more drinks daily) was associated with a greater risk of dementia.

is plenty of research that supports eating a wide variety of flavonoid-rich foods, which can include red wine. Bottom line: if you currently drink red wine in moderation, enjoy it. We know the alcohol it contains is good for your heart and most likely its flavonoid content provides additional health benefits.

Your Daily Quota

For ultimate health women should have no more than one drink per day and men no more than two drinks.

ONE DRINK	5 oz (145 mL) wine
	12 oz (350 mL) beer
	1.5 oz (45 mL) spirits/liquor

QUESTION OF THE DAY
"I don't usually drink alcohol during the week, but I tend to drink a lot on the weekends. Is this still beneficial for the heart?" For optimal heart health, drinking small amounts of alcohol regularly and with meals appears to offer the best protection—especially for reducing the risk of blood clots. Consuming four or five drinks within four hours (common weekend social drinking for many people) is associated with an increased risk of stroke—especially for people who are already at high risk.

A Word of Caution

» You don't need alcohol to be healthy. A diet rich in foods like whole grains, beans, nuts, fish, fruits, and vegetables provides excellent protection against disease (without any risks!).

» To reduce breast cancer risk, women who consume alcohol should make folate-rich foods, including 7 to 10 servings of colourful fruits and vegetables, a regular part of their diet. A folate-rich diet may also reduce colon cancer risk in moderate drinkers.

» Post-menopausal women taking hormones and women with a history of breast cancer may want to avoid alcohol altogether.

ULTIMATE FOODS FOR ULTIMATE HEALTH

If you choose to drink alcohol (wine, beer, liquor), eat a folate-rich diet. Women should consume no more than one drink per day and men no more than two drinks per day. Red wine may provide additional health benefits.

GOOD ADVICE

We don't know if there's a "safe" dose of alcohol that can be consumed by pregnant women. In a study from Washington University, researchers found that just two alcoholic drinks was enough to kill some of the developing brain cells in an unborn child. The only responsible advice to women who are pregnant or who could become pregnant (as many as 50% of pregnancies are unplanned) is to avoid alcohol entirely.

GOOD ADVICE

If you want to manage your waistline, watch your alcohol intake. Drink alcohol only in moderate amounts and be careful of its ability to rev up your appetite. One study found that having one alcoholic drink before a meal caused people to eat an average of 200 extra calories—on top of the added calories from the drink itself.

RESEARCH HIGHLIGHT

In a Harvard review of eight studies from five countries involving almost 500,000 men and women, drinking more than three alcoholic drinks per day was linked to a 40% higher risk of colon cancer.

DON'T FORGET THE CHOCOLATE!

FOR ULTIMATE HEALTH

» Enjoy chocolate in small quantities.

» Use chocolate to make healthy foods taste better.

» Choose cocoa or chocolate products that contain higher amounts of beneficial plant compounds.

CHOCOHOLICS UNITE!

There's food—and then there's chocolate. Based on a North American study, chocolate is craved by more people (especially women) than any other food. Seventy-five percent of chocolate-cravers also claim that when they have a yearning for chocolate, no other food will do. The sensory reward of chocolate is exceptional—the sweet aroma, the melt-in-your-mouth texture, and the rich flavour. But could this food, which is very high in fat and calories, possibly have a place in a healthy diet?

Good-For-You Chocolate

Exciting research on the potential health benefits of chocolate continues to accumulate. Here's what we know. The cocoa bean (from which chocolate and cocoa are made) is extremely rich in plant compounds called flavanols (they belong to a larger class of compounds called flavonoids). Flavanols are also found in tea, red wine, and certain vegetables and fruit. They protect health by acting as powerful antioxidants and preventing damage to body cells. The cocoa bean is unique in that it contains especially high quantities of a specific type of flavanol called proanthocyanidins. Proanthocyanidins are made up of two or more flavanol units joined together. These compounds are also found in apples, blueberries, cranberries, grape juice, red kidney beans, and cinnamon. It's these larger sized compounds that appear to have the strongest antioxidant potential, as well as the greatest ability to protect health.

QUOTE OF THE DAY
Chocolate is a food that's been loved by people for hundreds of years. The following is a note written by a mother to her daughter around 400 years ago: "If you are not feeling well, if you have not slept, chocolate will revive you. But you have no chocolate pot! I think of that again and again. How will you manage?"

RESEARCH HIGHLIGHT
The Kuna Indians live on a series of islands off the coast of Panama and drink three to four cups of flavanol-rich cocoa daily. They have remarkably healthy blood pressure levels and don't experience the age-related increases in blood pressure so common to people in other parts of the world. Kuna Indians who move to the mainland and no longer drink cocoa experience much higher rates of heart disease and cancer.

Heart Healthy Flavanols

Research indicates that chocolate flavanols help protect the heart by:

» preventing damage to LDL (bad) cholesterol (when LDL becomes damaged or oxidized, it's more likely to result in the formation of plaque on the artery wall)

» reducing platelet aggregation and adhesion, or "stickiness" of the blood (which diminishes the likelihood of heart attacks)

» regulating and increasing the production of nitric oxide (a compound that's critical to blood vessel health and dilation)

» decreasing inflammation (plaque is more likely to rupture and cause a heart attack or stroke if there's an inflammatory environment within the body)

More Cocoa Means More Flavanols

Generally, the more cocoa a product contains, the higher the flavanol content. Research from the United States Department of Agriculture ranked cocoa and chocolate products based on their antioxidant capacity and flavanol levels. Natural cocoa powder contained the highest amounts of these beneficial compounds, followed by unsweetened baking chocolate, "dutch" cocoa powder, dark chocolate, semi-sweet chocolate baking chips, and finally, milk chocolate. White chocolate doesn't contain cocoa and therefore isn't a source of flavanols. The cocoa content of dark chocolate bars is often listed on the label (some bars go as high as 99% cocoa). Hershey's has developed a seal to identify products, such as their Extra Dark chocolate bar, that are higher in cocoa.

Preserving Flavanols

Although products that contain more cocoa generally contain more flavanols, the way chocolate is processed is also important. Manufacturing processes, such as the fermentation and roasting of the cocoa bean, can destroy many of the flavanols. Mars Incorporated, the makers of products such as M&M's, has been a leader in our understanding of cocoa flavanols and their impact on health. Certain Mars products carry the "Cocoapro" logo. This logo communicates that the chocolate has been processed to maximize the retention of naturally occurring cocoa flavanols. A significant amount of the chocolate research to date has been done using Mars products, including the Dove Dark Chocolate Bar, M&M's Semi-Sweet Baking Bits, and their CocoaVia line of products. Ideally, all companies will eventually list the flavanol content of their chocolate on product labels (currently only the CocoaVia line carries this information).

RESEARCH HIGHLIGHT
In a Tufts University study, 20 men with high blood pressure ate either a dark chocolate bar containing 88 mg of flavanols or a white chocolate bar containing no flavanols for 15 days. Dark chocolate was linked to a decrease in both blood pressure and LDL (bad) cholesterol, as well as an improvement in artery wall dilation and insulin sensitivity (less insulin required to clear sugar from the bloodstream).

RESEARCH HIGHLIGHT
As much as 90% of beneficial flavanols can be lost during the harvesting and processing of cocoa and chocolate.

RESEARCH HIGHLIGHT
In a six-month study involving rabbits with high cholesterol levels, the antioxidant, heart-protective effect of cocoa flavanols was superior to vitamin C and vitamin E.

RESEARCH HIGHLIGHT
In the ORAC test—considered the gold standard for measuring the antioxidant power of foods—a dark chocolate bar scored higher in antioxidants than black tea, green tea, or ½ cup (125 mL) of blueberries.

Don't Sacrifice Your Waistline

For ultimate health enjoy chocolate in small quantities, ideally to make healthy foods taste better. Enjoy no more than one small serving daily.

Chocolate is a food that can come with a heavy price tag: lots of calories and fat in a small package. If you're having trouble managing a healthy body weight, be sure to choose the smaller serving size and consider the guidelines below.

ONE SERVING OF CHOCOLATE	½ to 1 oz (15 to 30 g) dark chocolate
	1 to 2 Tbsp (15 to 30 mL) cocoa
	1 to 2 Tbsp (15 to 30 mL) semi-sweet baking bits

» Enjoy chocolate primarily to make healthy foods taste better. Add semi-sweet chocolate baking chips, such as M&M's Semi-Sweet Baking Bits, to trail mix, whole-grain pancakes, and whole-grain muffins. One tablespoon (15 mL) of baking bits contains 73 calories and 4 grams of fat.

» Cocoa is flavanol-rich (if processed properly) and low in fat, making it one of the healthiest ways to get your daily chocolate fix. Enjoy a hot cocoa beverage made with low-fat milk or soy milk. Mairlyn's Frozen Cocoa beverage, page 270, is possibly one of the most delicious, nutritious cocoa drinks you'll ever taste. You can also add cocoa to your recipes or baked goods. One tablespoon (15 mL) of cocoa contains 20 calories and 0.5 grams of fat. Regular chocolate milk isn't rich in flavanols, but it's still a great way to enjoy a glass of milk!

» One half ounce (15 g) of dark chocolate or two small squares of most chocolate bars contains about 80 calories and 5 grams of fat.

CAFFEINE

QUESTION OF THE DAY
"Isn't chocolate high in caffeine?" A small milk chocolate bar (1.5 oz/45 g bar) contains about 10 mg of caffeine. A small dark chocolate bar (1.5 oz/45 g bar) contains about 30 mg of caffeine. A glass of chocolate milk generally contains less than 5 mg of caffeine— about the same as a cup of decaffeinated coffee. Current research supports limiting caffeine to about 300 to 400 mg daily. Bottom line: the caffeine content of chocolate shouldn't be a concern when it's consumed in small amounts as part of a healthy diet.

Get Your Flavanols!

For ultimate health choose cocoa and chocolate that contains higher amounts of flavanols.

» Buy natural or non-alkalinized cocoa instead of "dutch" cocoa. The process of alkalinization or "dutching" can significantly reduce the flavanol content.

» Buy dark chocolate that contains at least 60 to 70% cocoa (even though for most bars you don't know if the cocoa has been processed to preserve flavanols, a higher cocoa content generally means more of these beneficial compounds).

» Buy products that have been processed to preserve the flavanol content, including the Dove dark bar (only available in the United States) and M&M's Semi-Sweet Baking Bits.

» The CocoaVia line of products (www.cocoavia. com) is the ultimate line of products for heart health. These products (currently available only in the United States) contain flavanol-rich chocolate combined with plant sterols, which help lower blood cholesterol levels. At this time there's no recommended daily intake for cocoa flavanols. However, Mars—the chocolate research leader—designed their CocoaVia product line to contain 100 mg of flavanols per serving.

ULTIMATE FOODS FOR ULTIMATE HEALTH

If you love chocolate, enjoy it in small quantities. Use chocolate to make healthy foods taste better—like whole grain muffins, pancakes, and trail mix. Choose products that have a higher cocoa content and have ideally been processed to preserve the flavanol content.

JUST A TASTE

GOOD ADVICE
Remember that for most people, just a taste of chocolate is often as satisfying (and certainly better for the waistline) as a full-fledged chocolate binge. If you find it difficult to consume chocolate without overindulging, consider avoiding chocolate altogether or limiting yourself to a once-a-week chocolate treat.

PILL POPPING FOR ULTIMATE HEALTH

FOR ULTIMATE HEALTH

» Ensure that your vitamin and mineral needs are met.

» Optimize your intake of those vitamins and minerals that may be challenging to get enough of through food.

LET FOOD BE THY MEDICINE

If you'd like to roll out of bed each morning and pop a magic pill—one that promises optimal health, eternal youth, and protection from disease—you're not alone. I have good news and bad news. First, the good. You can dramatically influence your health, disease risk, longevity, and the overall quality of your life. The bad news. You're not going to do it with a pill. For ultimate health, you need food glorious food (and an active lifestyle). The complex, disease-protective power of nutrient-rich, fibre-rich, omega-3-rich, antioxidant-rich, and plant-compound-rich foods like vegetables, fruit, beans, fish, flax, nuts, and whole grains just can't be beat. The question is: can a pill or supplement, along with a healthy diet, assist in your quest for a healthy life?

Make It a Multi

For ultimate health take a multivitamin/mineral supplement each day, especially if you're female, or over the age of 50.

Here are my six top reasons for making a multivitamin a regular part of your day:

1 Inexpensive Insurance

Although the eating plan in this book was developed to optimize your intake of essential nutrients, taking a multivitamin pill is an easy and low-cost way to make sure this goal is met.

2 Do No Harm

Taking a multivitamin, rather than high doses of individual vitamins, is definitely your safest option when it comes to supplements. Vitamins and minerals interact with each other in a very delicate balance. Too much of one nutrient can interfere with the absorption and use of another nutrient. For example, too much zinc interferes with the

RESEARCH HIGHLIGHT
In a study from Denmark, 43 healthy men and women were given either 6 servings of fruits and vegetables a day, or a vitamin and mineral supplement to replace the nutrients found in the vegetables and fruit. After 25 days, researchers measured how well each diet protected against oxidative damage (damage from free radicals). Not surprisingly, the fruit and vegetable diet provided significantly more antioxidant protection than supplements alone.

absorption of both copper and iron. And too much beta-carotene can affect blood levels of lycopene. Many nutrients are also toxic when taken in high doses—especially vitamin A, vitamin B6, iron, zinc, copper, manganese, and selenium. Lastly, many nutrients work synergistically in the body (they work best together). For example, the B vitamins work as a team, as do many of the antioxidant vitamins such as vitamin E and selenium.

3 Women Need It

Iron deficiency is the most common nutrient deficiency among women of childbearing age. Even mild iron deficiency is linked to impaired learning ability, reduced work performance, and a lower resistance to infections. Before menopause, women have higher iron requirements because they lose significant amounts of iron each month during their period. Getting enough iron from food can be a challenge, especially if red meat isn't a major part of your diet (as is the case with the eating plan in this book). That's why a multi makes sense.

4 Over Fifty

Research shows that your ability to absorb and use certain nutrients decreases as you get older. For example, due to decreases in gastric acid secretion, as many as 30% of older adults are unable to absorb vitamin B12 in the form that it's naturally found in food (bound to protein). That's why the most recent nutrient recommendations from the National Academy of Sciences state that adults 51 years of age and older should get the majority of their vitamin B12 from a supplement or from a food that contains added vitamin B12, such as soy milk. As we get older, many of us (depending on our activity level) also eat less food in order to manage our waistlines. Less food means less nutrition and a greater chance that nutrient needs won't be met.

5 Disease-Fighting Folic Acid

Folic acid, referred to as folate when it occurs naturally in food, is a B vitamin. Its greatest claim to fame is its ability to prevent devastating birth

QUOTE OF THE DAY
"What you can buy in a bottle doesn't come close to providing you with the wealth of benefits that come automatically when those nutrients are present in the form of food."
—Linda Van Horn, Research Nutritionist, Northwestern University

QUESTION OF THE DAY
"I've heard that men and older women should not take supplements high in iron. Is this true?" While women of childbearing age often don't get enough iron due to losses from menstruation, post-menopausal women and men should consider a formula that's lower in iron (5 mg or less). Excess iron can damage body cells and is linked to a higher risk of some cancers, heart disease, and type 2 diabetes.

defects involving the spinal cord and nervous system. Because many women don't get enough folate through diet alone, a multivitamin containing 0.4 mg of folic acid helps ensure needs for this important nutrient are met. Long-term use of a multivitamin containing folic acid is also linked to a lower risk of colon cancer. As an added bonus, folic acid (the synthetic form found in supplements) is absorbed twice as well as the folate found in food.

6 Hard-to-Get-Nutrients

Even with a well-balanced diet, some nutrients, including magnesium, vitamin E, vitamin D, and zinc are hard to get enough of. A multi will boost your intake of these nutrients to complement the amount you get from food.

Choosing a Multivitamin

Trying to decide what brand of multivitamin to buy can be an overwhelming decision. Use these guidelines to help you in your choice:

1 Cover all the bases. Choose a multi that contains a complete mix of vitamins and minerals. A complete formula should contain 25 essential vitamins and minerals.

2 It's okay to buy store-brand and generic products. They still do the job.

3 Post-menopausal women and all men should consider a formula that's lower in iron (5 mg or less). Too much iron may generate free radicals that can damage body cells.

4 Avoid multis that contain more than 3,000 IU of vitamin A. Too much of this nutrient can be bad for bones.

5 Minerals such as calcium and magnesium are too bulky for a single multivitamin to contain 100% of your daily requirement. Choose a multi that contains at least 50 mg of magnesium and ideally closer to 100 mg. Depending on the amount of dairy in your diet you may need to take an additional supplement containing calcium (see calcium section).

6 Don't look to your multi to get much in the way of nutrients like potassium, vitamin K, lutein, or lycopene. Most multivitamins contain only small amounts of these, if any. To meet your needs for potassium, enjoy foods like bananas, potatoes, sweet potatoes, dried fruits, winter squash, cantaloupe, kiwi, orange juice, prune juice, and beans (including soy). For both vitamin K and lutein, dark leafy greens are your best ticket for a daily dose of these nutrients. As for lycopene, processed tomato products are what you need, although watermelon, guava, and pink grapefruit can also contribute.

MULTIVITAMINS

RESEARCH HIGHLIGHT
In the Harvard Nurses' Health Study involving about 80,000 women, those who had been taking a multivitamin for 15 years were 75% less likely to develop cancer of the colon. Folic acid was identified as the key nutrient in multivitamins responsible for this major reduction in risk.

QUESTION OF THE DAY
"When is the best time to take a multivitamin?" To get the most out of your multi, take it with meals to maximize absorption and minimize stomach upset. If you take it at the same time each day, you'll be more likely to remember to take it consistently.

GOOD ADVICE
Choose a multivitamin that contains no more than 3000 I.U. of vitamin A. Why? Too much vitamin A may be bad for your bones. In a study from the University Hospital in Sweden involving more than 2,300 men, high blood levels of vitamin A were linked to a 64% higher overall fracture risk and more than double the risk of a hip fracture.

7 Ignore the extras. Don't think that multivitamins with added herbs, such as ginseng or ginko biloba, are any better. There's little evidence that the amount contained in a multivitamin provides any benefit.

8 Use the chart below to pick a multi that's most suited to your nutrient needs. Be especially sure to find one that best meets your needs for the B vitamins (including folic acid for all women who may become pregnant, and B12 if you're over 50), iron, vitamin D, zinc, and the antioxidant nutrients (vitamin E, vitamin C, selenium). Never take supplements that contain more than the upper safe limit of any nutrient. Centrum is a brand I generally recommend.

NUTRIENT	RECOMMENDED DAILY INTAKE	UPPER SAFE LIMIT
Beta-carotene	none determined Most multivitamins contain about 3,000 to 5,000 IU and research suggests that the upper safe limit in a supplement is about 15,000 IU.)	none determined
Vitamin A	Women: 2,300 IU, Men: 3,000 IU	10,000 IU
Vitamin E	22 IU	1,500 IU
Vitamin C	Women: 75 mg, Men: 90 mg (Smokers require an additional 35 mg/day.)	2,000 mg
Folic Acid (folate)	0.4 mg (0.6 mg during pregnancy)	1 mg
Thiamin (vitamin B1)	Women: 1.1 mg, Men: 1.2 mg	none determined
Riboflavin (vitamin B2)	Women: 1.1 mg, Men: 1.3 mg	none determined
Niacin	Women: 14 mg, Men: 16 mg	35 mg
Pyridoxine (vitamin B6) over age 50	1.3 mg Women: 1.5 mg, Men: 1.7 mg	100 mg
Vitamin B12	2.4 mcg	none determined
Vitamin D over age 50 over age 70	200 IU 400 IU 600 IU	2,000 IU
Vitamin K	Women: 90 mcg, Men: 120 mcg	none determined
Biotin	30 mcg	none determined
Pantothenic Acid	5 mg	none determined
Calcium over age 50	1,000 mg 1,200 mg	2,500 mg
Phosphorus	700 mg	4,000 mg
Iodine	150 mcg	1,100 mg

chart continues on next page

NUTRIENT	RECOMMENDED DAILY INTAKE	UPPER SAFE LIMIT
Iron over age 50	**Women: 18 mg, Men: 8 mg** 8 mg (27 mg during pregnancy)	45 mg
Magnesium	**Women: 320 mg, Men: 420 mg** (The upper safe limit for magnesium applies only to intake from a supplement and doesn't include intake from food and water.)	350 mg
Copper	**0.9 mg**	10 mg
Manganese	**Women: 1.8 mg, Men: 2.3 mg**	11 mg
Potassium	**4,700 mg**	none determined
Chromium over age 50	**Women: 25 mcg, Men: 35 mcg** Women: 20 mcg, Men: 30 mcg	none determined
Molybdenum	**45 mcg**	2,000 mcg
Selenium	**55 mcg**	400 mcg
Zinc	**Women: 8 mg, Men: 11 mg**	40 mg

Source: National Academy of Sciences, Dietary Reference Intakes

Please Note

The nutrient recommendations listed in this chart are for adults over 18 years old.

There's currently no recommended intake determined for nickel, silicon, tin, or vanadium.

MULTIVITAMINS

QUOTE OF THE DAY
"There are few things in medicine that are not only good for your health, but also are safe and cheap. It is foolish not to take a multivitamin."
—Robert Fletcher, MD, Harvard University

QUOTE OF THE DAY
"Clearly we can improve the overall nutrient composition of most diets with a simple, once-daily multivitamin/multi-mineral pill."
—Jeffrey Blumberg, PhD, Tufts University

Protect Your Bones with Calcium

For ultimate health take a calcium supplement if you don't consume 3 to 4 servings of milk products daily.

Calcium is critical for bone health. Consuming at least 3 servings of milk products daily, or products fortified with calcium like soy milk, provides enough calcium for most adults. Adolescents (age 9 to 18) and men and women over the age of 50 need at least 4 servings to meet daily calcium needs. This can sometimes be a challenge, especially for older adults. A calcium supplement can help fill in the gaps. A supplement containing 300 mg of calcium should be taken for every serving of dairy missing from the diet. Calcium carbonate, found in products like Tums, is the least expensive form of supplemental calcium. Take it with meals, and take no more than 500 mg at a time for maximum absorption. Calcium citrate is a supplement that can be taken between meals.

Vitamin D: The Sunshine Vitamin

For ultimate health all people—especially those over the age of 50, those who live in Canada and the northern United States, and those with dark skin colouring—should consider taking a daily supplement of vitamin D.

Vitamin D is truly an amazing nutrient. It helps your body absorb and deposit calcium in bones and teeth. When vitamin D is lacking, calcium absorption decreases by as much as 65%. Vitamin D is a powerful inhibitor of abnormal cell growth. It's linked to a lower risk of many cancers, including breast, prostate, and colon cancer. Studies also suggest that people who get plenty of vitamin D are less likely to suffer from arthritis, multiple sclerosis, both type 1 and type 2 diabetes, and have stronger immune systems. Research shows that the majority of people in North America aren't getting enough of this nutrient. For most people to get enough, a vitamin D supplement is required. Bottom line: if you're interested in getting all-star protection from disease, optimizing your intake of this nutrient, which includes taking a supplement, should be a priority.

How Do You Get Vitamin D?

When sunlight strikes your skin, your body makes vitamin D. Ten to fifteen minutes of sunlight on your arms and face about three times per week helps you meet your daily requirement. However, if you live in Canada or the northern half of the United States (above 37° latitude), you could sit naked on your roof from mid-October to mid-April and your production of vitamin D would still be minimal, if any at all. Sunscreens that protect us from the damaging ultraviolet rays of the sun also interfere with our ability to make vitamin D. So does pollution. If you have dark skin pigmentation,

VITAMIN D

QUESTION OF THE DAY
"I was told that one type of vitamin D supplement was better than another. What should I look for?" Vitamin D supplements can be purchased in one of two forms, either as D2 (also known as ergocalciferol) or D3 (also known as cholecalciferol). The better and more potent form is D3—this is the one you should buy.

RESEARCH HIGHLIGHT
In a study from the University of California in San Diego involving 1,400 women, those with the highest blood levels of vitamin D had a 50% lower risk of breast cancer. However, only a small number of women achieved high blood levels.

Researchers believe that in order to get blood levels high enough to provide protection, most women would need to take a daily supplement containing 1,000 IU of vitamin D.

you make significantly less vitamin D. It can take someone with dark skin six times as long to make the same amount of vitamin D in the sun compared to someone with lighter skin colouring. Lastly, our body's ability to produce vitamin D decreases significantly with age, requiring a higher intake of vitamin D.

What About Food Sources?

Very few foods are naturally good sources of vitamin D. Higher fat fish, like salmon, are an exception. However, we don't eat fish every day. In Canada and the United States vitamin D is added to milk and most soy milk. It's added in smaller quantities to margarine and some yogurts. In the United States it's also added to some cereals and orange juice. One glass of milk (or fortified soy milk)—your best daily source of vitamin D from food—contains 100 IU of this necessary vitamin. Vitamin D isn't added to cheese or ice cream.

Current recommendations for vitamin D are 200 IU daily for adults, 400 IU if you're over the age of 50, and 600 IU if you're over the age of 70. However, many experts believe that current recommendations for vitamin D are too low and that getting at least 800 IU, and probably more, is what's necessary for full protection from disease. More research is needed to determine the optimal amount of vitamin D required. What's my advice? At the very least make sure that you take a multi every day that contains at least 400 IU to complement the amount you get from food. In addition, I believe that taking an additional 400 to 1000 IU may provide additional benefit. Don't take more than 2,000 IU in a supplement as this is considered the safe upper limit. Lastly, please note that a vitamin D supplement (400 IU) should also be given to all babies who are exclusively breast-fed.

Get Antioxidants from Food

For ultimate health don't take high doses of antioxidant nutrients, like vitamin E, vitamin C, beta-carotene, or selenium.

Certain nutrients, including vitamins E and C, beta-carotene, and selenium are believed to act as antioxidants within the body. Researchers believe that antioxidants reduce the risk of disease and even slow down the aging process by stopping nasty free radicals from damaging body cells. While it's clear that eating foods rich in antioxidants—like fruits and vegetables—helps prevent heart disease, cancer, and Alzheimer's, the link between high doses of antioxidant supplements and disease hasn't been promising. A research review completed by the National Academy of Sciences involving more than 40 leading scientists concluded that there's insufficient evidence to support taking mega-doses of antioxidants to prevent chronic disease. In one of

ANTIOXIDANT SUPPLEMENTS

RESEARCH HIGHLIGHT
In a study by the National Eye Institute involving 3,600 men and women, taking high doses of vitamin C (500 mg), vitamin E (400 IU), beta carotene (25,000 IU), and zinc (80 mg) daily reduced vision loss in people with early signs of macular degeneration.

If you're at high risk for this disease, this is one time when an antioxidant supplement may be beneficial. Discuss with your doctor. For most people high dose antioxidant supplements aren't recommended, and may do more harm than good.

RESEARCH HIGHLIGHT
A research review by an expert panel from the American Heart Association concluded that there's too little evidence to recommend taking antioxidant supplements to reduce the risk of heart disease. Instead, the panel advises getting plenty of antioxidants from food sources, such as fruits, vegetables, whole grains, and nuts.

the largest studies involving over 9,000 people with heart disease or diabetes—the HOPE study (Heart Outcomes Prevention Evaluation Study)—no benefit was reported from taking vitamin E supplements (400 IU) for heart disease or cancer. In the Alpha-Tocopherol, Beta-Carotene (ATBC) Lung Cancer Prevention Study, involving more than 29,000 male smokers, taking vitamin E (100 IU) and beta-carotene (33,000 IU) supplements didn't decrease lung cancer risk. More importantly, both of these studies reported potential harm. In the HOPE trial, vitamin E supplements were linked to a higher risk of heart failure and in the ATBC study, beta-carotene supplements were associated with an 18% higher lung cancer risk. A few studies have also linked selenium supplements (200 mcg) to a higher risk of non-melanoma skin cancer. What's my advice? Eat plenty of antioxidant-rich foods, along with a multivitamin, to optimize your intake of nutrients like vitamin E, C, beta-carotene, and selenium, but don't take high doses of antioxidant supplements.

Here are your best food sources of vitamin E, C, beta-carotene, and selenium:

Vitamin E

almonds, sunflower seeds, hazelnuts, vegetable oils (including the canola oil and extra virgin olive oil recommended in this book), margarine, most omega-3 eggs

Vitamin C

citrus fruits and juices, sweet peppers, kiwi, papaya, guava, broccoli, dark green leafy greens, strawberries

Beta-carotene

sweet potatoes, carrots, cantaloupe, pumpkin, red peppers, dark leafy greens

Selenium

Brazil nuts, seafood, poultry, meat, sunflower seeds

ULTIMATE FOODS FOR ULTIMATE HEALTH

Take a multivitamin/mineral supplement each day, especially if you're female or over the age of 50. If you don't consume 3 to 4 servings of milk products daily (or fortified soy milk), take a calcium supplement containing 300 mg of calcium for every serving missed. Most people should consider a supplement for vitamin D (400 to 1000 IU). For most people high doses of antioxidant nutrients, like vitamin E, vitamin C, beta-carotene, and selenium aren't recommended.

RESEARCH HIGHLIGHT

A research review of 38 studies by the Southern California Evidence-Based Practice Center concluded that taking vitamin C or vitamin E supplements doesn't help prevent or treat cancer.

QUESTION OF THE DAY

"Can vitamin C supplements prevent or treat the common cold?" A researcher from the Australian National University reviewed 55 studies from the past 65 years to determine whether doses of 200 mg or more of vitamin C daily reduces the incidence, duration, or severity of the common cold. He concluded that for most people vitamin C has no effect on whether or not you catch a cold, but may have a minor effect on the duration of a cold. My advice: Skip the supplements and eat your 7 to 10 servings of fruits and vegetables daily, including plenty of vitamin C-rich produce like orange juice, red peppers, kiwi, strawberries, and broccoli.

GET OFF THE COUCH!

FOR ULTIMATE HEALTH

» Make physical activity, including both lifestyle activities and regular planned exercise, a part of your daily routine.

» Optimize the amount and type of exercise you do in order to reduce your risk of disease and help you achieve and maintain a healthy body weight.

PARTICIPATION—NOT OPTIONAL!

Do you remember the fruit and vegetable chapter—the part where I wanted to jump, yell, and do triple back-flips just to be sure you were paying attention? Guess what? I'm back! Ready to scream, sing, dance from the rooftops, and generally do whatever it takes to communicate a message I know you've heard a million times (maybe a trillion zillion times!). Regular physical activity is essential to good health (I'm talking critical, fundamental, and so very very important!). Our bodies were built to move.

Move Your Body

I figure that if I'm going to scream, sing, and dance about physical activity, I'd better give you a whole bunch of great reasons why I think absolutely everyone needs to be active.

55 Incredible Reasons to Move Your Body

» Live longer (and have a less bumpy, more enjoyable ride along the way)

» Slash your risk of death from all causes

» Enjoy a better quality of life

» Feel better about yourself

» Look better

» Have more energy

» Reduce your risk of a heart attack

» Decrease the likelihood of a stroke

» Fall asleep faster and sleep more soundly (like a baby)

QUOTE OF THE DAY
"If exercise were a drug, it would be the most prescribed medicine in the world."
—National Institute of Aging

QUOTE OF THE DAY
"Inactivity is about the same risk factor as smoking in terms of health."
—Allan Rock, Minister of Health, Canada

- » Build and strengthen your muscles
- » Build bigger, stronger bones
- » Strengthen your joints
- » Lower your blood pressure
- » Lower your LDL (bad) cholesterol and increase your HDL (good) cholesterol
- » Lower your triglycerides
- » Improve the ability of your blood vessels to expand and constrict as needed
- » Reduce inflammation and plaque build-up on artery walls
- » Decrease the likelihood of a clot forming within a blood vessel
- » Improve brain cell communication
- » Enhance new brain cell growth
- » Improve your ability to think and remember
- » Increase your attention span
- » Boost your immunity
- » Prevent stress-induced suppression of your immune system
- » Decrease your chance of catching a cold
- » Improve your balance
- » Build your stamina
- » Be more productive at work
- » Breath easier
- » Maintain healthy blood sugar levels
- » Slash your risk of type 2 diabetes
- » Improve your sensitivity to insulin (less insulin is needed to lower blood sugar)
- » Smile more
- » Feel more relaxed and less anxious
- » Don't yell or get mad easily
- » Reduce stress
- » Decrease the likelihood of suffering from depression
- » Drive down your risk of colon and breast cancer
- » Lose weight
- » Maintain your weight
- » Prevent middle-age weight gain
- » Rev up your metabolism
- » Store less fat around your belly (the most dangerous place to store fat)
- » Look better in your bathing suit

QUOTE OF THE DAY
"Regular physical activity is probably as close to a magic bullet as we will come in modern medicine; if everyone were to walk briskly 30 minutes a day, we could cut the incidence of many chronic diseases by 30% to 40%."
—Dr. JoAnn Manson, Chief of Preventive Medicine, Harvard's Brigham and Women's Hospital

RESEARCH HIGHLIGHT
Get fit! Researchers from the Cooper Institute in Dallas looked at the fitness habits of over 21,000 men. They found that men who were fit but overweight had a lower death rate than men who were lean but unfit. Men who were fit and lean had the lowest death risk of all.

RESEARCH HIGHLIGHT
In the Aerobic Center Longitudinal Study involving almost 5,000 women, those who were the most fit were 70% less likely to develop diabetes than those who were the least fit. For every additional minute on the treadmill, there was a 14% reduction in the risk of developing diabetes. No wonder they call type 2 diabetes "inactivity syndrome."

» Look better in your little black dress (or slim-fitting tuxedo)

» Keep your mind sharp as you age

» Protect yourself against fractures later in life

» Prevent declines in muscle strength that occur naturally with age

» Remain independent as you get older

» Avoid disabilities in your later years

» Lessen your chance of Alzheimer's

» Reduce your risk of falling and hurting yourself when you're older

» Cut your risk of gallstones

» Strengthen your cartilage and lower your risk of osteoarthritis

» And last, but certainly not least . . . prevent bloating and get rid of gas (as Shrek said "better out than in")

The Bottom Line

An active lifestyle, along with a healthy diet, is the greatest gift you can give yourself.

We're a Sit-in-Your-Car & Stare-at-Your-Computer-Screen Society

For ultimate health increase the amount of time and energy spent in activities of daily living.

It's almost unavoidable to be lazy. We live in an environment where it's much easier to sit than to move. We drive, we don't walk. We take elevators, not stairs. Many of us spend endless hours at jobs that require moving little more than the computer mouse. We have remotes or timers for everything from garage doors, to TVs, to coffee machines. Why, it even takes less energy to fluff a duvet than to make a bed. We live in an environment that's completely opposite of the one that shaped human evolution and optimizes good health. The solution? We have to build activity back into our lives.

Top Twelve Easy Ways to Build Activity into Everyday Life

1 If you see stairs, take them. Pretend you have a serious allergy to elevators and escalators. If you live or work on the 23rd floor, consider taking the stairs for at least three flights each day and an elevator for the rest of the ride.

2 Don't spend 15 minutes circling the parking lot looking for the spot closest to the door of the mall or supermarket. Park farther away and walk.

RESEARCH HIGHLIGHT
A Harvard review of 23 international studies concluded that highly active people slash their risk of stroke by 27% and moderately active people by 20%. Jogging 15 to 20 minutes on most days was considered "highly active." Walking briskly for 30 minutes on most days was considered "moderately active."

RESEARCH HIGHLIGHT
In a study from Penn State University College of Medicine, which followed 12-year-old girls for 10 years, physical activity was found to be the most important factor for the development of strong bones. Weight-bearing activities such as walking, running, dancing, tennis, gymnastics, and lifting weights all help to strengthen bones. Even stretching helps build a strong skeleton because the muscles stress the bones by pulling on them.

3 Put on loud music in your house and dance, dance, dance. (Singing loudly is also an option.) Dance with your family. Dance by yourself. Dancing is incredibly fun and good for the soul.

4 Keep the car in the driveway and walk. Walk to the corner store. Walk to the mailbox. Walk to the restaurant. Get off your bus one stop early and walk home.

5 Smile and say to yourself with enthusiasm, "I love cleaning my house." Then vacuum that rug. Dust those shelves. Clean those toilet bowls. (Okay, forget the smile for the toilet bowls.)

6 Have a great garden. Spend time in your garden—planting, weeding, watering, and pruning.

7 Cut your grass (but not by riding on top of a giant lawnmower!).

8 Shovel the snow from your driveway.

9 When you go grocery shopping, walk up and down every single aisle.

10 When watching your kid's soccer or hockey game, walk around the field or the arena at least two or three times.

11 Wear or take walking shoes with you to work. Have walking meetings. Take "three-minute mini walking breaks" around the office each hour. Go for a walk at lunch—even if it's only for 5 or 10 minutes.

12 Don't get too comfortable on that couch! Cut back on sitting-down time and TV time. Clean out a closet. Call a friend with your portable telephone and walk while you talk. Play a game like Twister. If you must watch TV, use commercial time to do a few sit-ups, push-ups, or simply stretch that body of yours.

Each and every time you do one of these activities, give yourself a huge pat on the back. It all adds up and really makes a difference!

Put It in Your Calendar (then just do it!)

For ultimate health a minimum of 30 minutes to 1 hour of planned, moderate-to-vigorous physical activity on most (preferably all) days of the week is recommended. For optimal weight loss and weight maintenance, 1 to 1½ hours of daily activity may be required.

Fourteen Top Tips for "Planned" Activity

Making an effort to be physically active pays big dividends, including disease prevention, lifting of your spirits, and the achievement of a healthy body weight. But knowing you should do something and actually doing it aren't one and the same. Here are some tips to make being active every day easier:

1 For many people, getting started is the biggest hurdle. If you lack motivation, start by making a list (the longer the better!) of all the reasons that moving your body is well worth it to you. Focus on that list—especially on the days when you severely lack willpower. One woman found it motivating to hang a little black dress in front of her treadmill. Another man committed to being able to run a marathon by the end of the year. For me, maintaining a healthy weight and focusing on how great exercise makes me feel helps get me on my feet (trust me, I get grumpy when I'm not active). Figure out what motivates you.

2 Start slow. You can't expect to go from couch potato to elite athlete in one day, or even one month. If you try too hard, you'll pay the price with a body that feels like it was hit by a truck, not to mention you increase your risk of injury and even heart attack. A couple of times around the block really can be a major achievement—especially if the last time you got off the couch was many moons ago. Just remember, this is your starting place. By the end of the year I want you running circles around your friends!

RESEARCH HIGHLIGHT

What do 6,000 people who have lost at least 30 pounds and kept it off for at least one year have in common? Based on data from the National Weight Control Registry they:

- follow a low-calorie, low-fat diet
- watch less than 10 hours of TV per week (much less than the national average)
- eat fast food less than once a week and eat out at restaurants of any kind no more than three times a week
- eat breakfast regularly, which helps control hunger and prevents binge eating later in the day
- maintain a consistent eating pattern throughout weekdays and weekends
- weigh themselves frequently and record what they eat on a regular basis in order to catch weight fluctuations early and act quickly to correct them
- burn about 2,700 calories a week in physical activity—the equivalent of about one hour of moderately intense activity every single day

Moral of the story: you've got to eat healthy stuff and move it to lose it!

RESEARCH HIGHLIGHT
Women who are physically active the year before pregnancy and throughout pregnancy are significantly less likely to develop high blood pressure and gestational diabetes during pregnancy.

3 Don't expect miracles. If you expect to look like Angelina Jolie or Brad Pitt by the end of the month, you're delusional. If your clothes feel a little less tight, your muscles a bit more firm, or you just plain feel better, know that you're doing great.

4 Work out with a friend. Women especially benefit from the buddy system. A buddy makes exercising more fun, and decreases the likelihood that you'll skip a day or slack off. Having more than one exercise buddy is ideal: if one of your buddies can't make it, you've always got someone else to call.

5 Commit to working out regularly for at least six months (more than half of people drop out by this time), as this will increase your likelihood of getting hooked for life. It becomes a habit that just feels too good to give up.

6 Determine what activities you enjoy most and which ones fit most easily into your lifestyle. Men tend to like organized sports like hockey. Women, especially women with children, tend to prefer activities such as walking close to home. But don't limit yourself to one activity. Research shows that people who participate in a wider range of activities are more likely to stay active.

7 Work out at the same time every day. Studies show that this is a top strategy for sticking with an exercise plan. When it's programmed into daily life, just like eating, sleeping, and brushing your teeth, you'll find you really miss it when circumstances force you to skip a day or two.

8 Exercising close to home or work increases the odds of making fitness a habit. The simpler your life, the better.

9 If exercising all at one time is too hard, break it up into manageable chunks. You still reap all the incredible benefits. For example, you could walk for half an hour in the morning before work, go for a 10-minute walk at lunchtime, and enjoy another 20-minute stroll after dinner.

10 Fact: people exercise significantly longer and enjoy it far more when they listen to great music. It's a phenomenal motivator. Another option is to enjoy audio recordings of the latest bestselling book or your favourite motivational speaker (it was Tony Robbins who inspired me to write my first book).

11 Get a dog and walk it! They're called man's best friend for a multitude of reasons. Keeping you active is one of the best.

EXERCISE YOUR MIND

RESEARCH HIGHLIGHT

A study from the San Francisco Veterans Administration Medical Center involving about 6,000 women reported that exercise keeps your mind sharp as you age. Cognitive skills (thinking skills) were 40% higher in the aging women who were most active.

RESEARCH HIGHLIGHT

One of the best ways to say good-bye to anxiety and depression is with a regular dose of physical activity. In a study from Duke University Medical Center, people suffering from depression were put either on a regular exercise program or treated with an antidepressant. Not only did exercise work just as well at reducing or eliminating symptoms of depression, it did a better job than medication of preventing the depression from returning.

12 If you're thinking of joining a health club, choose a good one. The extra money is usually well worth it. If you're new to the health club scene, take the beginner and orientation classes. (Taking an advanced step class on your first day is definitely not a good idea!) Booking a few sessions with a personal trainer is also a super way to get started.

13 If you're going to buy exercise equipment for your home, consider a good-quality treadmill (it's most likely to be used long term), plus some weights. Exercise videos are also very convenient and highly recommended. To order a great catalogue of exercise videos, phone Collage Video at 1-800-433-6769 or check out their website at www.collagevideo.com. Some of my favourite instructors are Gin Miller, Kathy Smith, and Kari Anderson.

14 Don't stop because of your age. There are 80-year-old men and women out there who could put your average 40-year-old to shame at the gym. It's never too late to move your body and reap the rewards of an active lifestyle.

Recommended Activities

For ultimate health brisk walking and resistance exercises (lifting weights) are recommended.

Walk This Way

Brisk walking is so easy. It's extremely convenient. And most people really enjoy it. It also offers tremendous health benefits. Research shows walking can reduce the risk of a heart attack as much as vigorous exercises such as jogging, biking, and swimming. In the Nurses' Health Study, women who walked briskly for 3 hours each week reduced their risk of a heart attack by 30 to 40%. Those who walked briskly for five hours or more each week cut their heart attack risk by about half. Walking also prevented the development of type 2 diabetes as effectively as more vigorous exercise. Just remember, I'm talking about brisk walking, not a leisurely stroll.

Lift It

You have more than 600 muscles throughout your body. Every move you make involves muscles. Resistance exercise (working out with weights) builds muscular strength and endurance. It's good for your heart, improves insulin sensitivity, helps keep your bones healthy, and your mood lifted. It reduces your risk of falls and fractures and helps you remain independent as you get older. Pound for pound, muscle burns three times more calories to sustain itself than fat. This means the more muscle mass you have, the more efficiently and quickly you burn calories, even at rest. As you get older, you can lose up to half a pound (0.25 kg) of muscle

RESEARCH HIGHLIGHT
A four-year study from the National Institute on Aging found that inactive older people were twice as likely to become limited in their mobility than those who were active. Women who walked an average of four miles per week (6½ km) were 54% less likely to be sidelined by a health-related condition. Men were 72% less likely. As little as two hours of walking a week was helpful.

GOOD ADVICE
It you don't already own one, buy a pedometer today! It's a wonderful little gadget that clips onto the waist of your pants and calculates how many steps you take. Studies show that people who wear them are motivated to be significantly more active. It's like having your own personal "coach" attached to your body. Aim for a minimum of 7,000 steps each day—ideally 10,000 steps or more.

RESEARCH HIGHLIGHT
In a study from Johns Hopkins University, resistance training (working out with weights) boosted metabolism (calorie-burning) for 2 hours after working out, while the increase in calorie burning from aerobic exercise like jogging lasted for less than an hour afterward. A good exercise plan includes both aerobic and resistance training exercise.

mass a year if you don't keep your muscles challenged. The result is middle-age waistline expansion (also referred to as middle-age spread). Aim for at least one and ideally two to three sessions per week. Initially, get a demonstration video or work with a personal trainer to make sure you're using proper technique.

We Owe It to Our Children

We owe it to our children to keep them active. At an International Obesity Conference, researcher Professor Seideel said, "How we deal with childhood obesity is the biggest single public health challenge of this century." The waistlines of children around the world are expanding at an alarming rate. For the first time in history, record numbers of overweight children are being diagnosed with type 2 diabetes as early as age 10 (this disease typically hits closer to age 45 or 50). Sedentary lifestyles and poor diets are to blame. As a parent, I believe you can make a difference, and have the responsibility to do so.

Keep Kids Moving Tips

1 Limit total computer time and TV time to one to two hours a day.

2 Make family time active time. Go to the playground, go biking, go skiing, go hiking.

3 Encourage your children to learn a variety of different sports such as swimming, soccer, baseball, and skating. They'll be much more likely to carry these skills with them into adulthood and stay active.

4 Monkey see, monkey do. Children of active parents are much more likely to be active themselves. Be a good role model.

THE ULTIMATE EXERCISE PLAN

Increase the amount of time and energy spent on daily living activities (take the stairs, not the elevator). Enjoy a minimum of 30 minutes to 1 hour of planned, moderate-to-vigorous physical activity on most (preferably all) days of the week. For optimal weight loss and weight maintenance, 1 to 1½ hours may be required. Brisk walking and resistance exercises (lifting weights) are highly recommended activities.

RESEARCH HIGHLIGHT
The same daily physical activity that whittles your waistline, keeps heart disease at bay, and staves off diabetes also helps protect against viruses that cause sore throats, colds, and other respiratory infections.

RESEARCH HIGHLIGHT
In the Harvard Nurses Health Study involving almost 70,000 women, every two hours of TV watched daily was associated with a 23% increase in obesity and a 14% increase in the risk of type 2 diabetes. Moral of the story: turn off the tube!

QUOTE OF THE DAY
"No matter how far the science goes, though, there's one finding that will remain indisputable: any amount of exercise is better than none."
— Steven Blair, President of the Cooper Institute

PUTTING IT ALL TOGETHER

ULTIMATE EATING PLAN CHECKLIST

(Make a photocopy of the checklist and use it to keep track of your daily choices.)

HEALTHY FATS
3 to 6 servings daily

❏ ❏ ❏ ❏ ❏ ❏

ONE FAT SERVING	1 tsp (5 mL) canola oil or extra virgin olive oil
	1 tsp (5 mL) heart-healthy margarine
	1 tsp (5 mL) full-fat mayonnaise or salad dressing
	1 Tbsp (15 mL) light or low-fat mayonnaise or salad dressing

» Choose a margarine that's non-hydrogenated (trans fat free), low in saturated fat (2 g or less per serving), and contains at least 0.4 grams of omega-3 fats per serving.

» Look for salad dressings and mayonnaise made with canola oil or extra virgin olive oil.

FRUITS & VEGETABLES
7 to 10 servings daily

❏ ❏ ❏ ❏ ❏ ❏ ❏ ❏ ❏ ❏

ONE SERVING FRUITS AND VEGETABLES	1 medium-sized vegetable or fruit
	½ cup (125 mL) raw, cooked, or frozen fruit or vegetable
	½ cup (125 mL) juice
	1 cup (250 mL) salad
	¼ cup (60 mL) dried fruit

» Limit fruit juice to no more than 1 cup (250 mL) each day.

» Eat a wide variety of brightly-coloured, dark green, orange, red, and purple/black fruits and vegetables.

» For maximum disease protection, have each of the following at least three times per week: apples, berries, broccoli, pomegranate juice, spinach, and tomato-based foods.

HERBS, SPICES, ONIONS, & GARLIC

» Increase your intake of a wide variety of herbs and spices, especially cloves, cinnamon, oregano, and turmeric.

» Make onions and garlic a regular part of your diet.

» Lower your sodium intake by adding less salt to foods and reducing your intake of high-sodium processed, packaged, and fast foods.

GRAINS

5 to 8 servings of grain products daily (most, and ideally all, should be whole grain)

❑ ❑ ❑ ❑ ❑ ❑ ❑ ❑

ONE SERVING OF GRAINS	1 slice bread
	1 small muffin
	½ hamburger bun, English muffin, small bagel, pita bread
	one 6-inch (15-cm) tortilla
	½ cup (125 mL) cooked brown rice, barley, bulgur, pasta, quinoa
	5 small crackers
	one 4-inch (10-cm) pancake
	¾ cup (175 mL) cooked cereal
	1 oz (30 g) ready-to-eat cereal—that's about ¾ to 1 cup (175 to 250 mL) of most cereals

» Start most days with a bowl of high fibre, whole grain cereal.

» If you eat refined grains, limit your intake to no more than 1 to 2 servings daily.

MILK PRODUCTS

3 to 4 low-fat servings daily

❑ ❑ ❑ ❑

ONE SERVING MILK PRODUCTS	1 cup (250 mL) milk
	½ cup (125 mL) evaporated milk
	¾ cup (175 mL) yogurt
	2 slices (1½ oz or 45 g) hard cheese
	⅓ cup (175 mL) shredded cheese
	½ cup (125 mL) ricotta cheese
	2 oz (55 g) processed cheese
	4 Tbsp (60 mL) grated Parmesan cheese
ONE HALF SERVING MILK PRODUCTS	¾ cup (175 mL) ice cream
	½ cup (125 mL) frozen yogurt
	1 cup (250 mL) cottage cheese

» Choose milk and yogurt, especially a "probiotic" yogurt, more often than cheese.

» Fortified soy milk can be used as an alternative to cow's milk.

MEAT & MEAT ALTERNATIVES

Consume 2 to 3 servings of meat or meat alternatives daily.

MEAT ALTERNATIVES	fish
	eggs
	beans (including soy)
	nuts

BEANS (INCLUDING SOY)

1 to 2 servings at least four days of the week

ONE SERVING OF BEANS	½ cup (125 mL) any type of bean
	4 Tbsp (60 mL) hummus
	1 cup (250 mL) fortified soy milk
	3 Tbsp (45 mL) roasted soy nuts
	½ cup (125 mL) tofu or tempeh
	½ cup (125 mL) soy meat alternative
	3 Tbsp (45 mL) miso
	1 veggie burger

» Fortified soy milk can be counted as an alternative to meat or to milk.

FISH

2 servings of higher fat fish (like salmon, mackerel, herring, rainbow trout) each week

ONE FISH SERVING	3 oz (85 g) fish (deck of cards serving size)
	¾ cup (175 mL) flaked or canned fish

» People suffering from heart disease, high triglycerides, depression, or inflammatory disorders should consider a fish oil supplement in consultation with their doctor.

MEAT

Limit red meat to 2 to 3 servings weekly. Choose chicken, fish, or meatless meals like beans more often.

ONE SERVING OF MEAT	2 to 3 oz (55 to 85 g) lean meat or poultry (deck of cards serving size)
	2 slices lean cold cuts (2 oz/55 g)

» Choose only lean meat and poultry (skin removed) and cook to minimize the formation of cancer-causing compounds.
» Choose fresh meat over processed meat whenever possible.

EGGS

Buy omega-3 eggs and have no more than one egg daily and about 3 to 4 eggs each week.

ONE SERVING OF EGGS	one egg

FLAX

1 to 2 servings daily

❏ ❏

ONE FLAX SERVING	1 Tbsp (15 mL) ground flaxseed

NUTS

½ to 1 serving five or more days a week

ONE SERVING OF NUTS	1 oz (30 g) nuts—a small handful or about ¼ cup (60 mL)
	1 oz (30 g) seeds—about 2 to 3 Tbsp (30 to 45 mL)
	2 Tbsp (30 mL) peanut butter—about the size of a ping-pong ball

TEA

3 to 6 cups of green or black tea daily

❏ ❏ ❏ ❏ ❏ ❏

» For better health protection, choose green tea more often.

WATER

at least 4 to 6 cups (1 to 1.5 L) of water daily

❏ ❏ ❏ ❏ ❏

ALCOHOL (WINE, BEER, LIQUOR)

If you choose to drink, limit your daily intake to no more than two drinks for men and one drink for women

❏ ❏

ONE DRINK	5 oz (145 mL) wine
	12 oz (350 mL) beer
	1.5 oz (45 mL) 80-proof spirits/liquor

CHOCOLATE

no more than 1 small serving daily

❏

ONE SERVING OF CHOCOLATE	½ to 1 oz (15 to 30 g) dark chocolate
	1 to 2 Tbsp (15 to 30 mL) cocoa
	1 to 2 Tbsp (15 to 30 mL) semi-sweet chocolate baking bits

» Use chocolate to make healthy foods taste better (add to whole grain muffins, pancakes, and trail mix).
» Choose products that have a higher cocoa content and have ideally been processed to preserve the flavanol content.

VITAMIN & MINERAL SUPPLEMENTS

Take a multivitamin and mineral supplement each day, especially if you're female or over the age of 50.

❏

If you don't consume 3 to 4 servings of milk products daily (or fortified soy milk), take a calcium supplement containing 300 mg of calcium for every serving missed.

❏

Most people should consider a supplement for vitamin D (400 to 1,000 IU).

❏

Don't take high doses of antioxidant nutrients, like vitamin E, vitamin C, beta-carotene, or selenium.

A Few Reminders Before You Get Started

» Most women, especially older women and those trying to lose weight, should choose the lower number of servings within each category. Active men should generally choose the higher number. Most others should choose somewhere in between.

» This plan can be used with children. If under the age of nine, children need only about 5 to 6 servings of fruits and vegetables daily, 4 to 5 servings of whole grains, 2 servings of milk products, and smaller servings of meat or alternatives.

» Before starting any new eating plan or exercise program, be sure to check with your family doctor. It's also a great idea to get your blood pressure, blood cholesterol, triglycerides, and weight checked at this time so you can see what a difference healthy eating makes for you (see pages 312–13 for guidelines for healthy weight, blood pressure, blood cholesterol, and triglyceride levels).

» Take it slow, one step at a time. Don't feel you have to adopt every single aspect of the eating plan overnight. You may want to start by adding more fruits, vegetables, and whole grains to your diet and then slowly introduce other foods like flax and beans. This slow progress is especially important if your current diet falls into the less-than-healthy category. It takes time for your body to adjust to all these healthy foods, including the higher amounts of fibre.

» Don't forget your water! Because the recommended eating plan is high in fibre, it's very important to drink lots of water each day in order to keep things moving along (if you know what I mean).

SEVEN-DAY EATING PLAN FOR ULTIMATE HEALTH

To help you get started, here are seven days of recommended meals and snacks.

MEAL	SUNDAY	MONDAY	TUESDAY
Breakfast	½ Ruby Red Grapefruit, 1 tsp (5 mL) Sugar *French Toast, 1 tsp (5 mL) Margarine 3 Tbsp (45 mL) Light Syrup *Spiced Green Tea (made with cinnamon sticks & cloves)	¾ cup (175 mL) Oatmeal (made with 1 cup/250 mL milk, ½ tsp/ 2 mL cinnamon, ¼ cup/60 mL raisins, 1 Tbsp/15 mL flax, 1 tsp/5 mL sugar) ½ cup (125 mL) Orange Juice *Spiced Green Tea	1 cup (250 mL) General Mills Cheerios, ⅓ cup (75 mL) Kellogg's All-Bran Buds, 1 Tbsp (15 mL) Flax, 2 tsp (10 mL) Sugar, 1 cup (250 mL) Skim Milk ½ cup (125 mL) Orange Juice ½ cup (125 mL) Berries *Spiced Green Tea
Morning Snack	*Purple Pomegranate Smoothie (with 1 Tbsp/15 mL added flax) *Spiced Green Tea	*Big Breakfast Cookie Kiwi *Spiced Green Tea	Probiotic Yogurt Plum *Spiced Green Tea
Lunch	*Broccoli and Cheddar Cheese Soup Whole Grain Toast, 1 tsp (5 mL) Margarine Apple *Spiced Green Tea	4 Tbsp (60 mL) Hummus, ½ Whole Grain Pita Bread (with sliced tomato & cucumber) 8 grape tomatoes 1 cup (250 mL) Skim Milk *Spiced Green Tea	Turkey Sandwich (made with 1 Tbsp/15 mL light mayo) Small Caesar Salad (with light Caesar dressing) 1 cup (250 mL) Skim Milk *Spiced Green Tea
Afternoon Snack	Caffe Latte (made with skim milk) Dark Chocolate (2 small squares)	Probiotic Yogurt	3 Tbsp (45 mL) Roasted Soy Nuts ½ cup (125 mL) Pomegranate Juice
Dinner	*Terrific Salmon Teriyaki ½ cup (125 mL) Brown Rice (make extra rice for Wednesday dinner) *Basic Family-Style Steamed Spinach *Carrots with Raisins & OJ 1 cup (250 mL) Skim Milk	*Marvellous Mexican Beans *Corn and Diced Red Peppers Steamed Asparagus (4 spears) 1 tsp (5 mL) Margarine 1 cup (250 mL) Skim Milk	*Sensationally Simple Stir-Fried Rice 2 cups (500 mL) Spinach (with 2 Tbsp/30 mL *Antioxidant All-Star Dressing) 1 cup (250 mL) Skim Milk
Evening	3 cups (750 mL) Low-Fat Microwave Popcorn (drizzled with 1 tsp/5 mL Margarine) Herbal Tea	12 Almonds Apple Herbal Tea	½ cup (125 mL) Cantaloupe (drizzled with Lime Juice & 1 tsp/5 mL Honey) Herbal Tea

Please Note

» Those items with an asterix (*) refer to specific recipes featured in this book.
» Drink 4 to 6 cups (1 to 1.5 L) of water each day.
» Each day provides about 1,800 calories, which is an appropriate level for most women. Most men can simply add another ½ serving of nuts to each day, along with another 1 to 2 servings of grains.
» Be sure to use a heart-healthy, non-hydrogenated margarine.

WEDNESDAY	THURSDAY	FRIDAY	SATURDAY
1½ cups (375 mL) Nature's Path Flax Plus MultiBran Cereal, 2 tsp (10 mL) Sugar, 1 cup (250 mL) Skim Milk ½ cup (125 mL) Orange Juice ½ cup (125 mL) Berries *Spiced Green Tea	1 cup (250 mL) Kellogg's Mini-Wheats, ½ cup (125 mL) Kellogg's All Bran, 1 Tbsp (15 mL) Flax , 2 tsp (10 mL) Sugar, 1 cup (250 mL) Skim Milk ½ cup (125 mL) Orange Juice ½ cup (125 mL) Berries *Spiced Green Tea	1¼ cup (310 mL) General Mills Fibre 1 Honey Clusters, 1 Tbsp (15 mL) Flax, 2 tsp (10 mL) Sugar, 1 cup (250 mL) Skim Milk ½ cup (125 mL) Orange Juice ½ cup (125 mL) Berries *Spiced Green Tea	*Whole Wheat Blueberry Buttermilk Pancakes 1 tsp (10 mL) Margarine 3 Tbsp (45 mL) Light Syrup ½ cup (125 mL) Orange Juice *Spiced Green Tea
*Banana Chocolate Chip Muffin *Spiced Green Tea	Trail Mix (2 Tbsp/30 mL peanuts, 2 Tbsp/30 mL dried cranberries, 1 Tbsp/15 mL M&M's Semi-Sweet Baking Bits) *Spiced Green Tea	3 Tbsp (45 mL) Roasted Soy Nuts Kiwi *Spiced Green Tea	*Super Banana Chocolate Shake (with 1 Tbsp/15 mL Flax) *Spiced Green Tea
½ cup (125 mL) Marinated Bean Salad Whole Wheat Roll, 1 tsp (5 mL) Margarine 1 cup (250 mL) Skim Milk 6 Baby Carrots *Spiced Green Tea	*Sandwich made with Ultimate Salmon Salad Filling 1 cup (250 mL) Skim Milk 6 Baby Carrots *Spiced Green Tea	4 Tbsp (60 mL) Hummus, ½ Whole Grain Pita Bread (with sliced tomato & cucumber) 8 grape tomatoes 1 cup (250 mL) Skim Milk *Spiced Green Tea	Toasted Egg & Tomato Sandwich (2 tsp/10 mL margarine) 1 cup (250 mL) Skim Milk 6 Baby Carrots *Spiced Green Tea
¼ cup (60 mL) Mixed Nuts 1 cup (250 mL) low-sodium Tomato Juice	Apple	3 Tbsp (45 mL) Sunflower Seeds ½ cup (125 mL) Pomegranate Juice	Mango
*Grilled Herb Chicken *Quinoa Pilaf ½ cup (125 mL) Steamed Broccoli (with 1 Tbsp/15 mL light cheese sauce) Red Pepper & Onion Skewers (tossed with 1 tsp/5 mL olive oil and grilled on BBQ) 1 cup (250 mL) Skim Milk	*Blazin' Black Bean Chili 2 cups (500 mL) Spinach with 2 Tbsp (30 mL) Honey Mustard Dressing 1 cup (250 mL) Skim Milk	*Kid Friendly Spaghetti Sauce 1½ cups (325 mL) Whole Wheat Pasta 2 cups (500 mL) Baby Greens (with 2 Tbsp/30 mL *Unbelievably Delicious Raspberry Dressing) 1 glass Red Wine	*Pork Tenderloin (Jamaican Spiced Marinade) ½ cup (125 mL) Wild Rice ½ cup (125 mL) Steamed Broccoli, 1 tsp (5 mL) Margarine 1 cup (250 mL) Skim Milk
*Basic Fantastic Frozen Yogurt (raspberry) Herbal Tea	Whole Grain Toast (with 1 tsp/ 5 mL Margarine and 1 tsp/5 mL Honey) Herbal Tea	*Frozen Cocoa Herbal Tea	Apple Herbal Tea

LIFE IN THE FAST LANE

Does your life consist of a never-ending whirl-wind of activities that leaves you starved for time and dog-tired? If so, you're not alone. Most of us live life in the fast lane, with little time to spare. A busy lifestyle, however, is no excuse for a lousy diet. Neglecting our health, no matter how busy we are, is simply not an option. Healthy eating takes less time and effort than most people realize—and the payoffs are enormous. Here are my top tips for eating healthy in a hurry.

Top 10 Tips for Healthy Eating in a Hectic World

1 Decide on Dinner. Planning a week's worth of meals is ideal and highly recommended. If this isn't an option, at least decide one day in advance what you're going to cook. By making this decision you're significantly less likely to dine out or grab take-out on the way home. This is important, because the food most people eat at home is nutritionally better in every way than the food they eat outside the home.

2 Keep the House Stocked with Quick-to-Fix Menu Staples. Do a major shop at the grocery store at least once a week. Buy fresh food to use earlier in the week. Keep your freezer filled with frozen vegetables and fruit (especially berries), salmon fillets, and chicken breasts. Pack your cupboards with canned beans, peanut butter, nuts, canned fruit, brown rice, whole grain pasta, and tea. Purchase low-fat and low-sodium sauces, salad dressings, and marinades. At the very least, make sure your refrigerator contains milk, orange juice, pomegranate juice, tomato juice, yogurt, pre-washed bagged salads (including spinach), baby carrots, broccoli, and apples. It's also more convenient to buy pre-ground flaxseed than to grind it yourself.

3 Read the Labels on Frozen Dinners. If you're going to buy frozen dinners, you need to be an avid label reader (see page 137 in the label reading chapter). Dinners made with lean chicken or beans are generally your best choice. Many frozen dinners lack in whole grains and skimp when it comes to veggies. Serve them with microwaved veggies on

the side and a piece of whole grain bread. Don't forget the glass of milk!

4 Be a Snack Packer. Never leave home without packing healthy snacks in your briefcase, purse, or knapsack. Easy to pack options include apples, bananas, pears, mandarins oranges, or clementines, canned fruit cups, grapes, baby carrots, red or green pepper strips, cherry or grape tomatoes, nuts, and whole grain muffins. If you have a fridge at work, keep it stocked with yogurt and low-sodium tomato juice. With healthy snacks on hand you'll be less likely to play vending-machine roulette and reach for foods that provide little or no nutritional value.

5 Have Breakfast or Lunch for Dinner. Don't feel like cooking? A peanut butter sandwich is a great fast food alternative. Sandwich wraps or pita pockets filled with lean meat or hummus are other simple options. Kids love to build their own sub sandwiches, and French toast or pancakes for dinner are always a hit. Cereal can make a great meal at any time of day. An egg served with whole grain toast, a piece of fruit, and a glass of milk is about as easy as it gets.

6 Cook Once, Eat Twice. Doubling recipes is an easy way to cut down on kitchen prep time. Use leftovers for packed lunches or freeze them for instant dinners. I consistently make double batches of muffins. When it comes to spaghetti sauce, the bigger the batch, the fuller my freezer, the more meals I have without delay.

7 Have the Right Tools. A hand-held electric blender is a must-have for super quick and delicious smoothies and shakes. A countertop grill, like the George Foreman grill, cooks lean meat or fish in mere minutes. A slow cooker does the cooking while you're off working.

8 Pit-Stop at the Deli-Counter. Pre-roasted chicken (ditch the skin!) is healthy and fast. Marinated bean salads, whole-grain salads, roasted veggies, and sushi are also healthy take-home fare. Ready-to-serve veggie and fruit platters are a great addition to any meal. Pass on the potato or pasta salads made with mayo—the amount of mayo they contain is generally more than you need.

9 Get Ready for Tomorrow Today. Taking a few minutes at the end of each day to start preparing the next day's meals pays huge dividends. Make lunch the night before. Take out key ingredients for tomorrow's dinner, and if possible, do some of the prep the day ahead too. For example, marinate lean meat or chicken breasts overnight.

10 Try Mairlyn's Recipes. They were designed to be fast and easy. Check out the leftover brown rice recipes, including Smith's House Recipe for the Harried Mother (page 184). Try the Jazzy Beans (page 213) and Marvellous Mexican Beans (page 215), the Terrific Salmon Teriyaki (page 233), and Poached Salmon with Mairlyn's World-Famous Lime Mayo (page 230). Quick and easy shakes include the Purple Pomegranate Smoothie (page 268) and Super Banana Chocolate Shake (page 266). Enjoy!

The Dining Out Dilemma

If you dine out regularly, the news isn't good. Meals away from home, especially fast food meals, generally contain a lot of calories, sodium, sugar, and fat, including artery-clogging saturated fat and trans fat. They're less likely to contain fruit, vegetables, whole grains, and milk, and they lack in vitamins, minerals, and fibre. Not surprisingly, people who dine out often, especially if they make regular pit stops at fast food outlets, are also significantly more likely to be overweight and are at a higher risk for developing type 2 diabetes. My advice: make the effort to eat at home as often as possible. When you do dine out, follow my top tips for healthier choices.

Top 10 Healthy Dining Out Tips
(including words of advice for fast food survival)

Please Note

As you read some of the fat and calorie numbers below, keep in mind that most of us need no more than 1,800 to 2,000 calories and 55 to 65 grams of fat for an entire day.

1 Go on-line before you dine. People consistently underestimate the calories, fat, and sodium in a typical restaurant meal. Don't make that mistake. Most restaurants today, especially fast food outlets, coffee houses, and donut shops, provide full nutritional information for all of their products on their websites. You need to know what you're eating (use my label reading tips on pages 137–39 to guide you). Print off the nutrition information from the places you eat most often and keep a copy in your car. Get your kids involved—they need to learn how to make healthy choices too.

2 Super-sized portions equal super-sized people. Bigger portions on a plate encourage people to eat as much as 50% more calories. That's why it's so important to downsize, not super-size. The smallest portions available, including those intended for children, are generally the best size for everyone. A small hamburger may ring in at only 250 calories

and 8 grams of fat, but a double patty mega-burger can set you back 700 calories and 40 grams of fat. A small order of fries might contribute 230 calories and 11 grams of fat, but go for large and we're talking 600 calories and 30 grams of fat or more. Another way to downsize is to share your entrée with a friend or enjoy an appetizer as a main course meal.

3 Go for greens, but dress them properly. Salads are a super part of any meal, as long as you're wary of calorie-laden dressings and fatty extras like cheese or bacon. A fully dressed large caesar salad may cost you over 500 calories and more than 50 grams of fat. Slash the calories and fat by ordering light or low-fat dressings. Get the dressing on the side so you control how much you use. Always opt for salads made with darker greens like spinach or romaine, rather than less nutritious iceberg lettuce. Add beans, lean grilled chicken, or fish if you want a main meal salad.

4 Deep-fried is dangerous. Avoid deep-fried foods as much as possible. They're loaded with calories and fat, which often includes nasty trans fats. Donuts, fries, onion rings, nacho chips, chicken nuggets or strips, and breaded fish or chicken are all foods that are generally cooked by deep frying. They're definitely not good for your waistline and if they contain trans fats, they're also bad for your heart.

5 Build a better sandwich. A 6-inch sub sandwich made with fatty cold cuts like salami, plus cheese and mayo, can hit you with more than 600 calories and 40 grams of fat. A 6-inch turkey breast sandwich made with lean turkey, lettuce, tomatoes, onions, and mustard provides less than 300 calories and 5 grams of fat. When ordering a sandwich, request whole grain bread. Stick to lean protein choices like turkey or ham (both are unfortunately still high in sodium). A vegetarian sandwich made with hummus is an even healthier option. Stuff your sandwich with lots of veggies. Hold the mayo or choose low-fat or light mayo if

available. Consider sharing larger sandwiches with a friend. For example, most bagels today contain the equivalent of three to four slices of bread. If your sandwich is made with a bagel or large bun, half is all you need.

6 The two slice pizza rule. I've yet to meet a person who doesn't like pizza. It's one of those universally loved foods. The problem—it doesn't fit easily into a healthy diet. How do you make it fit? Go thin crust (whole wheat or multi-grain), light on the cheese, no fatty meat toppings, and always limit yourself to two slices. For example, two large slices of veggie lover's thin crust pizza will cost you about 350 calories and 14 grams of fat. Not a low-fat meal, but it's reasonable. If two slices doesn't fill you up, enjoy it with a salad on the side (low-fat dressing of course!). Compare that to a deep dish, meat lover's pizza topped with bacon, sausage, and pepperoni. Two large slices rings in at about 700 calories and 40 whopping grams of fat (most is the artery-clogging saturated kind!).

7 Choose chicken, fish, or beans—not ribs, wings, or alfredo. Grilled chicken or fish (especially salmon with those incredible omega-3 fats), chili, bean soups, veggie-loaded stir-fries, and pasta with tomato sauce are all great menu options. A side order of grilled or roasted veggies is always a wise idea. If it's beef you want, a small filet mignon or sirloin steak is your best bet. Steer clear of chicken wings, ribs, and cream-based pasta sauces like alfredo—they're called heart-attack-on-a-plate for good reason.

8 Avoid liquid candy and calorie-laden shakes and smoothies. For many people, beverages have become a major source of calories in the diet. A large soft drink (24 oz/730 mL) provides more than 300 calories and 20 teaspoons of sugar. A large milkshake, McFlurry, or blizzard-type drink can contain from 800 to more than 1,300 calories, 27 to more than 50 grams of fat, and as much as 35 teaspoons of sugar per serving. I believe in "everything in moderation," but these concoctions

are outrageous—way beyond moderation. Even smoothies, which many think of as the ultimate health drink, can push the limit with over 600 to 700 calories per serving (the best type of smoothies are the homemade kind, made with real fruit and low-fat milk or soy milk). So, what should you drink with your meal? How about a glass of milk, some water, or an unsweetened iced tea. Sparkling water or mineral water with lime or a touch of fruit juice is also light and refreshing. Chocolate milk for the kids is a much better option than pop. And for alcoholic beverages, a light beer or wine spritzer helps keep calories under control.

9 Be cautious at the coffee counter. Large size specialty coffees, iced coffees, and hot chocolates made with syrups, whipped cream, and full-fat milk or cream can clock in at more than 500 calories and 16 grams of fat. That's not a beverage, that's a meal. Specialty teas made with whole milk, like some Chai teas, aren't much better, containing almost 300 calories and 16 grams of fat. If you have a large muffin, scone, or giant-sized cookie with your beverage, count on adding another 400 to 500 calories or so and another 20 or more grams of fat. And some people do this every single day! If ever there was a time to keep it simple, that time is now. Your best bet: a latte or cappuccino made with skim milk or a simple green or black tea. If you must have a snack, consider a nature bar made with nuts and seeds, and share it with a friend.

10 Ditch dessert, take a walk. On occasion, a decadent dessert, shared with a friend, is perfectly acceptable (especially when it's made with chocolate!). More frequent dessert diners should consider low-fat frozen yogurt or fresh fruit, like seasonal berries. At fast food outlets, most berry parfaits are healthy and delicious. A small soft serve cone has less fat than most other options. But the truth is by the time most people get to dessert they've already had more calories than they need. My advice—instead of dessert, go for a walk and burn off those extra calories.

The Power of the Family Dinner

If you have children, no matter how busy life gets, make the effort to sit down as a family for dinner and other meals as often as you can. The following research is compelling. Studies show that kids who eat with their families eat healthier food, including more fruits, vegetables, and milk and are more likely to have a healthy body weight. In addition, the more frequently families eat together, the less likely kids are to smoke, drink, do drugs, suffer from depression or eating disorders, and consider suicide. Regular family meals are also linked to achieving better grades in school and a better vocabulary. Teenagers are more likely to delay sexual activity. The family meal is a time to communicate and connect—physically, mentally, and emotionally. Parents have the opportunity to serve as role models for healthy eating habits and to share their own morals and beliefs. Who would have ever thought that sitting down at a table could be so powerful? I think I'll have dinner with my family tonight!

USING FOOD LABELS TO MAKE HEALTHIER CHOICES

Reading food labels can sometimes seem complicated and confusing, but the more you do it, the easier it gets—and the more likely it is to become a habit. Here are some tips to help you focus on the most important information on the label.

Granola Bar Label

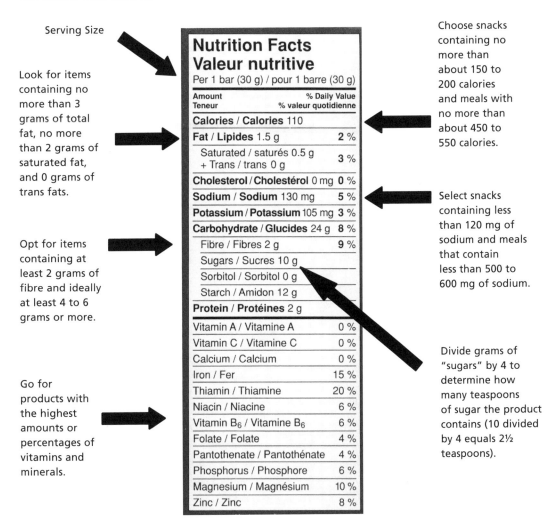

Serving Size

Look for items containing no more than 3 grams of total fat, no more than 2 grams of saturated fat, and 0 grams of trans fats.

Opt for items containing at least 2 grams of fibre and ideally at least 4 to 6 grams or more.

Go for products with the highest amounts or percentages of vitamins and minerals.

Choose snacks containing no more than about 150 to 200 calories and meals with no more than about 450 to 550 calories.

Select snacks containing less than 120 mg of sodium and meals that contain less than 500 to 600 mg of sodium.

Divide grams of "sugars" by 4 to determine how many teaspoons of sugar the product contains (10 divided by 4 equals 2½ teaspoons).

Nutrition Facts
Valeur nutritive
Per 1 bar (30 g) / pour 1 barre (30 g)

Amount Teneur	% Daily Value % valeur quotidienne
Calories / Calories 110	
Fat / Lipides 1.5 g	**2 %**
Saturated / saturés 0.5 g + Trans / trans 0 g	**3 %**
Cholesterol / Cholestérol 0 mg	**0 %**
Sodium / Sodium 130 mg	**5 %**
Potassium / Potassium 105 mg	**3 %**
Carbohydrate / Glucides 24 g	**8 %**
Fibre / Fibres 2 g	**9 %**
Sugars / Sucres 10 g	
Sorbitol / Sorbitol 0 g	
Starch / Amidon 12 g	
Protein / Protéines 2 g	
Vitamin A / Vitamine A	0 %
Vitamin C / Vitamine C	0 %
Calcium / Calcium	0 %
Iron / Fer	15 %
Thiamin / Thiamine	20 %
Niacin / Niacine	6 %
Vitamin B₆ / Vitamine B₆	6 %
Folate / Folate	4 %
Pantothenate / Pantothénate	4 %
Phosphorus / Phosphore	6 %
Magnesium / Magnésium	10 %
Zinc / Zinc	8 %

Check the Serving Size

» Always start by looking at the "serving size" on the nutrition label. Do you normally eat or drink more than the serving size listed? For example, a 16-oz (500-mL) bottle of pop may list the serving size as 8 oz (250 mL), which is half the bottle, but if you always drink the whole bottle, you need to multiply all of the nutritional information by two.

Balance Your Calories

» To maintain a healthy weight, it's important to balance the energy you take in (calories from food) with the energy you burn (physical activity).

» Most women need between 1,600 and 2,000 calories per day. Older, less active women (age 50 plus) and women trying to lose weight should be at the lowest calorie level, while younger, more active women at the higher calorie level. Most men need between 2,000 and 2,600 calories per day (same guidelines apply).

» Ideally we should have three meals and two to three snacks each day. A woman who needs 1,800 calories daily should aim for about 450 calories per meal and 150 calories per snack (based on 3 snacks daily). A man who needs 2,200 calories daily should aim for about 550 calories per meal and 180 calories per snack (based on 3 snacks daily). When looking at the amount of calories on the label, keep these guidelines in mind.

Limit Intake of Unhealthy Fats

» Choose products that contain mostly healthy fats, including polyunsaturated fats (especially the omega-3 fats) and monounsaturated fats.

» Choose lower fat products more often (no more than 3 g of fat per serving or no more than 3 g of fat for every 100 calories of food).

» Look for products that are low in saturated fat (2 g or less per serving) and trans fat free (0 g).

» Most women should have about 45 to 65 grams of total fat for an entire day, no more than about 12 to 16 grams of saturated fats, and as little trans fat as possible.

» Most men should have about 55 to 85 grams of total fat for an entire day, no more than 16 to 20 grams of saturated fat, and as little trans fat as possible.

Reduce Your Sodium (Salt) Intake

» Use your daily sodium limit of 2,300 mg as your benchmark.

» Look for soups or frozen dinners that contain less than 500 to 600 mg per serving (this is still not low sodium but is about as good as it gets). Choose snack foods like crackers, popcorn, or nuts that are unsalted or lower in sodium (120 mg per serving or less).

» Compare brands. Sodium content in the same food can vary tremendously from one brand to another.

» Many processed foods and fast food meals are very high in sodium.

Focus on Fibre

» Look for products that contain at least 2 grams of fibre per serving—ideally 4 to 6 grams of fibre or more.

Minimize Intake of Added Sugar

» Aim to have no more than about 10 teaspoons of added sugars each day (sugar contained in processed foods and the sugar you add to food). Ten teaspoons may seem like a lot of sugar. However, when you see how many foods contain added sugar (cereal, granola bars, fruit drinks, yogurt, jam), you'll see how quickly the teaspoons add up.

» To determine how many teaspoons of sugar a product contains, divide the grams of "sugars" listed on the food label by four. For example, if a granola bar contains 12 grams of sugars, that translates to 3 teaspoons of sugar per bar.

» Ingredients on food labels are listed by weight from most to least. If sugar is the first ingredient listed (or another word for sugar: glucose, fructose, dextrose, maltose), this indicates the product contains more sugar than any other ingredient.

Get More Vitamins & Minerals

» Choose products that contain the highest DV (daily value)—the highest percentage of vitamins and minerals. A food that has a DV of 15% or more for a specific nutrient, such as iron, would be considered high in iron.

Milk Products

» Choose milk products that are low in saturated fat and contain the highest amounts of calcium and vitamin D (highest % DV for these nutrients).

» Don't worry about the small amount of trans fats that are found naturally in milk products.

Grain Products

» Look for products that are 100% whole grain and high in fibre.

» Read the list of ingredients. Avoid products that contain "wheat flour," "enriched flour," "unbleached flour," or "untreated flour." Look for products that say "whole wheat flour." Rolled, instant, quick, or steel-cut oats all qualify as whole grain. Degerminated or degermed corn or cornmeal isn't a whole grain. Neither is pearled barley.

» The Whole Grains Council (www.wholegrains council.org) considers the following foods and flours as whole grain: amaranth, barley, brown rice, buckwheat, bulgur, corn and whole corn-meal, emmer, farro, kamut, millet, oatmeal and whole oats, popcorn, quinoa, sorghum, spelt, teff, triticale, whole rye, whole wheat, wheat berries, and wild rice.

Fruits & Vegetables

» Fresh fruits and vegetables don't require a nutrition label. They're always a healthy choice.

» When buying frozen or canned vegetables look for products that have no added salt or are low-sodium (less than 120 mg per serving).

» When buying canned or frozen fruit, look for products that contain no added sugars.

» Buy 100% fruit juice rather than fruit drinks, fruit punch, or sports drinks. Remember to limit fruit juice to no more than 1 cup (250 mL) daily (we should consume most of our fruits and vegetables whole).

Meat, Fish, Beans, & Nuts

» When buying meat, like chicken or beef, look for products that are lowest in saturated fat.

» Buy only extra lean ground beef or poultry and drain the fat.

» Compare brands and choose processed lean meat products, like cold cuts, that are lower in sodium.

» Remember to rinse canned beans before using them in a recipe. This will reduce the sodium content by almost half.

» Buy unsalted nuts and seeds.

SUPER NUTRITIOUS, INCREDIBLY DELICIOUS RECIPES

I love food. I love everything about food. I even love shopping for food. You want to see two kids in a candy store? Go with Liz and me the next time we hit our local Farmers' Market. There are fresh wild blueberries, just picked lettuces, hot off the tree peaches, pears, and apricots and every vegetable that can grow in Ontario. Liz is an absolute fresh pea fanatic, and I nearly have a cardiac arrest when I find the heirloom tomatoes. Yup, healthy, wonderful back-to-basics foods are fabulous. Food feeds not only our bodies but also our souls. We often rush out the door without a packed breakfast, lunch, or snack and end up eating fast food that doesn't taste like real food.

We need to get back to the basics. I know it may seem like a lot of work to prepare meals, but the results are worth it. Enlist your family, enjoy the process, and cook up foods that taste super nutritious and incredibly delicious.

Your long-term health and spirit depend on it.

Mairlyn Smith

WHAT THE HECK DOES UEPC MEAN?
It's the abbreviation for The Ultimate Eating Plan Checklist. Check how many servings of fat, fruits & vegetables, milk, beans, grains, and fish you're getting from each recipe serving. That way, you'll be able to count out your daily recommendations as you eat your way through the book.

Pantry List & Kitchen Toys

What do all great cooks have in common? A well stocked pantry—okay, and maybe a passion for food. You too can pull off a meal in minutes as long as you don't have to run out the door to buy an ingredient that should be in your pantry.

This list, although slightly daunting, will make your life simpler in the long run. Check to see what you already have and what you still need—then go shopping!

BAKING INGREDIENTS

Baking powder
Baking soda
Bran: wheat and oat
Brown sugar, dark
Chocolate chips, mini
Cocoa powder, natural
Dark bittersweet chocolate
Dried fruit
  Apricots
  Cranberries
  Currants
  Dates
  Prunes
  Raisins
Flaxseed, whole or ground
Honey
Icing sugar
M&M's mini baking bits
Maple syrup
Molasses
Prunes, strained baby food, no added sugar or starch, three 4.5 oz. (128 mL) jars
Pumpkin purée, pure canned
Rolled oats: large flake, quick-cooking, and Irish or Steel Cut
Vanilla extract, pure
Wheat germ
Whole wheat flour

COOKING INGREDIENTS

Anchovies, canned
Apricots, canned
Barley, pot
Beano
Beans in tomato sauce, canned
Beef broth, lower-sodium, canned, or in Tetra Pak
Black beans, canned
Brown rice: long and short grain
Cereal: Kellogg's All-Bran Buds, Post Cereal Spoon Size Shredded Wheat + Bran
Chicken stock, lower-sodium, canned, or in Tetra Pak
Evaporated milk, fat-free
Ginger, fresh
Kidney beans, canned
Leeks
Lentils, canned
Mushrooms, shiitake, dried

Nuts: almonds, cashews, peanuts, and walnuts
Oil: canola and extra virgin olive
Onions
Pasta, whole wheat: rotini and spaghetti
Peanut butter, natural, chunky or smooth
Plum tomatoes, canned, diced
Quinoa
Sockeye salmon, canned
Soy sauce, low-sodium
Shallots
Skim milk powder
Tapioca
Tea: black, green, and mint
Tomato paste, canned
Vinegar: apple cider, balsamic, red wine, and rice
Wheat berries
Worcestershire sauce

FROZEN INGREDIENTS

Banana, chunks
Blueberries
Corn
Cranberries
Edamame
Green beans
Mango

Orange juice, concentrate
Peas
Pineapple
Raspberry cocktail, concentrate
Raspberries
Strawberries

Pantry List & Kitchen Toys (cont'd)

REFRIGERATED INGREDIENTS

Baby spinach
Broccoli
Cheese, light, your choice
Dijon mustard: grainy and
  regular
Eggs, omega-3
Fresh Herbs, if you promise
  to use them
Fruits, your choice
Hot pepper jelly
Hot pickled peppers
Ketchup
Leeks
Lemons
Mango chutney
Margarine, non hydrogenated
Milk: skim and buttermilk
Mayonnaise, low-fat
Olives, kalamata
Pomegranate juice
Red peppers, roasted
Ribena
Salsa
Soy milk, your choice
Sun-dried tomatoes packed
  in olive oil
Vegetables, your choice
Wasabi paste
Yogurt, probiotic French
  vanilla, low-fat

HERBS & SPICES

Allspice
Basil
Black pepper
Cayenne
Chili powder
Cinnamon: ground and sticks
Cloves: ground and whole
Coriander
Cumin
Curry powder
Garlic powder
Nutmeg
Onion powder
Oregano
Paprika
Pepper: whole, cracked and
  ground black
Red pepper flakes
Salt
Summer Savory
Tarragon
Thyme
Turmeric

MUST-HAVE KITCHEN TOYS

Cocoa Whisk
Coffee bean mill (for grinding
  whole flaxseed)
Food processor
Garlic press
Hand-held immersion blender
Hand juicer
Ice cream scoop with release
  button: 1 tsp (5 mL) and
  ¼ cup (60 mL) size
Knife (make it a great one)
Meat thermometer
Parchment paper
Resealable plastic bags
Rice cooker
Salad spinner
Slow cooker
Tea leaf strainer
Tea pot, 4 cup (1 L) capacity
Zester

SALADS & SALAD DRESSINGS

Salad Dressings

Okay, you've committed to eating 7 to 10 fruits and veggies every day, and having a salad is a great way to add those raw nutrient-packed greens to your diet. You go out and spend money on tons of different types of salad greens only to let them turn to goo in the slimer drawer (aka vegetable drawer). What's a person to do? Go buy a bag or bin of greens. Look for "Spring Mix," which is an assortment of tender spring greens, or "Baby Spinach Leaves." Both are terrific and have a much longer refrigerator life than regular lettuces because they aren't constantly sprayed by water while in the produce section. Salad attack? Grab a handful of greens, wash well and spin them, pour on one of these terrific dressings, and you have lift-off.

Classic Favourite

Unbelievably Delicious Raspberry Salad Dressing

A quick and easy raspberry salad dressing that tastes unbelievably delicious.

⅓ cup (75 mL) **raspberry cocktail concentrate, thawed**
1 Tbsp + 1 tsp (20 mL) **canola oil**
1 **shallot, minced**
¼ tsp (1 mL) **freshly cracked pepper**
¼ tsp (1 mL) **paprika**
¼ tsp (1 mL) **Dijon mustard**

1 Whisk together all the ingredients. This dressing can be stored up to 1 week in the refrigerator. Tastes great with a plain green salad and some fresh raspberries thrown in for good measure.

Makes ½ cup (125 mL). Makes four 2-Tbsp (30-mL) servings.

WHERE THE HECK DO I FIND RASPBERRY COCKTAIL CONCENTRATE?
It's in the frozen juice aisle at your local grocery store.

WHAT THE HECK DO I DO WITH THE LEFTOVER RASPBERRY COCKTAIL?
Spoon out the amount that you need in its frozen state, and put the rest back into the freezer in its container for the next time you get a raspberry salad dressing attack. Warning: be sure to cover tightly. Spilled frozen raspberry concentrate is really hard to clean up. Words from experience.

ONE SERVING	75 Calories
	4.5 g Total Fat
	0 g Sat Fat
	0 g Trans Fat
	0 mg Sodium
	10 g CHO
	0 g Fibre
	0 g Protein
UEPC	1 Fat

Classic Favourite

Everyday House Dressing

I've been making this dressing for the past 20 years; it's a golden oldie. Chances are, if you're eating a salad at my house, you're getting this dressing.

¼ cup (60 mL) **balsamic vinegar**
1 Tbsp + 1 tsp (20 mL) **extra virgin olive oil**
2 tsp (10 mL) **grainy Dijon mustard**
2 tsp (10 mL) **honey**
1 **clove garlic, crushed**

1 Whisk together all the ingredients. Can be stored up to 1 week in the refrigerator.

Makes ½ cup (125 mL). Makes four 2-Tbsp (30-mL) servings.

ONE SERVING	60 Calories
	4.5 g Total Fat
	0.5 g Sat Fat
	0 g Trans Fat
	40 mg Sodium
	5 g CHO
	0 g Fibre
	0 g Protein
UEPC	1¾ Fat

New

Honey Mustard Salad Dressing

I created this for a dinner theatre fundraiser at my church. Everyone loved the recipe so much they came into the kitchen to write it down. The only problem was that version served 92 people. Hopefully they all knew math.

1 Tbsp (15 mL) **orange juice concentrate, thawed**
1 Tbsp (15 mL) **canola oil**
1 Tbsp (15 mL) **apple cider vinegar**
1 Tbsp (15 mL) **honey**
1 tsp (5 mL) **Dijon mustard**

1 Whisk all the ingredients together in a small bowl. Serve, or store in the refrigerator for up to 2 days.

2 Go ahead and double it. You can also 92 × the recipe. Think a really big crowd.

Makes ¼ cup (60 mL). Makes four 1-Tbsp (15-mL) servings.

ONE SERVING	50 Calories
	3.5 g Total Fat
	0 g Sat Fat
	0 g Trans Fat
	15 mg Sodium
	7 g CHO
	0 g Fibre
	0 g Protein
UEPC	¾ Fat

New

The Antioxidant All-Star Salad Dressing

Blackcurrants are antioxidant all-stars of the berry world.
Ribena is made with a ton of them. A blackcurrant
concentrate made in England, Ribena can be found in
either the juice aisle beside the lemon juice or, of all
places, in the pop aisle.

¼ cup (60 mL) **Ribena**
1 Tbsp + 1 tsp (20 mL) **extra virgin olive oil**
1 Tbsp (15 mL) **balsamic vinegar**
1 tsp (5 mL) **Dijon mustard**
¼ tsp (1 mL) **cracked pepper**
2 Tbsp (30 mL) **minced shallots**

1   Whisk all the ingredients together in a small bowl. Serve,
     or store in the refrigerator for up to 2 days.

Makes ½ cup (125 mL). Makes eight 1-Tbsp (15-mL) servings.

BIG COOKING TIP
All of the dressings are
smoother and creamier if
you give them a whirl with a
hand-held immersion blender.

ONE SERVING	47 Calories
	2 g Total Fat
	0 g Sat
	0 g Trans
	12 mg Sodium
	5 g CHO
	0 g Fibre
	0 g Protein
UEPC	½ Fat

New

California Spinach Salad

LOW-FAT CAESAR SALAD DRESSING? WHICH ONE DO I PICK?
Choose whichever one you love. Just make sure that it's made with canola or olive oil. Feel free to dress the salad with my House Dressing (see page 145), or the Unbelievably Delicious Raspberry Salad Dressing (see page 144). Both are excellent choices.

This is our house winter salad. Pink Lady and Granny Smith apples are both plentiful in the winter months and have that wonderful tartness that goes so well with walnuts.

1 **large Pink Lady or Granny Smith apple**
⅛ **of a medium red onion, diced**
6 cups (1.5 L) **baby spinach leaves**
3 Tbsp (45 mL) **low-fat caesar salad dressing**
2 Tbsp (30 mL) **chopped California walnuts**

1 Cut the apple into quarters. Remove the core and slice thinly.

2 Wash and dry the baby spinach leaves.

3 Toss together the apple, onion, spinach, and low-fat salad dressing.

4 Divide equally between 2 plates. Sprinkle each plate with walnuts.

Makes 2.

WHY THE HECK DO I HAVE TO BUY CALIFORNIA WALNUTS?
If you're lucky enough to be growing your own walnuts or have access to local walnuts, I'm so jealous. All the rest of us agricultural misfortunates have to buy them. I find the California walnuts are the best commercial product out there. They're never bitter, and they really do taste better than most other commercial ones. Buy them shelled and store them in the freezer to maintain freshness. They take only a couple of minutes to thaw.

ONE SERVING	210 Calories
	12 g Total Fat
	0.6 g Sat Fat
	0 g Trans Fat
	310 mg Sodium
	25 g CHO
	7 g Fibre
	3 g Protein
UEPC	1½ Fats
	4 Fruits & Vegetables
	½ Nut

Strawberry and Spinach Salad

I do most of my fruit and vegetable shopping in the spring, summer, and fall at my local farmers' market. I'm in heaven the week the local strawberries arrive. You can smell them as you cross the lawn from the parking lot. Nothing beats locally grown produce. I always recommend that you support your local farmers and frequent their markets as often as possible. In the winter? It's back to your local grocery store.

8 cups (2 L) **baby spinach leaves**
4 cups (1 L) **strawberries (about 24)**
½ cup (125 mL) **almonds, chopped**

Dressing
2 Tbsp + 2 tsp (40 mL) **extra virgin olive oil**
2 Tbsp + 2 tsp (40 mL) **balsamic vinegar**
2 Tbsp (30 mL) **dark brown sugar**
2 Tbsp (30 mL) **frozen raspberry concentrate, thawed**
½ tsp (2 mL) **paprika**
½ tsp (2 mL) **Worcestershire sauce**

1   Wash and dry the spinach. Store in the refrigerator, wrapped in a paper towel in a plastic bag, until ready to use.

2   Gently wash the strawberries and lay out on a cloth or paper towel until dry.

3   In a small bowl, whisk together all of the dressing ingredients. Set aside until serving time.

4   Slice the strawberries. Set aside until serving time.

5   Okay, it's finally serving time. You have 2 serving choices.

   Divide the spinach equally between the 4 plates, sprinkle equally with the sliced strawberries and salad dressing, then top with 2 Tbsp (30 mL) of chopped almonds (if using).

   Or toss everything together in a bowl and then divide equally between the 4 plates.

Serves 4.

ONE SERVING with almonds	260 Calories
	18 g Total Fat
	2 g Sat Fat
	0 g Trans Fat
	90 mg Sodium
	20 g CHO
	6 g Fibre
	5 g Protein
UEPC	2 Fat
	4 Fruits & Vegetables
	1 Nuts

BIG COOKING TIP

You can prep most of this salad up to 2 days in advance. A great choice for a dinner party.

Revised

Romaine with Feta and Blueberries

I love adding blueberries to salads. Try tossing in a handful of berries the next time you're making a regular salad with lettuce, cucumbers, tomatoes, onion, and celery, and you'll be surprised how that little hint of sweetness adds a huge hit of flavour. Adding feta along with the blueberries? Well, it's a major-league flavour burst that will wow your socks off.

1 **large head of romaine lettuce**
2 cups (500 mL) **fresh wild blueberries**

Dressing
⅓ cup (75 mL) **light feta cheese**
2 Tbsp (30 mL) **apple cider vinegar**
1 Tbsp-+ 1 tsp (20 mL) **extra virgin olive oil**
1 Tbsp (15 mL) **honey**
1 **small shallot, minced**

1   Wash romaine, spin dry, and wrap in paper towel. Put it into a plastic bag and store in the refrigerator for up to 2 days.

2   Use a hand-held immersion blender or mini food processor to purée the feta, vinegar, olive oil, honey, and shallot. Store this dressing in the refrigerator for up to 2 days.

3   On serving day, gently wash the blueberries. Drain well and dry on paper towels.

4   When ready to serve, tear or chop the romaine into bite-sized pieces. In a large bowl, toss the romaine with the dressing. Add the blueberries. Toss gently and serve.

Serves 4.

ONE SERVING	140 Calories
	6 g Total Fat
	1.5 g Sat Fat
	0 g Trans Fat
	120 mg Sodium
	19 g CHO
	3 g Fibre
	4 g Protein
UEPC	1 Fat
	2 Fruits & Vegetables

Almost as Good as Grandma's Coleslaw

According to my son, his grandma makes the best coleslaw around. He told me this is a close second. His grandma is a great cook. I count myself lucky to be the runner-up.

½ **medium red or green cabbage**
½ **medium red onion**
1 **red pepper**
4 **large carrots**

Dressing
½ cup (125 mL) **apple cider vinegar**
1 Tbsp (15 mL) **canola oil**
1 tsp (5 mL) **honey**

TIP
This is a great snack after school or work. Low in calories, high in flavour, and a wonderful way to get those servings of fruits and veggies.

1 To make your life easier, you need to make this with a food processor. If you don't own one, either thinly slice or grate the veggies, ask for a food processor as a gift, run out and buy one.

2 Let's assume you own a food processor. Using the thinnest slicing blade, slice the cabbage, red onion, and red pepper. Place the sliced veggies into a large bowl.

3 Change to the grater blade and grate the carrots. Add the carrot to the other veggies.

4 Whisk together all the dressing ingredients and pour over the veggies. Toss well.

5 Store in the refrigerator for up to 4 days.

Makes 8 cups (2 L). Makes eight 1-cup (250-mL) servings.

Kid Friendly

ONE SERVING	60 Calories
	2 g Total Fat
	0 g Sat Fat
	0 g Trans Fat
	30 mg Sodium
	11 g CHO
	3 g Fibre
	1 g Protein
UEPC	¼ Fat
	2 Fruits & Vegetables

Classic Favourite

Grape Tomato Salad

NO GRAPE TOMATOES?
Feel free to use cherry
tomatoes and cut them into
quarters. Or try strawberry
tomatoes for a real gourmet
treat.

**NOTE TO THE OLIVE
CHALLENGED**
Yes, you can omit them.

Let's face it, tomatoes only taste like tomatoes when they're in season. If you live north of the 49th parallel a tomato that rode on the bus from California in the middle of December isn't going to taste like a summer tomato. It may look like a tomato but that's where the similarities end, unless you find grape tomatoes. These little babies taste like summer no matter what time of year it is.

2 cups (500 mL) **grape tomatoes, halved**
1 Tbsp + 1 tsp (20 mL) **extra virgin olive oil**
1 **clove garlic, minced**
10 **fresh basil leaves, chopped**
6 **green olives, diced**
pinch **hot pepper flakes**

1   Mix all the ingredients together in a medium bowl. Let it sit for at least 1 hour and no longer than 3. Serve over lettuce, or eat alone as a vegetable side dish. Can be stored in the refrigerator for at least 2 days.

Makes 2 cups. Makes four ½-cup (125-mL) servings.

ONE SERVING	70 Calories
	6 g Total Fat
	0.5 g Sat Fat
	0 g Trans Fat
	60 mg Sodium
	4 g CHO
	1 g Fibre
	1 g Protein
UEPC	1 Fat
	1 Fruits & Vegetables

Baby Greens with Mandarins and Honey Mustard Dressing

A huge hit anytime I serve it. Store the unopened can of mandarins in the refrigerator. Cold tastes so much better when you're an orange.

Honey Mustard Salad Dressing

Yes, it's the same one as one page 145. Thought it would help you from flipping back and forth.

1 Tbsp (15 mL) **frozen orange juice concentrate, thawed**
1 Tbsp (15 mL) **canola oil**
1 Tbsp (15 mL) **apple cider vinegar**
1 Tbsp (15 mL) **honey**
1 tsp (5 mL) **Dijon mustard**

Salad
12 cups **baby spinach leaves or spring mix salad greens**
one 10-oz (284-mL) can **Mandarin oranges, whole segments, drained**
⅛ **medium red onion, diced**

1   Whisk together all the ingredients for the Honey Mustard Salad Dressing in a small bowl. Set aside.

2   Wash and dry the salad greens or baby spinach and divide between 4 plates.

3   Add ¼ of the mandarins to each plate (about 11 segments per serving).

4   Sprinkle ¼ of the red onion overtop the mandarins.

5   Drizzle each salad with 1 Tbsp (15 mL) of dressing. Serve.

Serves 4.

Kid Friendly

TIP
For a salad dressing with a bit more bite, add an extra 1 tsp (5 mL) of Dijon mustard.

ONE SERVING	110 Calories
	3.5 g Total Fat
	0 g Sat Fat
	0 g Trans Fat
	80 mg Sodium
	21 g CHO
	5 g Fibre
	3 g Protein
UEPC	¾ Fat
	3½ Fruits & Vegetables

New

Fresh California Guacamole

HOW THE HECK DO I PEEL AND CHOP AN AVOCADO?

There are more ways to do it than you'd think. Ask any chef and they'll have their own version. My way is to wash it first, cut it in half lengthwise, then twist off one half from the pit. I pry the pit from the other half with the sharp end of my knife. Once the pit is removed, I use a small knife to make shallow cuts into the avocado, first in one direction, then in the other—sometimes called cross hatching. Then I flip the peel inside out and the pieces of avocado are easily removed. Alternately, cut the avocado in half, remove the pit, and scoop out the avocado with a small spoon or tiny melon scoop.

I'm in love with avocados. They're one sexy little green powerhouse of nutrients and flavour. Remember, avocado fat calories tend to be high, so even though this is nutrient dense, it's calorie dense as well. See tips on buying and storing avocados on page 218.

1 **ripe Hass avocado, peeled and chopped (see sidebar)**
2 Tbsp (30 mL) **minced onion**
1 Tbsp (15 mL) **fresh lime juice**
1 **clove garlic, minced**
pinch **red pepper flakes (optional)**

1   Gently toss all ingredients with a fork. Serve immediately or store in the refrigerator for up to 10 hours.

Makes ¾ cup (175 mL). Makes five 2-Tbsp (30-mL) servings.

ONE SERVING	
	60 Calories
	4 g Total Fat
	1 g Sat Fat
	0 g Trans Fat
	0 mg Sodium
	3 g CHO
	0 g Fibre
	1 g Protein
UEPC	1 Fat

Walnut Pesto

Pesto is another culinary necessity for your refrigerator, and it comes in all flavours and forms. This one is more traditional and can be used as a sauce for hot or cold pasta, a sandwich spread, or as a homemade pizza topping. Beware, even though it's packed with wonderfully healthy ingredients, it's also packed with calories. A little goes a long way. I like to make this in the summer and freeze extras. So if you've had a bumper basil crop, feel free to double or quadruple the recipe.

1 cup (250 mL) **packed basil leaves**
2 **cloves garlic**
2 Tbsp (30 mL) **chopped walnuts (about 7 walnut halves)**
2 Tbsp (30 mL) **grated Parmigiano Reggiano**
2 Tbsp (30 mL) **extra virgin olive oil**

1   Pulse all the ingredients in a food processor until well blended. Store in the refrigerator for up to 2 days, or freeze in ice cube trays. Most ice cube trays hold 1 Tbsp (15 mL) per cube. Once frozen, pop them out and store in a freezer bag for up to 3 months.

2   Just add a frozen cube or two to your next pasta dish.

Makes ⅓ cup (75 mL). Makes five 1-Tbsp (15-mL) servings.

ONE SERVING	90 Calories
	9 g Total Fat
	1.5 g Sat Fat
	0 g Trans Fat
	50 mg Sodium
	1 g CHO
	1 g Fibre
	2 g Protein
UEPC	1 Fat

SOUPS

Broccoli and Cheddar Cheese Soup

I always laugh when parents tell me their kids love little trees with cheese sauce on them. Hey, I'd eat trees with cheese sauce on them. It's quite obvious it's the cheese sauce they love, which got me thinking. How about we purée the living daylights out of those little trees and add cheese to the rest of the recipe? Voila, a broccoli soup that kids will eat.

1½ cups (375 mL) **lower-sodium chicken broth**
2 **medium onions, diced**
4 **cloves garlic, minced**
6 cups (1.5 L) **chopped broccoli, about 2 average-sized bunches**
one 14-oz (385-mL) can **fat-free evaporated milk**
1 cup (250 mL) **shredded light aged cheddar cheese**
½ tsp (2 mL) **freshly ground black pepper**
½ tsp (2 mL) **Worcestershire sauce**
pinch **cayenne**

1   In a medium pot, add the chicken broth, onions, garlic, and broccoli, in that order. You want the onions and garlic cooking in the chicken stock with the broccoli sitting on top. Bring to a boil, then reduce the heat to medium-low. Cover and cook for 15 minutes, or until broccoli is tender.

2   Add the evaporated milk, pepper, Worcestershire sauce, and cayenne. Purée the soup using an hand-held immersion blender. Stir in the cheddar cheese. Mix until the cheese is melted.

3   Divide equally between 4 bowls. Serve.

Makes 6½ cups (1.6 L). Makes four heaping 1½-cup (375-mL) servings.

Kid Friendly

MUST HAVE KITCHEN TOYS
A hand-held immersion blender. Instead of pouring hot soup into a blender and then making a huge mess because you filled it too high and it exploded all over the wall, just put the hand-held immersion blender into the pot so the blades are beneath the surface of the soup—otherwise you may still have it all over the wall. It's easy, handy, and wonderful. Use it for soups, salad dressings, one-serving blender drinks, and the list goes on. I have one. You need one. Ask for it as a gift. They range anywhere from $45 to $75. It's one of the few things I wouldn't give up—and bear in mind that I've given up two husbands.

ONE SERVING	
	190 Calories
	2 g Total Fat
	1 g Sat Fat
	0 g Trans Fat
	350 mg Sodium
	28 g CHO
	4 g Fibre
	17 g Protein
UEPC	2 Fruits & Vegetables
	1 Milk

Immune Enhancing Shiitake Mushroom Soup

Hot chicken broth plus fresh garlic, red pepper flakes, and fresh ginger all help to clear your sinuses. This soup is a definite must-have the next time you catch a cold. When I was recipe testing I served this to my dear friend Joanne and her husband Mike. They both loved it so much she made it for her next dinner party. So whether you have a cold or not, it's a winner.

3 cups (750 mL) **lower-sodium chicken broth**
1 cup (250 mL) **dried shiitake mushrooms (see sidebar)**
4 **large kale leaves**
4 **cloves garlic, minced**
1 Tbsp (15 mL) **minced fresh ginger**
1 tsp (5 mL) **red pepper flakes**
1 cup (250 mL) **chopped fresh cilantro**
½ cup (125 mL) **sliced green onion**

1   Add the chicken broth to a medium pot and bring to a boil. Remove the pot from the stove and stir in the mushrooms. Cover and let sit for 15 minutes.

2   Meanwhile, remove the kale leaves from the stem. Discard stem. Thinly slice the kale leaves (chef lingo: chiffonade). See page 202.

3   Return the pot to the stove and heat over medium-low heat. Add the kale and stir well. You're only just cooking the kale.

4   Add the garlic, ginger, and red pepper flakes. Stir well. Remove from heat.

5   Divide the cilantro equally between two Asian-style soup bowls. Pour half the soup into each bowl. Top with the green onions. Serve.

Makes 4 cups (1 L). Makes two 2-cup (500-mL) servings.

BIG COOKING TIP
There are two camps in the cilantro story. One camp loves the stuff, the other thinks it tastes like old socks. I'm in the love-it camp. If you're in the opposing camp, omit it from the recipe and substitute with your favourite fresh herb.

ONE SERVING	115 Calories
	1.5 g Total Fat
	1 g Sat Fat
	0 g Trans Fat
	340 mg Sodium
	17 g CHO
	6 g Fibre
	10 g Protein
UEPC	3 Fruits & Vegetables

Jamaican Black Bean Pumpkin Soup

After months of eating stale bread, salted meat, dried peas, raisins, and copious amounts of beer, Christopher Columbus and his band of slightly-sloshed Spaniards landed on the island of Jamaica on May 4, 1492, ready for a really great meal. Among the array of exotic offerings, allspice became a big hit with the Spanish, who named it Jamaican pepper. The English, always up for a good game of nomenclature, renamed the exotic berry allspice because it has the aroma of cloves, pepper, cinnamon, and nutmeg.

1 Tbsp (15 mL) **extra virgin olive oil**
1 **medium onion, diced**
2 **stalks celery, diced**
2 Tbsp (30 mL) **minced fresh ginger**
3 **cloves garlic, minced**
2 tsp (10 mL) **thyme**
½ tsp (2 mL) **allspice**
¼ tsp (1 mL) **cinnamon**
3 cups (750 mL) **lower-sodium chicken broth**
2½ cups (625 mL) **canned pure pumpkin purée**
one 19-oz (540-mL) can **black beans, drained and rinsed**

1   Heat a large saucepan over medium heat. Add the olive oil, onion, and celery. Sauté for 4 minutes.

2   Add the ginger, garlic, thyme, allspice, and cinnamon. Sauté for 1 minute, stirring occasionally.

3   Pour in the chicken broth, then add the pumpkin and beans. Stir well. Bring to a boil, cover, and reduce the heat to low. Simmer for 20 minutes, stirring occasionally. Serve.

Makes 5½ cups (1.4 L). Makes four 1⅓-cups (325-mL) servings.

BIG COOKING TIP

Make sure that your herbs and spices are fresh. If you have dried spices and herbs that are older than six months, take my advice: throw them out. They don't have the same flavour as fresh ones. Here comes the Big Cooking Tip part. If you received a spice rack complete with spices as a wedding gift 15 years ago, hurl them out the window and immediately rush out to the store for new ones.

ADULT FRIENDLY TIP

Add hot sauce to yours and feel the love.

SIDEBAR

What the heck do I do with the 1 cup (250 mL) of pure pumpkin purée I have left from that huge can I had to buy? Make the Double Chocolate Muffins on page 283.

ONE SERVING	
	210 Calories
	4.5 g Total Fat
	1 g Sat Fat
	0 g Trans Fat
	400 mg Sodium
	40 g CHO
	13 g Fibre
	10 g Protein
UEPC	¾ Fat
	2 Fruits & Vegetables
	1 Bean

New

Leek and Lemon Soup

WHAT THE HECK IS A LEEK?
WHAT THE HECK IS A LEEK?
Leeks look like a really fat green onion that's been on steroids. You'll find them in the produce section; they're the ones with the roots and long green tops.

When my neighbours Tom and Evelyn were over for an official taste of this soup, I knew it was a hit when Evelyn starting licking her bowl. A light soup packed full of antioxidants, serve it hot or cold. When chilled, it packs a bigger lemon kick.

1 Tbsp (15 mL) **extra virgin olive oil**
½ cup (125 mL) **diced shallots**
2 **large leeks (see sidebar)**
3 cups (750 mL) **lower-sodium chicken or vegetable broth**
4 cups (1 L) **baby spinach leaves**
½ cup (125 mL) **loosely packed diced parsley**
zest of 1 **lemon**
⅓ cup (75 mL) **fresh lemon juice**

1 Heat a medium pot over medium heat. Add the oil, shallots, and leeks. Sauté for 3 minutes, stirring occasionally.

2 Add the broth and bring to a boil. Cover, reduce heat, and simmer for 10 minutes.

3 Remove from heat. Add the spinach, parsley, lemon zest, and lemon juice. Stir until the spinach wilts.

4 Purée gently with a hand-held immersion blender, food processor, or upright blender. You want the texture to be chunky, not silky-smooth. Serve.

Makes 5 cups (1.25 L). Makes four 1¼-cup (300-mL) servings.

HOW THE HECK DO I CLEAN A LEEK?
They are grown in sand, so you need to give them a really good bath. It's best to cut off most of the bitter dark green part. I usually save about 3 inches (8 cm) of the light green part, so the leek is about 6 to 8 inches (15 to 20 cm) long once I've discarded the really dark green part. Cut off the root end just above the root. Now the sand issue. What to do? I make a lengthwise cut from the bottom to the top, sometimes called a butterfly cut. Stick them in a sink of cold water, fan the leaves out, and swish them in the water. Finish by rinsing under running water. Sounds like a lot, but it's very simple once you get the knack of it. Learn something new every day.

ONE SERVING	
	100 Calories
	4 g Total Fat
	0.5 g Sat Fat
	0 g Trans Fat
	345 mg Sodium
	15 g CHO
	2 g Fibre
	4 g Protein
UEPC	¾ Fat
	2½ Fruits & Vegetables

Marvellous Minestrone

This quick and easy meal-in-a-bowl soup is packed with outstanding veggies: tomatoes, carrots, onions, kale, and whole grain pasta as well as heart-healthy extra virgin olive oil and cholesterol lowering beans. I made this on TV one morning and the crew gobbled it up. Eating beans at 8:00 a.m—the soup was either delicious, or the crew were out of their minds. I'm going with delicious.

1 Tbsp + 1 tsp (20 mL) **extra virgin olive oil**
1 **large onion, diced**
2 **large carrots, chopped**
4 **cloves garlic, minced**
one 28-oz (796-mL) **can diced tomatoes**
one 19-oz (540-mL) **can kidney beans, drained and rinsed**
2 cups (500 mL) **lower-sodium chicken broth**
1½ (375 mL) **cups water**
4 cups (1 L) **chopped kale leaves, stems removed or spinach**
¼ cup (60 mL) **whole wheat rotini**
½ tsp (2 mL) **red pepper flakes**
¼ tsp (1 mL) **pepper**
2 Tbsp (30 mL) **chopped fresh basil**
2 Tbsp (30 mL) **balsamic vinegar (optional)**

1   Heat a large pot over medium heat. Add the oil and onion. Sauté for five minutes, stirring often, or until the onion is a golden colour.

2   Add the carrots and garlic. Sauté for 3 minutes, stirring often.

3   Add the tomatoes, beans, chicken broth, and water.

4   Bring to a boil. Add the kale, rotini, red pepper flakes, and pepper. Bring back to a boil and cover. Reduce the heat and simmer for 10 to 12 minutes, or until the pasta is cooked.

5   Add the basil and vinegar, if using. Stir and serve. If desired, sprinkle with freshly grated Parmesan cheese.

Makes 10 cups (2.5 L). Makes six 1½-cups (375-mL) servings.

Kid Friendly

KID FRIENDLY TIP
Skip adding the pepper and the red pepper flakes to the pot. Add them to your own bowl when you serve. Sprinkle theirs with extra Parmesan.

BIG COOKING TIP
My friend Michale adds the balsamic vinegar and raves about how that little zip adds something wonderful to the soup. If you're keeping score, that's Michale two points, Mairlyn none. Refer to Spicy Salmon Cakes on page 234 for further clarification.

ONE SERVING	210 Calories
	4 g Total Fat
	0.5 g Sat Fat
	0 g Trans Fat
	490 mg Sodium
	33 g CHO
	10 g Fibre
	10 g Protein
UEPC	¾ Beans
	¾ Fat
	2½ Fruits & Vegetables
	¼ Grains

Mulligatawny Soup

BIG COOKING TIP

I make this soup in the order that the ingredients are listed. While the broth comes to a boil, I wash and cut the leeks and carrots. After adding those and waiting for it to boil, I prep the chicken and the remaining veggies. While the veggies and apple cook, I wash and chop the parsley. The next thing you know, the soup is ready.

HISTORY LESSON

While the Brits were out colonizing the world, they happened to come up with this soup while in hot sultry India. Sweating helps cool you down. Tell that to a menopausal women and see what happens.

I had my first bowl of this amazing soup when I was touring with Second City Comedy Troupe. We were out West eating at some smoky bar and mulligatawny soup was the only thing on the menu that wasn't deep fried. I tried it and was pleasantly flabbergasted. Slightly spicy and loaded with flavour—a stunning soup. Great served with 100% whole wheat rolls and a nice cold beer. Every one of my recipe testers licked the bowl on this one. Which just goes to show, you never know what you'll discover at your local drinking establishment.

4 cups (1 L) **lower-sodium chicken broth**
1 **large leek, sliced into ¼-inch (5-mm) rings**
1 **large carrot, cut in half lengthwise, then into ¼-inch (5-mm) half-moons**
14 oz (400 g) **skinless, boneless chicken breasts or thighs, cut into 16 pieces**
1 **red pepper, diced**
1 **stalk celery, diced**
1 **Granny Smith apple, unpeeled, cored, cut into 16 pieces**
1 tsp (5 mL) **curry powder**
¼ tsp (1 mL) **turmeric**
¼–½ tsp (1–2 mL) **red pepper flakes**
½ cup (125 mL) **loosely packed chopped parsley**

1. Boil the broth in a large pot over medium-high heat.

2. Add the leeks and carrots and return to a boil. Cover, reduce heat, and simmer for 5 minutes.

3. Add the chicken and return to a boil. Cover, reduce heat, and simmer for 10 minutes.

4. Add the red pepper, celery, apple, curry powder, turmeric, and red pepper flakes. Return to a boil. Cover, reduce heat, and simmer for 5 minutes.

5. Remove from heat. Add parsley and serve.

Makes 7 cups (1.75 mL). Makes four 1¾-cup (425-mL) servings.

Kid Friendly

ONE SERVING	240 Calories
	8 g Total Fat
	2.5 g Sat Fat
	0 g Trans Fat
	465 mg Sodium
	17 g CHO
	3 g Fibre
	25 g Protein
UEPC	2 Fruits & Vegetables
	1 Meat

Quick and Hearty Chicken Noodle Soup

This family friendly soup is one of the few things my cooking challenged sister makes. If Kathleen can make this, and trust me she takes no offence with this, any-one can.

4 cups (1 L) **lower-sodium chicken broth**
1 **onion, minced**
3 **cloves garlic, minced**
2 **large carrots, diced**
14 oz (400 g) **skinless boneless chicken breast**
1 cup (250 mL) **whole wheat rotini**
2 cups (500 mL) **chopped kale leaves, stems removed see page 187**

1   Pour the chicken broth into a medium saucepan. Add the garlic, onions, and carrots. Bring to a boil.

2   Meanwhile, slice the chicken into 1-inch (2.5-cm) pieces. When the broth has come to the boil, add the chicken, rotini, and kale. Bring to a boil. Cover and lower the heat. Simmer for 10 minutes, or until the chicken is cooked and the rotini is tender. Serve.

Makes 6 cups (1.5 L). Makes four 1½-cups (375-mL) servings.

Kid Friendly

ONE SERVING	300 Calories
	3 g Total Fat
	1 g Sat Fat
	0 g Trans Fat
	465 mg Sodium
	33 g CHO
	5 g Fibre
	37 g Protein
UEPC	1½ Fruits & Vegetables
	1 Grains
	1 Meat

Summer Fresh Puréed Pea and Mint Soup

Cold soups are an oxymoron as far as I'm concerned. Growing up on the West Coast it never got hot enough to want to make a cold soup. When I moved to the hot, humid East I revisited the whole cold soup thing. Quite frankly, anything cold is great when it's 42°C/ 107°F.

1 Tbsp (15 mL) **extra virgin olive oil**
½ cup (125 mL) **diced shallots (see sidebar)**
2 **stalks celery, diced**
3 cups (750 mL) **lower-sodium chicken or vegetable broth**
4 cups (1 L) **fresh or frozen peas, thawed**
4 cups (1 L) **fresh baby spinach leaves**
1 cup (250 mL) **loosely packed fresh mint leaves, diced**
¼ cup (60 mL) **chopped fresh chives**
2 cups (500 mL) **low-fat plain probiotic yogurt**

1   Heat a medium saucepan over medium heat. Add the oil, shallots, and celery. Sauté for 3 minutes or until the shallots are a golden colour.

2   Pour in the broth. Add the peas. Bring back to a boil and cover. Reduce heat and simmer for 10 minutes.

3   Remove from heat and add the spinach. Stir until wilted. Add the mint leaves.

4   Purée using a hand-held immersion blender, food processor, or upright blender. Chill the soup in the refrigerator about 2 hours or until cold.

5   At serving time, stir in the yogurt and chives. Serve.

Makes 8 cups (2 L). Makes six 1⅓-cup (325-mL) servings.

Kid Friendly

ONE SERVING	
	190 Calories
	4 g Total Fat
	1 g Sat Fat
	0 g Trans Fat
	290 mg Sodium
	29 g CHO
	9 g Fibre
	12 g Protein
UEPC	½ Fat
	2½ Fruits & Vegetables
	½ Milk

VEGETABLES

New

Asian-Style Eggplant

VEGETABLE RULES
Rule #1
Always wash veggies really well under running water before cutting or chopping.

KID FRIENDLY VERSION
Reduce diced ginger to 1 Tbsp (15 mL).

HOW THE HECK DO I DICE A PIECE OF GINGER?
Remove the peel (the outer brown layer) with a small knife, peeler, or a small spoon. I use a small spoon, scraping the peel off with the bowl of the spoon. Once peeled, cut the ginger in half so you have a flat surface to work with. Lay the flat side on the cutting board and begin making tiny slices. Continue until you have a mound of thinly sliced ginger. Then rock the knife back and forth over the mound until the slices are just tiny pieces. Voila, you have minced a ginger root.

ONE SERVING	50 Calories
	1.5 g Total Fat
	0 g Sat Fat
	0 g Trans Fat
	160 mg sodium
	9 g CHO
	3 g Fibre
	2 g Protein
UEPC	¼ Fat
	2 Fruits & Vegetables

The first time I visited New York I had an eggplant dish in Chinatown so amazing that I ate most of it myself. Unfortunately, I was sitting at a table of eight and they were all slightly appalled that I could snarf down a dish meant to feed 10.

1 lb (500 g) **Asian eggplant**
½ cup (125 mL) **lower-sodium chicken broth**
2 Tbsp (30 mL) **diced fresh ginger**
3 **cloves garlic, minced**
1 Tbsp (15 mL) **low-sodium soy sauce**
1 tsp (5 mL) **canola oil**
½ tsp (2 mL) **red pepper flakes**

1   Wash the eggplant. Chop off the top and bottom. Don't peel it. Slice the remaining eggplant into ¼-inch (5-mm) thick medallions.

2   Heat a large pan with a tight-fitting lid over medium heat and add the eggplant. That's right, there isn't any oil in the pan, you're toasting the eggplant, not frying it. Flip and toast the medallions for 7 to 10 minutes, or until brown on both sides.

3   Mix together the chicken broth, ginger, garlic, soy sauce, canola oil, and red pepper flakes in a small bowl.

4   Add this sauce to the eggplant and cover the pan with a lid. When you add the sauce it's going to bubble up. Don't worry, just get the lid on fast. Reduce the heat to medium-low and continue cooking about 2 to 3 minutes, or until the eggplant is soft. Serve.

Makes 2 cups (500 mL). Makes four ½-cup (125-mL) servings.

WHAT THE HECK IS ASIAN EGGPLANT?
Just to make matters confusing, Asian eggplant is sometimes called Japanese or Chinese eggplant. They're milder and sweeter than the bigger Italian eggplants. They also have thinner skins, are longer and skinnier, and are a violet colour instead of deep purple. Readily available in larger supermarkets, you'll definitely find them in an Asian produce store. Store them uncovered in the refrigerator (not in the plastic bag you bought them in) and use within one week of purchasing.

Asparagus

Asparagus is one of my ultimate favourite vegetables. Buy dark green spears with compact purplish tips. Most stores sell them standing in water to maintain their freshness. Choose crisp looking stalks, not wilted ones. The thickness is totally your choice. I like the thinner stalks for stir-frying and the thicker ones for grilling.

BIG COOKING TIP
Snap off the woody ends of the asparagus before cooking.

New
Asparagus Stir-Fry

When asked what the harbinger of spring is, most people would say a daffodil poking its stalk out of the dark soil, a robin digging for juicy worms, or the first crop of local asparagus. In my neighbourhood the first sign of spring is a skunk bomb that drifts through the air and makes you bolt to close all the windows before you gag to death. Given a choice, I prefer the first asparagus sighting.

2 tsp (10 mL) **extra virgin olive oil**
1 lb (500 g) **asparagus, cut into 1-inch (2.5-cm) pieces**
1 **red pepper, diced**
2 **cloves garlic, minced**
2 tsp (10 mL) **low-sodium soy sauce**
½ tsp (2 mL) **red pepper flakes**
4 **green onions, cut into ½-inch (1-cm) pieces**

1   Heat a medium frying pan over medium heat. Add the oil, asparagus, and red pepper. Sauté 3 to 4 minutes, or until vegetables are tender-crisp.

2   Whisk together the garlic, soy sauce, and red pepper flakes in a small bowl. Pour this sauce over the vegetables and stir-fry for 30 seconds.

3   Toss in the green onions and heat through. Serve.

Makes 4 cups (1 L). Makes four 1-cup (250-mL) servings.

ONE SERVING	100 Calories
	3 g Total Fat
	0 g Sat Fat
	0 g Trans Fat
	200 mg Sodium
	16 g CHO
	5 g Fibre
	5 g Protein
UEPC	½ Fat
	2 Fruits & Vegetables

New

Grilled Asparagus

All you need is a barbecue and about 4 minutes. If you don't have either, rethink your life.

1 lb (500 g) **asparagus**
1 Tbsp (15 mL) **fresh lime juice**
1 tsp (5 mL) **extra virgin olive oil**

1   Preheat the barbecue to medium.

2   Grill the asparagus for 2 minutes. Turn the asparagus and grill for another 2 minutes. Remove from the grill and place on a clean platter.

3   Whisk together the lime juice and oil. Sprinkle this sauce over cooked asparagus. Serve.

Serves 4.

ONE SERVING	40 Calories
	1.5 g Total Fat
	0 g Sat Fat
	0 g Trans Fat
	0 mg Sodium
	5 g CHO
	2 g Fibre
	3 g Protein
UEPC	¼ Fat
	2 Fruits & Vegetables

Grilled Veggie Salad

I make this grilled salad every summer. It's so simple (especially if you get someone else to stand over the barbecue while you lollygag in the lake sipping a cool cocktail—the Pomegranate Martini on page 275 would be an excellent choice).

2 **red peppers, quartered**
1 **orange pepper, quartered**
1 lb (500 g) **asparagus**
1 tsp (5 mL) **canola oil**

Dressing
1 Tbsp (15 mL) **balsamic vinegar**
1 tsp (5 mL) **extra virgin olive oil**
1 tsp (5 mL) **Dijon mustard**
1 tsp (5 mL) **honey**
1 **small garlic clove, crushed**
¼ cup (60 mL) **diced fresh basil**

1   Preheat the barbecue to medium. In a large bowl or plastic bag, toss the peppers and asparagus with the 1 tsp (5 mL) canola oil (or coat with canola spray).

2   Place the veggies on the grill and close the lid.

3   Grill about 3 minutes, or until slightly blackened on the underside. Turn them over and continue grilling until slightly blackened all over. Remove from the grill.

4   Cut each cooked pepper quarter into 4 pieces. Cut each asparagus spear into 3 pieces.

5   Whisk together the balsamic vinegar, olive oil, mustard, honey, and garlic.

6   Pour this dressing over the veggies and toss. Add the basil and stir until coated. Serve at room temperature.

Makes 4 cups (1 L). Makes four 1-cup (250-mL) servings.

ONE SERVING	90 Calories
	3 g Total Fat
	0 g Sat Fat
	0 g Trans Fat
	25 mg Sodium
	16 g CHO
	3 G Fibre
	4 g Protein
UEPC	¼ Fat
	2½ Fruits & Vegetables

Brussels Sprouts
(aka the Wee Baby Cabbages that no one eats)

STILL HATE BRUSSELS SPROUTS?
Okay, at least you tried.

My mother and her mother decimated Brussels sprouts by cooking them for a minimum of 30 minutes. I thought they were supposed to be grey blobs of mush and I kept trying to like them, but to no avail. Imagine my delight and total amazement the first time I ate the wee baby cabbages when they were the brilliant colour of emerald green, cooked to a tender-crisp texture, and tasted—well—great. This couldn't be the same vegetable that mom cooked. They've since become a personal favourite—but only when cooked correctly.

ONE SERVING	45 Calories
	3 g Total Fat
	0 g Sat Fat
	0 g Trans Fat
	50 mg Sodium
	4 g CHO
	2 g Fibre
	2 g Protein
UEPC	¼ Fat
	1 Fruits & Vegetables

Revised
Basic Brussels

2 cups (500 mL) **Brussels sprouts (about 15 large or 30 small)**
1 Tbsp (15 mL) **non-hydrogenated margarine**
juice **1 lemon**

1   Wash Brussels sprouts and cut off woody ends. Place 1 cup (250 mL) of water in the bottom of a medium-sized pot. Place the sprouts in a steamer basket, place the steamer basket in the pot, cover, and bring the water to a boil.

2   Steam for 5 minutes or until they're a bright emerald green. Remove from the pot, place in a bowl, and toss with the margarine. Squeeze the fresh lemon juice over top. Serve.

Makes 2 cups (500 mL). Makes four ½-cup (125-mL) servings.

ONE SERVING	60 Calories
	3 g Total Fat
	0 g Sat Fat
	0 g Trans Fat
	50 mg Sodium
	7 g CHO
	2 g Fibre
	2 g Protein
UEPC	¼ Fat
	1 Fruits & Vegetables

Brussels with Maple Syrup

Basic Brussels + 1 Tbsp (15 mL) **maple syrup**

Add the syrup after you've added the margarine (omit the lemon juice). Toss and serve.

Butternut Squash

Butternut squash is a winter squash that hits the markets around late August. By far the most popular of all the squashes, it looks like a bowling pin and has a golden butter-coloured interior and sweet flavour.

Classic Favourite

Butternut Squash with Brown Sugar and Cinnamon

My rule of thumb is never to buy anything bigger than my head. This applies to all veggies and water-bras (something I didn't adhere to back in the 1980s). Bigger doesn't mean better in the vegetable world, unless you're out to win Biggest Gourd at your local fall fair.

2 lb (1 kg) **butternut squash**
2 tsp (10 mL) **non-hydrogenated margarine**
2 tsp (10 mL) **brown sugar**
1 tsp (5 mL) **cinnamon**

1   Cut the squash into quarters using a large knife. Scoop out and discard the seeds.

2   Place the butternut squash into a microwave safe casserole dish. Dot with the margarine and the brown sugar. Microwave on high for 10 to 15 minutes or until soft.

3   When cooked through, scoop out the flesh and mash. Sprinkle with cinnamon. Serve.

Makes 3 cups (750 mL). Makes six ½-cup (125-mL) servings.

ONE SERVING	90 Calories
	1.5 g Total Fat
	0 g Sat Fat
	0 g Trans Fat
	25 mg Sodium
	19 g CHO
	3 g Fibre
	2 g Protein
UEPC	⅓ Fat
	1 Fruits & Vegetables

Carrots

A perennial favourite among kids and adults, carrots are one of the easiest vegetables to prepare. Just steam and go. Look for fresh carrots with the greens still on. Don't buy a hairy carrot, or anything else in the produce section with hair on it for that matter. Hairy vegetables mean they're way past their due date.

Classic Favourite
Honey-Glazed Carrots

When I found out that baby carrots were in fact large carrots mechanically shaped to look like baby carrots, I just about flipped. We consumers are demanding so many baby carrots the producers had to make them rather than grow them. If you want the real thing, you're going to have to grow them yourself or buy them at a farmers' market. The good news is these commercialized carrots are still carrots. They've just had a little cosmetic surgery.

2 cups (500 mL) **baby carrots**
1 Tbsp (15 mL) **non-hydrogenated margarine**
1 Tbsp (15 mL) **honey**

1   Place 1 cup (250 mL) of water in the bottom of a medium-sized pot. Place the carrots in a steamer basket, place the steamer basket in the pot, cover, and bring the water to a boil.

2   Steam for 3 to 5 minutes or until tender-crisp.

3   Remove from the steamer, place in a bowl, and toss with the margarine and honey. Serve.

Makes 2 cups (500 mL). Makes four ½-cup (125-mL) servings.

ONE SERVING	70 Calories
	3 g Total Fat
	0 g Sat Fat
	0 g Trans fat
	85 mg Sodium
	10 g CHO
	2 g Fibre
	1 g Protein
UEPC	¾ Fat
	1 Fruits & Vegetables

New

Carrots with Raisins and Orange Juice

The added sweetness of the raisins may entice a picky eater to try these—or not.

1 tsp (5 mL) **canola oil**
2 cups (500 mL) **peeled and thinly sliced carrots coins**
¼ cup (60 mL) **dark raisins**
½ cup (125 mL) **orange juice**
zest of 1 **orange**
2 tsp (10 mL) **dark brown sugar**

1   Heat a medium frying pan over medium heat. Add the canola oil and carrot coins. Sauté for 1 minute.

2   Add the raisins and orange juice. Cover and reduce the heat. Cook on low for 5 minutes.

3   Remove the lid and add the brown sugar and orange zest. Stir and cook until the liquid is almost gone. Serve.

Makes 2 cups (500 mL). Makes four ½-cup (125-mL) servings.

BIG COOKING TIP
Using organic carrots? No need to peel them; just give them a good wash.

ONE SERVING	90 Calories
	1.5 g Total Fat
	0 g Sat Fat
	0 g Trans Fat
	45 mg Sodium
	19 g CHO
	2 g Fibre
	1 g Protein
UEPC	¼ Fat
	1½ Fruits & Vegetables

Corn

That natural sweetness of freshly picked corn starts to turn to starch the moment it's picked. This is why just-picked corn from a farmer's field can taste a lot sweeter than corn you've had sitting in your refrigerator for four days. Most frozen vegetables have been picked at their peak of freshness and flash frozen within 2 to 4 hours of being harvested. This retains the nutrients as well as the sweet taste, making frozen corn a great way to get the sweet taste of just-picked corn. It's a staple in my house. Corn is a great source of the antioxidant lutein, which may lower the risk of macular degeneration, an age-related vision loss.

New
Corn and Diced Red Peppers

If you want to live on the razor's edge, try adding ½ cup (125 mL) salsa to the following recipe.

1 tsp (5 mL) **canola oil**
1 **red pepper, diced**
2 cups (500 mL) **fresh cooked or frozen corn, thawed (see page 204)**

1   Heat a medium frying pan over medium heat. Add the oil and red pepper. Sauté for 1 minute.

2   Toss in the corn. Stir and cook for about 3 minutes or until heated through. Serve.

Makes 2 cups (500 mL). Makes four ½-cup (125-mL) servings.

ONE SERVING	
	80 Calories
	1.5 g Total Fat
	0 g Sat Fat
	0 g Trans Fat
	45 mg Sodium
	16 g CHO
	3 g Fibre
	3 g Protein
UEPC	¼ Fat
	1½ Fruits & Vegetables

Spinach

Cooked spinach really rocks. It takes about 12 cups (3 L) of raw spinach to yield four servings, which means that for every ½ cup (125 mL) of cooked spinach, you're really getting three servings of this antioxidant hero. Now that's what I call major vegetable superstar.

Here is one basic recipe with two variations. They all make 2 cups (500 mL) and serve four. Go for it.

New

Basic Family-Style Steamed Spinach

It doesn't get much easier than this.

12 cups (3 L) **washed baby spinach leaves**
Or one 10-oz (284-g) **bag of spinach, washed**
1 **clove garlic, minced**
1 tsp (5 mL) **extra virgin olive oil**

1   Place spinach into a large pot. You don't need to add any extra water: the water clinging to the leaves is enough. Sprinkle with garlic and cover with a lid. Place over high heat and cook for about 3 to 5 minutes or until the spinach wilts.

2   Drain. Toss in olive oil. Serve.

Makes 2 cups (500 mL). Makes four ½-cup (125-mL) servings.

WHERE THE HECK DO I BUY BABY SPINACH?
Baby spinach is available in most grocery stores in bags or containers. It's pre-washed, but yes, you do need to wash it well before eating.

WHY BABY SPINACH?
Baby spinach is more tender than the larger leaves. It cooks quickly and is great to add to soups, omelets, or your favourite salad.

ONE SERVING	40 Calories
	1 g Total Fat
	0 g Sat Fat
	0 g Trans Fat
	70 mg Sodium
	8 g CHO
	3 g Fibre
	2 g Protein
UEPC	¼ Fat
	3 Fruits & Vegetables

WHAT THE HECK IS WRONG WITH THE BAGS OF BIG LEAVES OR THE FRESH BUNCHES?
Nothing. I just prefer the convenience of having one type of spinach in my refrigerator. The large leaves aren't as tender when they're cooked and there's a lot more grit to wash off from the bunches. For me, it really comes down to convenience.

ONE SERVING	45 Calories
	1 g Total Fat
	0 g Sat Fat
	0 g Trans Fat
	210 mg Sodium
	8 g CHO
	3 g Fibre
	2 g Protein
UEPC	¼ Fat
	3 Fruits & Vegetables

ONE SERVING	80 Calories
	3.5 g Total Fat
	1.5 g Sat Fat
	0 g Trans Fat
	120 mg Sodium
	10 g CHO
	3 g Fibre
	5 g Protein
UEPC	¼ Fat
	3 Fruits & Vegetables

Variations

#1 Asian-Style

Cook Basic Family-Style Steamed Spinach (page 174). Add 2 tsp (10 mL) low-sodium soy sauce when you add the olive oil.

#2 Spinach with Ricotta

Cook Basic Family-Style Steamed Spinach. Add ½ cup (125 mL) light ricotta cheese and ¼ tsp (1 mL) fresh ground pepper when you add the olive oil.

Roasted Garlic Potatoes

Here's my dream question on "Jeopardy":

MAIRLYN: "I'll take Vegetable Storing Questions for
$1,000.00, Alex."
ALEX TREBECK: "This is the only potato that loves to be
stored in the refrigerator."
MAIRLYN: "What is a new potato?"
ALEX: "You're right, and take the lead with $68,000.00."

Yes, the only type of potato that likes being in the
refrigerator is the new potato. Store them in an opened
plastic bag for up to one week. Then either steam them
or roast them.

20 new baby potatoes
1 Tbsp + 1 tsp (20 mL) extra virgin olive oil
¼ cup (60 mL) fresh lemon juice
2 Tbsp (30 mL) diced fresh rosemary (optional)
salt and pepper (optional)
8 cloves of garlic, unpeeled

1 Preheat the oven to 400°F (200°C).

2 Wash the potatoes and cut into quarters.

3 Toss the potatoes with the olive oil and 2 Tbsp (30 mL) of
   the lemon juice.

4 Line a 13- × 9-inch (3.5-L) pan with wet parchment
   paper (see page 260) or use tin foil. Dump in the
   potatoes and sprinkle with rosemary and salt and pepper
   (if using).

5 Place the pan in the oven and roast for 45 to 60 minutes
   or until cooked through.

6 While the potatoes are roasting, wrap the 8 unpeeled
   cloves of garlic in a piece of tin foil. Place the garlic alongside the pan of potatoes and roast for 30 minutes or until
   soft. Remove the garlic from the oven. Cool slightly.

7 Pop the roasted garlic out of its peel. Mash slightly, then
   add the lemon juice and mash until smooth. Set aside.

8 When the potatoes are cooked, dump them into a large
   bowl. Toss with the garlic/lemon mixture. Serve.

Makes 4 cups (1 L). Makes four 1-cup (250-mL) servings.

ONE SERVING	150 Calories
	4.5 g Total Fat
	1 g Sat Fat
	0 g Trans Fat
	10 mg Sodium
	25 g CHO
	2 g Fibre
	3 g Protein
UEPC	1 Fat
	2 Fruits & Vegetables

Sweet Potatoes

BIG COOKING TIP
Feel free to roast the sweet potatoes in the oven. Takes about 1 hour at 350 F/180 C. Then follow step 2.

Sweet potatoes are often called yams in the produce section, which is incorrect. I tried explaining the difference between sweet potatoes and yams to the produce manager at my local grocery store, and he now thinks I'm insane. Every time he sees me he beelines for the back. Sweet potatoes have yellow-orange to red-orange insides. Yams on the other hand have white insides. Note: two totally different interiors. Yams have scaly, rough looking skin. Sweet potatoes' skin is smooth. Note: two totally different exteriors. Get my point? Sweet potatoes, although listed in almost every store I've ever been in as a yam, are grown in North America. Yams are grown in Africa, Asia, and the Caribbean.

So to summarize, anyone who calls a sweet potato a yam isn't to be trusted.

Classic Favourite

Quickie Sweet Potatoes

A perennial classic at our house.

2 sweet potatoes
2 to 3 Tbsp (30 to 45 mL) **frozen orange juice concentrate, thawed**

1   Scrub the sweet potatoes and prick them with a fork. Wrap loosely in a dry paper towel. Microwave on high for 10 to 12 minutes, depending on their size.

2   Once they're soft, let them rest in a bowl for 5 minutes. This little "sweet potato rest time" makes it easy to peel them, which just happens to be the next step. Peel the sweet potatoes with a knife. You can also cut the potatoes in half and scoop out the insides with a spoon.

3   Mash the sweet potatoes with the thawed orange juice concentrate. For a subtle orange flavour, use only 2 Tbsp (30 mL) of the orange juice concentrate.

Makes 2 cups (500 mL). Makes four ½-cup (125-mL) servings.

ONE SERVING	120 Calories
	0 g Total Fat
	0 g Sat Fat
	0 g Trans Fat
	65 mg Sodium
	28 g CHO
	4 g Fibre
	2 g Protein
UEPC	1 Fruits & Vegetables

Sweet Potatoes (cont'd)

New
Roasted Sweet Potatoes

Buy the organic ones and you don't even need to peel them. Just give them a good wash.

6 cups (1 .5 L) **1 × 1 inch/2.5 × 2.5 cm cubed sweet potatoes**
2 Tbsp (30 mL) **canola oil**
1 Tbsp (15 mL) **chili powder**
1 tsp (5 mL) **onion powder**
1 tsp (5 mL) **garlic powder**
¼ tsp (1 mL) **granulated white sugar**

1   Preheat the oven to 350°F (180°C).

2   Line a 13- × 9-inch (3.5-L) metal pan with wet parchment paper. See page 260.

3   In a medium bowl, toss the sweet potatoes with the canola oil.

4   In a small bowl, mix together the chili powder, onion powder, garlic powder, and sugar.

5   Sprinkle this spice mixture over the sweet potatoes and toss until well coated. Pour into the pan and arrange the sweet potatoes in a single layer.

6   Roast for 45 minutes or until cooked through. Serve.

Makes 4 cups (1 L). Makes four 1-cup (250-mL) servings.

ONE SERVING	240 Calories
	7 g Total Fat
	0.5 g Sat Fat
	0 g Trans Fat
	130 mg Sodium
	42 g CHO
	7 g Fibre
	4 g Protein
UEPC	1½ Fat
	3 Fruits & Vegetables

New

Roasted Sweet Potatoes and Cranberries

This is one of those recipes that begs for wet parchment paper. If you don't have any, make sure you're nowhere near the kitchen when it's time to do the dishes.

2 lbs (1 kg) **sweet potatoes, peeled and cut into 1- × 1-inch (2.5- × 2.5-cm) cubes**
2 cups (500 mL) **fresh or frozen cranberries**
1 cup (250 mL) **orange juice**
¼ cup (60 mL) **maple syrup**

1 Preheat the oven to 450°F (230°C).

2 Line a 9- × 13-inch (3.5-L) metal pan with wet parchment paper. See page 260. Add the sweet potatoes and cranberries. Make sure the cranberries are evenly distributed.

3 Drizzle the orange juice and maple syrup over top.

4 Roast for 40 to 45 minutes or until the sweet potatoes are tender and you can pierce them easily with a fork. Serve.

Makes 4 cups (1 L). Makes four 1-cup (250-mL) servings.

ONE SERVING	150 Calories
	0 g Total Fat
	0 g Sat Fat
	0 g Trans Fat
	65 mg Sodium
	36 g CHO
	5 g Fibre
	2 g Protein
UEPC	2 Fruits & Vegetables

GRAINS

Make It Once, Eat It All Week Brown Rice

WHAT THE HECK DO I DO WITH ALL THAT LEFTOVER BROWN RICE?
I've created four different recipes for you to try as an alternative to simply reheating the rice.

MUST-HAVE KITCHEN TOY
A rice cooker. Basically, add rice and water, cover, turn on, and walk away. It shuts itself off when the rice is cooked. Brilliant.

If you think brown rice is boring, do I have some recipes for you. Sure, cooking up a pot of brown rice with water can be a tad bland, but add a little of this and a dash of that, and bingo, you've got nirvana in a pot. Make this big pot of rice and then check out the four recipes on the next page. It'll make you a brown rice convert.

2 cups **long- or short-grain brown rice**
4 cups **water or lower-sodium chicken or vegetable stock**

1   In a medium heavy-bottomed pot with a tight fitting lid, add the rice and water (or stock). Bring to a boil. Cover and reduce heat to simmer. Cook for 40 to 45 minutes. Better yet, buy a rice cooker. See Must-Have Kitchen Toys (page 142).

2   Cooked rice can be stored in the fridge for up to 5 days, or you can freeze it for up to 2 months.

Makes 7 to 8 cups (1.75 to 2 L).

Awesome Lentil and Rice Salad

Okay, there are a lot of ingredients in this salad, but it's not as scary as it looks. I've made the method a one bowler, meaning, throw all the ingredients into one bowl and toss. Too easy. The best part is that it's a complete meal in one bowl.

1 Tbsp (15 mL) **lemon zest**
¼ cup (60 mL) **fresh lemon juice**
2 Tbsp (30 mL) **extra virgin olive oil**
1 tsp (5 mL) **Dijon mustard**
¼ tsp (1 mL) **cinnamon**
pinch **cayenne**
one 19-oz (540-mL) can **lentils, drained and rinsed**
2 cups (500 mL) **cooked long- or short-grain brown rice**
1 cup (250 mL) **coarsely chopped fresh parsley, loosely packed**
¾ cup (175 mL) **diced red onion**
½ cup (125 mL) **currants**
½ cup (125 mL) **dried cranberries**
1 Tbsp (15 mL) **finely chopped fresh mint**

1   In a large bowl, whisk together the lemon zest, lemon juice, olive oil, Dijon, cinnamon, and cayenne. Add the lentils and toss.

2   Toss in the brown rice until just combined.

3   Add the parsley, red onion, currants, dried cranberries, and mint. Toss until just combined. Serve. Cover and store any leftovers in the fridge for up to 3 days.

Makes 5 cups (1.25 L). Makes four 1¼-cup (310-mL) servings.

ONE SERVING	400 Calories
	8 g Total Fat
	1 g Sat Fat
	0 g Trans Fat
	200 mg Sodium
	65 g CHO
	14 g Fibre
	12 g Protein
UEPC	1½ Fat
	1 Bean
	1 Grain
	1½ Fruits & Vegetables

Sensationally Simple Stir-Fried Rice

CHANGE IT UP

Add 1 chopped red pepper when you sauté the onion. Garnish with ½ cup (125 mL) finely chopped fresh chives and ½ cup (125 mL) finely chopped fresh cilantro.

HOW THE HECK DO I THAW FROZEN VEGETABLES?

For the quick method, put them in a colander and pour boiling water over them. Voila—thawed.

My son took Foods and Nutrition class and not only learned how to make a wicked stir-fry but also how to plan a meal. I believe that one of the reasons our nation is getting fatter is because no one knows how to cook. We dash to the store and buy convenience foods. Open package, heat, eat.

Here's a novel idea—let's make Foods and Nutrition a mandatory class. Not only will there be a generation of people who know what a frying pan is, but they'll know how to use it. Brilliant.

2 tsp (10 mL) **canola oil**
1 **large onion, diced**
4 **cloves garlic, minced**
2 **omega-3 eggs**
2 cups (500 mL) **cooked long- or short-grain brown rice**
2 cups (500 mL) **frozen peas and carrots, thawed**
3 Tbsp (45 mL) **low-sodium soy sauce**
1 Tbsp (15 mL) **Thai style chili sauce optional**
½ cup (125 mL) **cashews, chopped**

1 Heat a medium frying pan over medium heat. Add the oil and onion and sauté for 3 minutes or until onion is just cooked through. Add the garlic and the eggs. Stir until eggs are cooked through. Make sure to break the egg into smaller pieces. You don't want one big blob of cooked egg.

2 Add the rice, vegetables, soy sauce, and Thai-style chili sauce (if using). Stir well.

3 Cover and reduce the heat to low. Cook for 5 minutes or until the vegetables are heated through.

4 Sprinkle with cashews and serve.

Makes 6 cups (1.5 L). Makes four 1½-cup (375-mL) servings

ONE SERVING	330 Calories
	14 g Total Fat
	2 g Sat Fat
	0 g Trans Fat
	540 mg Sodium
	42 g CHO
	5 g Fibre
	12 g Protein
UEPC	½ Fat
	½ Egg
	1 Grains
	1 Fruits & Vegetables
	1 Nut

New

The Smith's House Recipe for the Harried Mother

I make this when I'm tired, starving, or slightly crabby. According to my teenage son, this is most days.

2 cups (500 mL) **cooked long- or short-grain brown rice**
2 Tbsp (30 mL) **water**
2 cups (500 mL) **fresh cooked or frozen peas, thawed**
¼ cup (60 mL) **light peanut sauce**
½ cup (125 mL) **unsalted peanuts**
¼ cup (60 mL) **chopped green onion**

1 Put the rice in a large microwaveable container with a lid and sprinkle with water. Cover and microwave on medium-high for 3 minutes, or until hot. Stir in peas and peanut sauce. Microwave for 2 more minutes, or until hot.

2 Divide rice equally between 4 plates. Sprinkle each with 2 Tbsp (30 mL) peanuts. Sprinkle each with 1 Tbsp (15 mL) green onion. Serve.

Makes 5 cups (1.25 mL). Makes four 1¼-cup (310-mL) servings

WHERE THE HECK DO I FIND LIGHT PEANUT SAUCE?
It's usually in the condiment aisle, but you can also try the Asian or international foods aisle. Once you've found it, memorize its location. You'll be back.

ONE SERVING	280 Calories
	12 g Total Fat
	2 g Sat Fat
	0 g Trans Fat
	80 mg Sodium
	36 g CHO
	6 g Fibre
	10 g Protein
UEPC	1 Grain
	1 Fruits & Vegetables
	1 Nut

New

Japanese Brown Rice Salad

BIG COOKING TIP
Want a bigger wasabi hit? Add an extra 1 tsp (5 mL) wasabi paste to the dressing. Be prepared to have your sinuses cleared.

I've been greatly influenced by Japanese cuisine. I love the clean flavours, the attention to detail, the unique use of ingredients, and most of all I'm really into their dishes. You can't find a plate bigger than your head—a good thing when it comes to portion control.

2 cups (500 mL) **cooked long- or short-grain brown rice**
½ **English cucumber, diced (unpeeled)**
2 **carrots, diced**
2 **stalks celery, diced**
1 **red pepper, diced**
4 **green onions, finely chopped**
½ **avocado, diced**

Dressing
1 Tbsp + 1 tsp (20 mL) **rice vinegar**
1 Tbsp (15 mL) **water**
2 tsp (10 mL) **low-sodium soy sauce**
1 tsp (5 mL) **canola oil**
1 tsp (5 mL) **wasabi paste (see sidebar page 239)**

1 In a large bowl, toss together the rice, cucumber, carrots, celery, red pepper, and green onion.

2 In a small bowl, whisk together the rice vinegar, water, soy sauce, oil, and wasabi paste.

3 Pour the dressing onto the salad and toss until the salad is well coated. Store in the fridge. When ready to serve, take out of the fridge and gently toss in the avocado.

Makes 5 cups (1.25 mL). Makes four 1¼-cup (310-mL) servings.

ONE SERVING	200 Calories
	6 g Total Fat
	1 g Sat Fat
	0 g Trans Fat
	160 mg Sodium
	34 g CHO
	4 g Fibre
	4 g Protein
UEPC	½ Fat
	1 Grain
	2 Fruits & Vegetables

Brown Rice with Dried Cranberries and Orange

If you attend a cranberry festival and get caught up in the frenzy of cranberry lust and happen to purchase a 20-lb (9-kg) bag of cranberries, like my friend Vivien did, then you're going to love this recipe.

You can either freeze those cranberries, or buy a food dehydrator and dry your own. Drying your own may be a bit Martha-esque, but it's your call. Personally, I say freeze the entire bag and buy dried cranberries at the grocery store for this recipe. Next thing to do is vow never to buy anything larger than your truck, unless of course it's chocolate.

IS IT BROTH OR IS IT STOCK?
Depending on the company who makes it, it's either one or the other. Bottom line: they're interchangeable.

1 cup (250 mL) **long-grain brown rice**
2 cups (500 mL) **lower-sodium chicken broth**
¼ cup (60 mL) **minced shallots**
½ cup (125 mL) **dried cranberries**
zest of 1 **orange**

1   In a medium pot, mix together the brown rice, chicken broth, and shallots. Bring to a boil. Cover with a tight fitting lid and reduce the heat to simmer. Cook for 40 minutes.

2   Add the dried cranberries. Cover and continue cooking for 5 minutes, or until the rice is tender. Remove from the heat and fluff the rice gently with a fork or a rice paddle. Let stand for 5 minutes. Add the orange zest, fluff, and serve.

Makes 3 cups (750 mL). Makes six ½-cup (125-mL) servings.

ONE SERVING	140 Calories
	1 g Total Fat
	0 g Sat Fat
	0 g Trans Fat
	155 mg Sodium
	30 g CHO
	2 g Fibre
	4 g Protein
UEPC	1 Grains
	¼ Fruits & Vegetables

Revised

Short-grain Brown Rice Risotto with Kale and Squash

SO WHAT THE HECK DOES KALE
LOOK LIKE ANYWAY?
Tucked away with all the other less popular greens, kale is found in the produce section. It has dark green, frilly leaves and is usually sold in bunches. It's a member of the cabbage family but has a far milder taste than its stronger tasting cousins. The smaller frilly leaves are the most tender. Always remove the leaves from the stalk before cooking, as the stalk tends be bitter. Whenever I serve kale to my son's friends, my son always tells them it doesn't taste like anything. Kid translation: it doesn't taste awful.

All you risotto lovers are going to take one look at this recipe and say, "No way, Smith. There isn't a hope anywhere on this earth that this is going to be creamy and delicious like a real risotto."

Well here's the scoop: when stirred, short-grain brown rice becomes creamy, especially when you add butternut squash.

3 cups (750 mL) **lower-sodium chicken broth**
1 **large leek, chopped into ¼-inch (5-mm) slices (see page 159)**
4 **cloves garlic, minced**
1 cup (250 mL) **short-grain brown rice**
3 cups (750 mL) **peeled and cubed butternut squash (1-inch/
2.5-cm cubes)**
4 cups (1 L) **chopped kale leaves (see sidebar)**
¼ cup (60 mL) **grated really good Parmesan cheese (see
sidebar below)**

1   In a medium-sized, heavy bottomed pot with a tight fitting lid, mix together the chicken broth, leeks, garlic, brown rice, and squash. Bring to a boil. Stir and cover. Reduce the heat to low and simmer for 40 minutes.

2   When the squash and rice mixture is ready, stir in the kale. Wilting the kale will look impossible, but be tenacious. It's going to wilt.

3   Simmer for 10 more minutes, stirring occasionally.

4   Sprinkle each serving with 2 tsp (10 mL) Parmesan.

Makes 4 cups (1 L). Makes six ¾-cup (175-mL) servings.

Kid Friendly

ONE SERVING	230 Calories
	3 g Total Fat
	1.5 g Sat Fat
	0 g Trans Fat
	390 mg Sodium
	45 g CHO
	5 g Fibre
	8 g Protein
UEPC	2 Fruits & Vegetables
	1 Grains

SO WHAT THE HECK IS REALLY GOOD PARMESAN?
Well, it's not the stuff that comes out of a container. My favourite is Parmigiano Reggiano, which comes from, you guessed it, Italy. It has a sharp, rich flavour. A little goes a long way. Available at the deli or cheese counter in most supermarkets. It comes as a block and you grate it as you need it. Store it in the fridge.

Barley and Brown Rice Pilaf with Mushrooms

Mention you're serving a barley dish to a Scot, or anyone on my dad's side of the family, and they'll be waiting with their glass in hand. Go ahead and tip a glass of whiskey or beer, but remember that barley is better for you when you have to chew it.

½ cup (125 mL) **dried shiitake or porcini mushrooms**
1 cup (250 mL) **boiling water**
½ cup (125 mL) **pot barley**
½ cup (125 mL) **short-grain brown rice**
3 cups (750 mL) **lower-sodium chicken broth**
½ cup (125 mL) **diced shallots**
1 cup (250 mL) **fresh or frozen peas, thawed**
~~½ cup (125 mL) **unsalted cashews**~~

1   Put the water in a medium pot and bring to a boil. Add the mushrooms and let stand for 15 minutes.

2   Add the pot barley, brown rice, chicken broth, and shallots. Bring to a boil. Cover and reduce the heat to simmer. Cook for 50 minutes, or until the rice is cooked.

3   Remove from heat and fluff with a fork. Let it sit for 5 minutes.

4   Add the peas and cashews. Serve.

Makes 5 cups (1.25 L). Makes four 1¼-cup (310-mL) servings.

ONE SERVING	390 Calories
	10 g Total Fat
	2 g Sat Fat
	0 g Trans Fat
	350 mg Sodium
	61 g CHO
	8 g Fibre
	18 g Protein
UEPC	1 Grain
	1 Fruits & Vegetables
	1 Nut

Quinoa 101

Make this dish vegetarian by substituting low-sodium vegetable stock for the chicken stock. To eliminate most of the sodium, make this with water instead.

And now for a grain lesson (you never know when you'll need to know this): quinoa (pronounced keen-wah) is an ancient cereal that was eaten by the Incas centuries ago. They called it the Mother Grain. Quinoa is so high in protein (13%) that the United Nations classified it as a super crop. This tiny, nondescript grist has the nutritional clout of an Olympic athlete.

Quinoa grains are naturally coated with a bitter resin called saponin. This resin can be removed by washing but is often removed by mechanical polishing. Unfortunately for us, this process makes quinoa less nutritious by removing the germ as well. Choose whole grain quinoa and rinse it well before cooking.

1 cup (250 mL) **whole grain quinoa**
¼ cup (60 mL) **minced shallots**
2 cups (500 mL) **lower-sodium chicken broth**

1   Place quinoa in a strainer and rinse well. Put rinsed quinoa in a medium pot and add shallots and chicken broth. Bring to a boil. Cover and cook over medium heat for 18 to 20 minutes, or until the quinoa is cooked.

2   Fluff with a fork. Remove from the heat and let stand for 5 minutes. Serve.

Makes 3 cups (750 mL). Makes six ½-cup (125-mL) servings.

Kid Friendly

ONE SERVING	
	120 Calories
	2.5 g Total Fat
	0 g Sat Fat
	0 g Trans Fat
	150 mg Sodium
	32 g CHO
	3 g Fibre
	9 g Protein
UEPC	1 Grain

New

Quinoa Pilaf

I have a huge peeve with the supermarket people.
I can't find anything. I'm fairly convinced there's a plot
to make you go on a scavenger hunt every time you go
to a different location. One store will have quinoa in,
say, the cereal aisle, because, hello, it's a cereal. Another
store will have it in the baking section. Why? I have no
idea. Is it because if you grind it up it would be flour?
It's all enough to make a girl want to yell at the produce
guy. Oh wait, I've already done that (see Sweet Potatoes
page 177). Oh dear, off on another tangent . . .

TIP
Make this dish vegetarian
by substituting low-sodium
vegetable broth for the
chicken broth.

1 cup (250 mL) **whole grain quinoa**
2 tsp (10 mL) **cumin**
1 tsp (5 mL) **coriander**
2 **stalks celery, diced**
2 **large carrots, diced**
1 **medium onion, diced**
2 cups (500 mL) **lower-sodium chicken broth**

1   Place the quinoa in a strainer and rinse well. Put rinsed
    quinoa in a medium pot with a tight fitting lid.

2   Add the cumin, coriander, celery, carrots, onion, and
    chicken broth. Bring to a boil. Cover and reduce the heat
    to medium. Simmer for 15 to 20 minutes. Remove from
    the heat and fluff with a fork. Cover and let stand for 5
    minutes. Serve.

Makes 4 cups (1 L). Makes eight ½-cup (125-mL) servings.

Kid Friendly

ONE SERVING	110 Calories
	1.5 g Total Fat
	0 g Sat Fat
	0 g Trans Fat
	120 mg Sodium
	20 g CHO
	3 g Fibre
	5 g Protein
UEPC	1 Grain
	½ Fruits & Vegetables

Revised

Barley Risotto

In my humble culinary opinion, risotto is the ultimate Italian comfort food. Its creamy consistency and rich flavours of garlic and Parmesan are delicious and comforting. On a cold winter night, not many things beat a great dish of risotto. Okay, if pressed, I can think of a couple of things. But I digress.

Barley is an underused grain just waiting to be discovered. So embrace the grain and start barley risotto-ing.

2 tsp (10 mL) **extra virgin olive oil**
2 **medium onions, diced**
2 **large portabello mushrooms, coarsely chopped**
3 **cloves garlic, minced**
¾ cup (175 mL) **pot barley**
2½ cups (625 mL) **lower-sodium chicken broth**
¼ cup (60 mL) **Parmigiano Reggiano (see sidebar page 187)**

1 Heat a medium saucepan that has a tight fitting lid over medium heat. Add the oil and onions. Sauté for 1 minute.

2 Add the mushrooms and garlic. Sauté for 1 minute.

3 Add the pot barley and chicken broth and stir. Bring to a boil. Reduce the heat, cover, and simmer for 50 minutes, or until the barley is cooked.

4 Remove from heat. Gently stir in the Parmesan and serve.

Makes 4 cups (1 L). Makes eight ½-cup (125-mL) servings.

ONE SERVING	100 Calories
	3 g Total Fat
	1 g Sat Fat
	0 g Trans Fat
	240 mg Sodium
	22 g CHO
	1 g Fibre
	4 g Protein
UEPC	¼ Fat
	¼ Fruits & Vegetables
	½ Grains

Blueberry Wheat Berry Salad

What are wheat berries? And where the heck do you find them? On a wheat bush?

Wheat berries are whole wheat kernels that haven't been milled, polished, or heat treated. This unadulterated, virgin wheat is the real deal, and remember that the closer we get to the real deal, the healthier it is. Wheat berries taste very nutty and have a slightly dense texture. They're well worth the hour it takes to cook them.

You can find wheat berries in any health food store and in most major supermarkets in the cereal aisle or the health food section. There are generally two kinds of wheat berries available at natural foods stores: hard and soft. I prefer the hard.

1 cup (250 mL) **wheat berries**
2½ cups (625 mL) **water**
3 cups (750 mL) **tightly packed fresh parsley**
1 cup (250 mL) **tightly packed fresh mint leaves**
6 **green onions, sliced thinly**
2 oz (55 g) or ½ cup (125 mL) **crumbled light feta cheese**

Dressing
¼ cup (60 mL) **fresh lemon juice**
2 Tbsp (30 mL) **extra virgin olive oil**
1 tsp (5 mL) **Dijon mustard**
3 cups (750 mL) **wild blueberries, fresh or frozen (see sidebar)**

WHY WILD BLUEBERRIES?
I really love tiny wild blueberries much more than the larger commercial ones. See Liz's "Are blueberries the best to eat?" on page 30. If fresh blueberries are out of season, use the frozen wild ones. Add them to this salad while still frozen and let them thaw on the way to a picnic or BBQ—a great way to keep your salad cold. Just a little warning: when you use frozen blueberries, the salad will turn purple the day after. Don't worry. It still tastes excellent. The kids may even be intrigued to try a purple food.

ONE SERVING	92 Calories
	3 g Total Fat
	0.5 g Sat Fat
	0 Trans Fat
	250 mg Sodium
	14 g CHO
	3 g Fibre
	3 g Protein
UEPC	½ Fats
	½ Fruits & Vegetables
	½ Grain

WHERE DO I FIND FRESH MINT?
In the produce section. I find it can be pricey unless you buy it at a local green grocer in bunches. I grow my own. It's a cinch. I know, I know, I'm such a foodie. A lot of gardeners treat it like a weed, but I let it run amuck in my garden. In the spring I transplant it into pots and either cook with it or add it to my green tea.

WHY THE HECK DOES THIS RECIPE MAKE 8 CUPS? CAN'T I CUT THE RECIPE IN HALF?
Sure you can, but this dish tastes so amazing, you'll kick yourself for halving it.

WHY CAN'T I JUST PULSE THE PARSLEY AND THE MINT TOGETHER AT THE SAME TIME?
They have different structures and if you pulse them together in the food processor you'll end up with puréed parsley and a hint of mint soup.

1 Mix together the wheat berries and water in a medium pot. Bring to a boil. Cover and reduce the heat to low. Simmer for 1 hour. This should yield about 3 cups (750 mL).

2 Meanwhile, mince the parsley with a knife, or pulse it in a food processor until minced. Transfer to a large bowl.

3 Either mince the mint with a knife or pulse in the food processor. Add to the parsley.

4 Add the green onion and crumbled feta. Toss together and store in the fridge until the wheat berries are finished cooking.

5 When the wheat berries are cooked, drain any excess water, and let them cool to room temperature.

6 Toss cooled wheat berries into the parsley and mint mixture.

7 Whisk together the dressing and pour over the salad. Gently mix in the blueberries and serve.

Makes 8 cups (2 L). Makes sixteen ½-cup (125-mL) servings.

Kid Friendly

Wonderful Waldorf Wheat Berry Salad

The grande dame of hotels, the Waldorf Astoria in NYC, was the first to introduce room service. In my opinion, room service is the main reason you stay in a great hotel. I love being able to order what I want, have it appear at my door, and have someone whisk it away when I'm finished.

½ cup (125 mL) **wheat berries**
1½ cups (375 mL) **water**
2 **large red skinned or Granny Smith apples**
1 cup (250 mL) **diced celery**
½ cup (125 mL) **dried cranberries**
½ cup (125 mL) **walnut halves, coarsely chopped**

Dressing
3 Tbsp (45 mL) **low-fat mayonnaise**
3 Tbsp (45 mL) **low-fat plain probiotic yogurt**
3 Tbsp (45 mL) **apple cider vinegar**

1 Mix together the wheat berries and water in a medium pot. Bring to a boil. Cover and reduce heat to low. Simmer for 1 hour.

2 When the wheat berries are cooked, drain any excess water and let them cool to room temperature.

3 Wash and core the apples. Cut into eighths and then chop into small pieces about the size of a grape. Place in a medium bowl.

4 Add the celery. Toss in dried cranberries.

5 Pour in the dressing and toss in the wheat berries. Store in the fridge until ready to serve.

6 Just before serving, toss in the walnuts.

Makes about 6 cups (1.5 L), depending on the size of the apples. Makes eight ¾-cup (175-mL) servings.

Kid Friendly

ONE SERVING	165 Calories
	6 g Total Fat
	0.7 g Sat Fat
	0 Trans Fat
	57 mg Sodium
	25 g CHO
	4 g Fibre
	3 g Protein
UEPC	½ Fat
	1 Fruits & Vegetables
	½ Grain
	½ Nut

PASTA & SAUCES

Adults Only Pasta Sauce

You looked at the anchovies in the ingredient list and you're thinking, "Aren't they those teeny fishy things I pick off pizza?" You'd be correct, oh great foodie expert, you. Those tiny little fish are a staple in the Mediterranean diet and they're loaded with those amazing omega-3 fatty acids Liz keeps raving about. They melt in the pan, which renders them impossible to pick out, and their flavour is so unique, no one will ever figure it out. Yup, the secret ingredient in this terrific pasta sauce is anything but mundane.

HOW THE HECK DO I COOK WHOLE WHEAT PASTA?

Use a large pot with plenty of water. Bring the water to a boil, add the pasta, stir, bring back to a boil, and cook with the lid off for 8 to 10 minutes or until al dente.

4 **anchovy fillets, drained and diced**
6 **cloves garlic, minced**
one 28-oz (796-mL) can **diced tomatoes**
24 **kalamata olives, pitted**
1 cup (250 mL) **dry red wine**
¼ to ½ tsp (1 to 2 mL) **red pepper flakes**

1   Make sure you have all your ingredients prepped and ready to go.

2   Heat a large frying pan over medium heat. Add the anchovies and garlic and stir quickly. Don't let it burn. Sauté for 1 minute.

3   Add the tomatoes, olives, red wine, and red pepper flakes. Bring to a boil. Reduce the heat and simmer for 20 minutes.

4   Serve over cooked pasta.

Makes 3 cups (750 mL). Makes four ¾-cup (175-mL) servings.

ONE SERVING	
	160 Calories
	4 g Total Fat
	1 g Sat Fat
	0 g Trans Fat
	500 mg Sodium
	12 g CHO
	2 g Fibre
	4 g Protein
UEPC	¾ Fat
	1½ Fruits & Vegetables

New

Kid Friendly Spaghetti Sauce

Grape juice, or what I like to call unfermented wine, is a fabulous ingredient to add to a pasta sauce. Not only are you adding antioxidants to your diet, you're also adding a slightly sweet ingredient that makes this sauce totally kid friendly. Liz and I always say that any healthy recipe a kid will eat is worth making.

2 Tbsp (30 mL) **extra virgin olive oil**
1 **large onion, diced**
one 370-mL jar **roasted red peppers, drained and diced**
Or 3 **whole roasted red peppers, diced**
4 **cloves garlic, minced**
two 28-oz (796-mL) **can plum tomatoes**
1 cup (250 mL) **Concord or purple grape juice**
½ tsp (2 mL) **red pepper flakes (optional)**

1 Heat a large pot over medium heat. Add the oil and onion and sauté for about 5 minutes or until well cooked.

2 Add the roasted red peppers and garlic. Sauté for 1 minute.

3 Add the plum tomatoes and grape juice. Press the tomatoes using a potato masher.

4 Bring to a boil. Reduce heat to medium and cook for 30 minutes. Stir often.

5 Add the red pepper flakes, if using. Pour over cooked whole wheat pasta and serve. You can freeze this sauce for up to 2 months.

Makes 6 cups (1.5 L). Makes twelve ½-cup (125-mL) servings.

Kid Friendly, of course

ONE SERVING	80 Calories
	2.5 g Total Fat
	0 g Sat Fat
	0 g Trans Fat
	55 mg Sodium
	12 g CHO
	2 g Fibre
	2 g Protein
UEPC	½ Fat
	1¼ Fruits & Vegetables

Asian Noodle Salad

I look forward to summer every year with great expectations. I love the warmer weather, my perennial garden,
and going to my friend's cottage to make summer-only
recipes. This is one of those recipes. Make it the day
before and serve it well chilled on one of those hazy
summer days that's so hot you feel like melting.

4 oz (115 g) **uncooked whole wheat spaghetti**
4 cups (1 L) **shredded red cabbage (about ½ a medium
    cabbage)**
1 **large carrot**
1 **red pepper**
4 cups (1 L) **small broccoli florets**

Dressing
¼ cup (60 mL) **natural crunchy peanut butter**
2 Tbsp (30 mL) **rice vinegar**
2 Tbsp (30 mL) **water**
2 Tbsp (30 mL) **low-sodium soy sauce**
2 Tbsp (30 mL) **honey**
1 Tbsp (15 mL) **garlic chili sauce**
2 Tbsp (30 mL) **fresh lime juice**

¼ cup (60 mL) **unsalted peanuts**

Optional Toppings
1 cup (250 mL) **chopped fresh cilantro**
1 **green onion, chopped**

BIG COOKING TIP
Omit the peanuts and serve
with grilled or stir-fried
skinless, boneless chicken
breasts.

**WHAT IF I CAN'T FIND RICE
VINEGAR?**
Go ahead and use apple cider
vinegar.

ONE SERVING	350 Calories
	14 g Total Fat
	2 g Sat Fat
	0 g Trans Fat
	465 mg Sodium
	46 g CHO
	9 g Fibre
	14 g Protein
UEPC	4 Fruits & Vegetables
	1 Grains
	1 Nuts

WHAT THE HECK DOES 4 OZ
(115 G) OF UNCOOKED PASTA
LOOK LIKE?
It's one third of a 375-g (12-oz)
box of pasta.

KID FRIENDLY TIP
If your kids aren't into spicy
food, omit the garlic chili sauce.
At serving time, dish theirs out
and then add the garlic chili
sauce to the remainder. Toss
well and serve to the adults.
My son has been eating spicy
foods since he was 7. So don't
give up. Offer your kids some
of the spicy version from time
to time. One day they may just
surprise you and ask for it. The
older I get, the more I believe
in miracles.

1   Cook pasta according to the package directions.

2   While the pasta is cooking, grate the carrot and dice the red pepper. Toss shredded cabbage, broccoli florets, carrots, and red pepper in a large bowl. Set aside. This is a lot easier if you have a food processor to shred the cabbage and grate the carrot. If you don't have a food processor, slice the cabbage as thinly as possible by hand and grate the carrot using a hand grater.

3   Make the dressing. Combine the peanut butter, rice vinegar, water, soy sauce, honey, garlic chili sauce, and lime juice in a bowl. Whisk until blended.

4   Pour the dressing over the veggies. By this time, the pasta should be cooked. Drain the pasta and combine with the veggies. Toss until everything is well coated with the dressing.

5   Cover and refrigerate for 3 hours, or until well chilled.

6   When ready to serve, divide the salad equally between 4 plates. Sprinkle each serving with 1 Tbsp (15 mL) peanuts. If you decide on more of an Asian flavour, sprinkle each serving with ¼ cup (60 mL) of the cilantro and ¼ of the green onion.

Makes 8 cups (2 L). Makes four 2-cup (500-mL) servings.

Mairlyn's Amazing Tomato Sauce

This has, and always will be, my house sauce. It's multi-functional: you can serve it with some cheese, freeze it for later, use it in a lasagna recipe, or pour it over chicken and bake it in the oven. It will become your house sauce as well.

2 Tbsp (30 mL) **extra virgin olive oil**
1 **large onion, diced**
two 28-oz (796-mL) **cans whole plum tomatoes**
one 370-mL jar **roasted red peppers, drained and diced**
Or 3 whole roasted red peppers, diced
8 **cloves garlic, minced**
2 Tbsp (30 mL) **chopped fresh basil**

KID FRIENDLY TIP
Garlic alert! If you have really young children, they may find the garlic too intense. The kids that have loved this sauce are usually over 5 years old. So if you feel your child won't like the garlic, feel free to downgrade it to 4 cloves. Or just make the Kid Friendly Spaghetti Sauce on page 197.

1   Heat a large pot over medium heat. Add the oil and onion. Sauté for about 5 minutes or until cooked.

2   Add the plum tomatoes, roasted red peppers, and garlic. Mash with a potato masher. Bring to a boil. Reduce heat and simmer uncovered for 25 minutes, or until the sauce begins to thicken. Stir occasionally.

3   Add the fresh basil and remove from the heat. Serve over cooked whole wheat pasta. You can freeze this sauce for up to 2 months.

Makes 6 cups (1.5 L). Makes eight ¾-cup (175-mL) servings.

ONE SERVING	100 Calories
	4 g Total Fat
	0.5 g Sat Fat
	0 g Trans Fat
	300 mg Sodium
	16 g CHO
	5 g Fibre
	3 g Protein
UEPC	¾ Fat
	1½ Fruits & Vegetables

Revised

Rotini with Plum Tomatoes and Lentils

QUICK DINNER TIP
For a side dish, steam some broccoli after you add the pasta to the lentil mixture. The broccoli will be cooked by the time the lentils are ready.

My sister Kathleen doesn't like lentils. As a matter of fact, she hates them (as well as a whole bunch of other stuff). Several years ago she came for a visit. She arrived starving at 9:00 p.m. and the only thing I had in the refrigerator was my Rotini with Plum Tomatoes and Lentil dish. I heated it up. She took one look at them and said, "I'm not eating those things, Mair. You know I hate them." I convinced her that they were really very good, so she reluctantly gave them a taste. To her surprise—not mine—she loved them. She even had a second helping. If my picky sister loves them, this is a recipe worth trying.

1½ cups (375 mL) **uncooked whole wheat rotini**
2 tsp (10 mL) **extra virgin olive oil**
1 **onion, diced**
½ cup (125 mL) **chopped roasted red pepper**
one 28-oz (796-mL) can **diced tomatoes**
one 19-oz (540-mL) **can lentils, drained and rinsed**
2 Tbsp (30 mL) **tomato paste**
1 tsp (5 mL) **dried basil**
1 tsp (5 mL) **Worcestershire sauce**
¼ tsp (1 mL) **red pepper flakes**
1 **clove garlic, minced**
2 Tbsp (30 mL) **Parmesan cheese**
¼ cup (60 mL) **diced fresh parsley**

ONE SERVING	370 Calories
	4 g Total Fat
	1 g Sat Fat
	0 g Trans Fat
	550 mg Sodium
	64 g CHO
	15 g Fibre
	20 g Protein
UEPC	1 Beans
	¼ Fat
	2 Fruits & Vegetables
	1½ Grains

1 Put a medium pot of water on the stove to boil.

2 Heat a large skillet over medium heat. Add the olive oil and onions. Sauté for 3 minutes.

3 Add the roasted red peppers and tomatoes.

4 Add the lentils, tomato paste, basil, Worcestershire, red pepper flakes, and garlic. Bring to a boil. Cover and reduce the heat to simmer. Cook for 10 minutes, stirring occasionally.

5 Meanwhile, back to that pot of water. When it comes to a boil, add the rotini. Stir. Cook about 10 minutes, or until just cooked or as we like to call it—al dente.

6 When the pasta is cooked, drain. Add to the tomato-lentil mixture. Stir well and simmer for 5 minutes. Serve with 1 tsp (5 mL) Parmesan cheese and 1 Tbsp (15 mL) parsley on each serving.

Makes 7 cups (1.75 mL). Makes four 1¾-cup (425-mL) servings.

Revised

Rotini with Feta and Tomatoes

This recipe appeared in my first cookbook *Lick the Spoon!*, in 1998. I updated it a couple of years ago and I'm in love with this new version.

Because this sauce is basically raw, you aren't allowed to make it unless the tomatoes are perfect. Think a sunny day in Tuscany kind of perfect tomato. If you've never been there, open up a great bottle of red wine and start dreaming.

1½ cups (375 mL) **uncooked whole wheat rotini**
8 cups (2 L) **chopped luscious, ripe, bursting with flavour tomatoes**
¼ cup (60 mL) **minced shallots**
8 **kalamata olives, pitted**
¾ cup (175 mL) **crumbled light feta cheese**
¾ cup (175 mL) **fresh basil chiffonade (see sidebar)**
2 Tbsp (30 mL) **balsamic vinegar**

1   Open up a bottle of red wine. Let it breath. Put on Il Divo and dance around the kitchen. Pour wine to sip while cooking. Begin recipe.

2   Cook pasta according to the directions on the package, or check out How the Heck Do I Cook Whole Wheat Pasta, page 196.

3   While the pasta is cooking, cut each tomato into bite-sized pieces. Use a serrated knife; it's easier.

4   Gently toss together the tomatoes, shallots, olives, feta cheese, basil, and balsamic vinegar in a large bowl.

5   When the pasta is cooked, drain. Pour over the tomato mixture. Toss gently.

6   Crack on some fresh pepper and serve.

Makes 10 cups (2.5 L). Makes six 1½-cups (375-mL) servings.

WHAT THE HECK DOES CHIFFONADE MEAN?
A cheffy term that will impress the socks off your dinner guests. Chiffonade means to slice a fresh herb or leafy vegetable into thin ribbons. Either stack the leaves on top of one another and slice, or roll the leaves together and then slice, whichever is easiest. You'll end up with tiny ribbons of whatever it is you're chiffonading.

WHAT DOES 8 CUPS OF TOMATOES LOOK LIKE?
It looks like 4 really large tomatoes.

ONE SERVING	160 Calories
	3.5 g Total Fat
	1 g Sat Fat
	0 g Trans Fat
	270 mg Sodium
	27 g CHO
	3 g Fibre
	8 g Protein
UEPC	2½ Fruits & Vegetables
	½ Grains

BEANS

Japanese-Style Edamame and Corn Salad

The Japanese have been eating edamame (pronounced ey-dah-MAH-meh) for over two thousand years; I think they may be on to something here. These delicious beans, albeit mild tasting, can be found in the frozen vegetable or health food section in larger supermarkets, or at any Asian food store worth its salt in seaweed. These green soybeans, which are bought parboiled and flash-frozen, come either in the pod or shelled. Unless your idea of a really fun Saturday night is shelling beans (yikes), buy the shelled ones.

Enjoy the salad with one of the dressings below.

2 cups (500 mL) **frozen, shelled edamame**
1 cup (250 mL) **fresh cooked or frozen corn, thawed**
1 **red pepper, diced**
4 **green onions, thinly sliced**

Japanese Dressing
1 Tbsp (15 mL) **fresh lime juice**
1 Tbsp (15 mL) **low-sodium soy sauce**
1 Tbsp (15 mL) **rice vinegar**
2 tsp (10 mL) **miso paste**
1 tsp (5 mL) **canola oil**
2 **cloves garlic, minced**
1 Tbsp (15 mL) **minced fresh ginger**

Citrus Dressing
1 Tbsp (15 mL) **frozen orange juice concentrate, thawed**
1 Tbsp (15 mL) **canola oil**
1 Tbsp (15 mL) **rice vinegar**
1 Tbsp (15 mL) **honey**
1 Tbsp (15 mL) **fresh lime juice**
1 tsp (5 mL) **Dijon mustard**

HOW DO I THAW FROZEN CORN?

Place frozen corn in a colander. Drain the cooked edamame over the corn. Voila, thawed corn.

MAKE IT QUICKER

I love Japanese salad dressing. My favourite is a store-bought dressing called Miso, made by JC. It's made with canola oil and has only 40 calories and 3.5 g of fat per tablespoon (15 mL), and no saturated fat. For a really quick salad, try using JC Miso Dressing (or any other commercial Japanese-style salad dressing made with canola oil) instead of the Citrus or Japanese Dressing.

ONE SERVING using Japanese Dressing	
	170 Calories
	4.5 g Total Fat
	0 g Sat Fat
	0 g Trans Fat
	330 mg Sodium
	22 g CHO
	6 g Fibre
	11 g Protein
UEPC	1 Beans
	1 Fruits & Vegetables

BIG COOKING TIP
The beauty of this salad is that you have your choice of dressing. The Citrus Dressing is slightly sweet, which is great for kids, and the Japanese Dressing has an authentic miso flavour, which is stronger and more adult friendly. Try them both and see which you like best.

WHERE THE HECK DO I FIND MISO PASTE?
In the Asian section of most large grocery stores or at any Asian food store.

1 In a small pot, bring 1 cup (250 mL) of water to a boil. Add the edamame and bring back to a boil. Reduce heat and cover. Simmer for 4 minutes. Don't overcook, as they tend to go soggy. While they're cooking, make one of the dressings.

2 Whisk together the ingredients for your chosen dressing in a small bowl. Store covered in the fridge until ready to serve.

3 Hopefully making the dressing didn't take longer than 4 minutes. Drain the edamame.

4 In a medium bowl, toss together the edamame, corn, red pepper, and green onion.

5 Cover and store in the fridge for 1 to 2 hours, or until well chilled.

6 At serving time, remove the salad and dressing from the fridge and toss together. Serve.

Makes 4 cups (1 L). Makes four 1-cup (250-mL) servings.

Kid Friendly

ONE SERVING using Citrus Dressing	200 Calories
	7 g Total Fat
	0 g Sat Fat
	0 g Trans Fat
	75 mg Sodium
	26 g CHO
	6 g Fibre
	10 g Protein
UEPC	¼ Fat
	1 Beans
	1 Fruits & Vegetables

Out-of-this-World Chili

There are as many chili recipes out there as there are wannabe Texans. The original recipe originated in the Lone Star State and had no beans in it at all. It was just a big bowl of cooked meat with spices. I'm sure this recipe would send any Texan worth their weight in beef for a loop—it doesn't have any meat in it at all. Well, nothing that originated on four legs anyhow. There's a meaty look to it, but it comes from a soy meat replacement. I've been using this in my chili for years and no one has ever figured it out. Don't be soy challenged. Give it a go.

2 Tbsp + 2 tsp (40 mL) **extra virgin olive oil**
1 **onion, diced**
1 **carrot, diced**
1 **red pepper, diced**
3 **cloves garlic, minced**
one 19-oz (540-mL) can **black beans, drained and rinsed**
one 19-oz (540-mL) can **kidney beans, drained and rinsed**
one 28-oz (796-mL) can **diced tomatoes**
2 Tbsp (30 mL) **tomato paste**
¼ cup (60 mL) **salsa, mild, medium, or hot**
2 Tbsp + 1 tsp (35 mL) **chili powder**
1 tsp (5 mL) **cumin**
1 tsp (5 mL) **dried oregano**
1 tsp (5 mL) **dried basil**
one 12-oz (340-g) **package Yves Veggie Ground Round**

1 Heat a large pot over medium heat. Add the oil and onion. Sauté for 3 minutes or until the onion is translucent.

2 Add the carrots, red pepper, and garlic. Sauté for 2 minutes.

3 Add the black beans, kidney beans, tomatoes, tomato paste, salsa, chili powder, cumin, oregano, and basil. Bring to a boil. Reduce heat and cover. Simmer for 20 minutes or until the carrots are cooked.

4 Add the package of Yves Veggie Ground Round and heat through. Serve.

Makes 10 cups (2.5 L). Makes eight 1¼-cup (310-mL) servings.

Kid Friendly

ADULT VERSION
Want more spice? I add ¼ tsp (1 mL) red pepper flakes to the pot after I've dished out my son's portion.

IS IT SALSA OR A SALT LICK?
Make sure you're sitting down the next time you read the sodium content of most commercial salsas. With an average of 480 mg of sodium per ¼ cup (60 mL) of salsa, you're going to hit your sodium stratosphere in no time. Check out the labels and pick a salsa with around 260 mg of sodium per ¼ cup (60 mL). I found that most fresh salsas hit that number, along with reduced sodium bottled brands. Bottom line? Read your labels.

ONE SERVING	250 Calories
	5 g Total Fat
	0g Sat Fat
	0 g Trans Fat
	600 mg Sodium
	35 CHO
	13 g Fibre
	16 g Protein
UEPC	1½ Beans
	1 Fat
	1 Fruits & Vegetables

Blazin' Black Bean Chili

TIP
For all you carnivores, you can add ¾ lb (375 g) extra lean ground beef or turkey. Brown in a pan, drain off any excess fat, and add it in step #2.

Blazing Saddles, the classic cowboy movie from the '70s, has a tour de force campfire farting scene. I live with a smelly dog, a stinky partner, and a teenage son who all think a good toot is the funniest thing in the world. The old song, "Beans, beans, the musical fruit, the more eat the more you toot," is incorrect. The real version should be, "The more you eat on a regular basis, the less you'll toot." Not nearly as rhythmic, but true nonetheless. Start serving your family beans at least three times a week. There's that scary inaugural period, but after that it should be clear sailing.

2 cups (500 mL) **fresh cooked or frozen corn, thawed**
1 **large onion, diced**
two 19-oz (540-mL) **cans black beans, drained and rinsed**
one 28-oz (796-mL) **can diced plum tomatoes**
3 **cloves garlic, minced**
1 Tbsp (15 mL) **dried oregano**
2 tsp (10 mL) **chili powder**
2 tsp (10 mL) **cumin**
2 tsp (10 mL) **coriander**
1 tsp (5 mL) **dried basil**
¼ tsp (1 mL) **cracked pepper**
½ cup (125 mL) **pomegranate juice**
1 Tbsp (15 mL) **extra virgin olive oil**

ONE SERVING	240 Calories
	4 g Total Fat
	0 g Sat Fat
	0 g Trans Fat
	520 mg Sodium
	41 g CHO
	13 g Fibre
	12 g Protein
UEPC	1 Beans
	½ Fat
	1¾ Fruits & Vegetables

1   Heat a large pot over medium heat. Add the corn and onion. Yes, you read it correctly. There isn't any oil added. We want to blacken those veggies. Stir occasionally for 5 minutes, or until the corn and onion begin to turn dark brown.

2   Add the black beans, tomatoes, garlic, oregano, chili powder, cumin, coriander, basil, and cracked pepper. Stir well.

3   Bring to a boil. Reduce heat and cover. Simmer for 20 minutes, stirring occasionally.

4   Remove from heat. Stir in pomegranate juice and olive oil. Serve.

Makes 7 cups (1.75 mL). Makes seven 1-cup (250-mL) servings.

Kid Friendly

Summer Fiesta Chickpea Salad

Oh, the glamour of a cookbook author, holed up in
her kitchen for endless hours, creating food that either
tastes like a gift from the culinary gods, or not. This one
was definitely sent to me by those very helpful gods.
Bless their foodie hearts.

Dressing
1 Tbsp + 1 tsp (20 mL) **extra virgin olive oil**
1 Tbsp + 1 tsp (20 mL) **red wine vinegar**
1 Tbsp (15 mL) **Dijon mustard**
3 **cloves garlic, minced**
1 tsp (5 mL) **honey**

Salad
one 19-oz (540-mL) **can chickpeas, drained and rinsed**
1 **large red pepper, diced**
1 **large orange pepper, diced**
2 cups (500 mL) **grape tomatoes, cut into halves**
3 **green onions, finely chopped**
1 **stalk celery, thinly sliced**
2 Tbsp (30 mL) **diced fresh basil**

1   In a large bowl, whisk together the olive oil, red wine
    vinegar, Dijon, garlic, and honey.

2   Add the chickpeas, red pepper, orange pepper, grape
    tomatoes, green onion, celery, and basil. Toss well.
    Cover and refrigerate for 30 minutes. Lasts for 5 days
    in the fridge.

3   Serve as is, or over chopped romaine or baby spinach.

Makes 6 cups (1.5 L). Makes four 1½-cup (375-mL) servings.

ONE SERVING	260 Calories
	7 g Total Fat
	1 g Sat Fat
	0 g Trans Fat
	220 mg Sodium
	44 g CHO
	9 g Fibre
	9 g Protein

UEPC	1 Beans
	1 Fat
	2½ Fruits & Vegetables

Totally Terrific Taco-Taco Salad

TURN WHOLE WHEAT SOFT TORTILLAS INTO BAKED TORTILLAS

Preheat the oven to 400°F (200°C). Cut each tortilla into 4 pieces. Place on a metal baking pan and put into the preheated oven. Bake for 5 to 7 minutes or until lightly browned. Let cool on pan for 10 minutes. Serve with salsa or salad, if desired.

When my son was 11, he and I were at a fast food place (okay, it was Wendy's), and he ordered the Taco Salad. He loved it. Midbite he said, "Hey, mom, you should make this for your book." Well, I took his advice and here it is. A totally kid friendly fast meal that's ready in 20 minutes and devoured every time you serve it.

1 Tbsp + 1 tsp (20 mL) **extra virgin olive oil**
1 **medium onion, chopped**
2 **cloves garlic, minced**
7 oz (200 g) **ground turkey, extra lean**
1 Tbsp (15 mL) **chili powder**
1 tsp (5 mL) **cumin**
½ tsp (2 mL) **dried oregano**
¼ cup (60 mL) **tomato paste**
1 cup (250 mL) **water**
2 Tbsp (30 mL) **ketchup**
1 tsp (5 mL) **Worcestershire**
one 19-oz (540-mL) can **black beans, drained and rinsed**
1 **head of romaine**
1 **red pepper**
4 **large 100% whole wheat soft tortillas, trans fat free (optional)**

1   Heat a large frying pan over medium heat. Add the oil and onions and sauté until almost cooked, about 3 to 5 minutes. Add the garlic and sauté for 1 minute.

2   Add the ground turkey and brown. Drain any excess fat. Add the chili powder, cumin, and oregano. Stir well.

3   Add the tomato paste, water, ketchup, and Worcestershire. Stir well.

4   Stir in the beans and heat through. This will take about 3 to 5 minutes.

5   While you wait, wash, dry, then chop the romaine and red pepper into bite-sized pieces. Divide the lettuce equally between 4 plates.

6   When the bean mixture is hot, remove it from the heat and spoon equally over the four plates of lettuce. Sprinkle with the red pepper. Serve tortillas as is or baked (see sidebar). Watch your kids gobble this up. Make a mental note to serve this at least once a week until they move out.

Serves 4.

Kid Friendly

ONE SERVING without Tortillas	
	275 Calories
	7 g Total Fat
	1 g Sat Fat
	0 g Trans Fat
	360 mg Sodium
	35 CHO
	11 g Fibre
	22g Protein
UEPC	1 Beans
	1 Fat
	1½ Fruits & Vegetables
	½ Meat

Quickie Quesadillas that your family will love

I've discovered that the only people not running around losing their minds have a nanny, housekeeper, personal chef, tutor, massage therapist, and a shrink. Or they're copious list writers. As a Type A personality, I'm in the latter category. Without my blessed lists to keep me organized, I'd go nuts. This dinner is one of my classic favourites. I keep all the ingredients on hand so I can pull off this meal in minutes—to cheers and applause. Once an actor, always an actor.

TIP
Most canned refried beans are high in sodium. If you're really being careful about how much salt you're using, try my recipe for Cheater Refried Beans on page 212.

4 large 100% whole wheat soft tortillas, trans fat free
one 396-mL (14-oz) can low-fat or fat-free refried beans, mild, medium, or hot
½ cup (125 mL) shredded light Monterey Jack cheese
1 cup (250 mL) salsa, mild, medium, or hot

1   Preheat the oven to warm at 200°F (95°C).

2   Heat a large frying pan over medium heat.

3   Spread 2 Tbsp (30 mL) refried beans over half of the tortilla. Place the tortilla in the frying pan.

4   Sprinkle with 2 Tbsp (30 mL) of the cheese. Fold tortilla in half. Press down gently with a spatula.

5   Fry until the cheese is melted and the tortilla is golden brown on one side. Flip and heat 1 more minute, or until golden brown on both sides.

6   Remove from the frying pan. Keep warm in the oven until all tortillas are cooked. Cut into 4 triangles. Serve with salsa.

Serves 4.

Kid Friendly

ONE SERVING	200 Calories
	3.5 Total Fat
	2 g Sat Fat
	0 g Trans Fat
	520 mg Sodium
	37 CHO
	6 g Fibre
	15 g Protein
UEPC	1 Beans
	½ Fruits & Vegetables
	2 Grains
	½ Milk

Revised

Remarkable Refried Beans

Most canned refried beans are loaded with artery clogging lard, a big fat no-no. My low-fat heart healthy version has only 1 tsp (5 mL) of extra virgin olive oil in the entire recipe. Use the beans as a dip for vegetables, to spread on burritos and quesadillas, or add to a plate of nachos. This recipe keeps up to 5 days in the fridge—if it lasts that long.

1 tsp (5 mL) **extra virgin olive oil**
1 **onion, minced**
3 **cloves garlic, minced**
one 19-oz (540-mL) can **black beans, drained and rinsed**
1 Tbsp (15 mL) **chili powder**
½ cup (125 mL) **water**

1   Heat a large frying pan over medium heat. Add the oil and onion. Sauté for 1 minute, stirring constantly.

2   Add the garlic, black beans, chili powder, and water. Cover and simmer for 10 minutes.

3   Remove from heat. Transfer to a food processor or blender and purée, or mash with a potato masher. Store in the fridge until ready to use. Try it in the Quickie Quesadillas, page 210.

Makes 2 cups (500 mL). Makes eight ¼-cup (60-mL) servings.

ONE SERVING	80 Calories
	1.5 Total Fat
	0 g Sat Fat
	0 g Trans Fat
	100 mg Sodium
	13 g CHO
	5 g Fibre
	5 g Protein
UEPC	½ Beans

Cheater Refried Beans

The hardest part of this recipe is hauling the food processor out of the cupboard. It's so easy that if you actually wreck it, you'd better email me: we need to talk.

one 19-oz (540-mL) can **black beans, drained and rinsed**
1 Tbsp (15 mL) **chili powder (see sidebar)**
1 tsp (5 mL) **cumin**

1   Place all ingredients in a food processor. Pulse until smooth. Serve immediately or store in the fridge for up to 3 days.

Makes 2¼ cups (550 mL). Makes nine ¼-cup (60-mL) servings.

KID FRIENDLY TIP
These beans are fairly spicy. To make it kid friendly, reduce the chili powder to 1 tsp (5 mL).

ONE SERVING	60 Calories
	1 g Total Fat
	0 g Sat Fat
	0 g Trans Fat
	100 mg Sodium
	11 CHO
	4 g Fibre
	4 g Protein
UEPC	½ Beans

Take One Can of Beans

Three Ultimate Quick-and-Easy Recipes

Revised
Jazzy Beans

This recipe is definitely a candidate for a healthy eating award. Open a can of beans in tomato sauce, add some stuff, and you're eating dinner in about 15 minutes. Only prerequisite? You need a can opener or you're out of luck.

2 tsp (10 mL) **extra virgin olive oil**
1 **onion, diced**
1 **red pepper, diced**
1 **clove garlic, minced**
one 14-oz (398-mL) can **of beans in tomato sauce**
2 Tbsp (30 mL) **ketchup**
1 Tbsp (15 mL) **Dijon mustard**
1 Tbsp (15 mL) **molasses**

1 Heat a medium-sized saucepan over medium heat. Add the oil, onion, and red pepper. Sauté for 3 minutes.

2 Add the garlic, beans, ketchup, Dijon, and molasses. Cover and simmer for 10 minutes, stirring occasionally. Serve.

Makes 3 cups (750 mL). Makes four ¾-cup (175-mL) servings.

Kid Friendly

ONE SERVING	
	170 Calories
	3 g Total Fat
	0 g Sat Fat
	0 g Trans Fat
	500 mg Sodium
	33 g CHO
	7 g Fibre
	7 g Protein
UEPC	1 Beans
	½ Fat
	½ Fruits & Vegetables

New
Kindergarten Curry

This recipe is for all you RCC's (rookie curry cooks), who haven't quite made it to the big kid side of the curry playground.

2 tsp (10 mL) **extra virgin olive oil**
1 **onion, diced**
2 tsp (10 mL) **curry powder**
1 tsp (5 mL) **dried ginger (optional)**
½ tsp (2 mL) **cumin**
¼ tsp (1 mL) **cinnamon**
pinch **allspice**
1 **clove garlic, minced**
one 14-oz (398-mL) can **of beans in tomato sauce**
3 Tbsp (45 mL) **ketchup**

1   Heat a medium-sized saucepan over medium heat. Add the oil and onion. Sauté for 2 minutes.

2   Add the curry powder, ginger (if using), cumin, cinnamon, and allspice. Stir well and cook for 1 minute.

3   Add the garlic, beans, and ketchup. Cover and simmer for 10 minutes, stirring occasionally. Serve.

Makes 2½ cups. Makes four ⅔-cup (150-mL) servings.

Kid Friendly

ONE SERVING	160 Calories
	3 g Total Fat
	0 g Sat Fat
	0 g Trans Fat
	520 mg Sodium
	29 g CHO
	7 g Fibre
	7 g Protein
UEPC	1 Beans
	½ Fat

New

Marvellous Mexican Beans

If you want your kids to eat healthy, you need to offer them healthy choices. Here's a tip: offer them two choices. Tell them they can choose between Mexican Beans or Flambéed Frog's Legs. Funny thing, they usually choose the beans.

2 tsp (10 mL) **extra virgin olive oil**
2 **large red peppers, chopped**
1 **onion, diced**
1 **clove garlic, minced**
one 14-oz (398-mL) can **of beans in tomato sauce**
1 cup (250 mL) **salsa, mild, medium, or hot**
½ cup (125 mL) **diced cilantro (optional)**

1   Heat a medium-sized saucepan over medium heat. Add the oil, red pepper, and onion. Sauté for 3 minutes.

2   Add the garlic, beans, and salsa. Cover and simmer for 10 minutes, stirring occasionally. Sprinkle with cilantro if desired. Serve.

Makes 3 cups (750 mL). Makes four ¾-cup (175-mL) servings.

Kid Friendly

ONE SERVING	185 Calories
	3 g Total Fat
	0 g Sat Fat
	0 g Trans Fat
	600 mg Sodium
	33 g CHO
	8 g Fibre
	7 g Protein
UEPC	1 Beans
	2 Fruit and Vegetables
	½ Fat

Revised
Jerk Black Beans

This is one of my favourites in the book for its flavour and ease of preparation. This is a mild version of jerk flavour, like a jerk flavour in training. If you want to turn up the heat, add another ¼ tsp (1 mL) cayenne. Remember, no emails on this: I did warn you.

2 tsp (10 mL) **extra virgin olive oil**
1½ tsp (7 mL) **thyme**
1 tsp (5 mL) **allspice**
¼ tsp (1 mL) **cinnamon**
¼ tsp (1 mL) **nutmeg**
¼ tsp (1 mL) **cayenne**
1 **bunch green onions, chopped into 2-inch (5-cm) pieces**
   (include the white part)
3 **cloves garlic, minced**
one 19-oz (540-mL) can **of black beans, drained and rinsed**
½ cup (125 mL) **water**

1 Heat a large frying pan over medium heat. Add the olive oil, thyme, allspice, cinnamon, nutmeg, and cayenne. Stir until the flavours hit you in the face. You'll know when that happens. It might be a good idea to turn on the stove's exhaust.

2 Add the chopped green onions and garlic. Stir until they're coated with the spice mixture.

3 Add the black beans and the water. Stir. Bring to a boil. Cover and reduce heat to simmer. Cook for 10 minutes. Serve with brown rice and steamed, baked, or micro-waved sweet potatoes.

Makes 3 cups (750 mL). Makes four ¾-cup (175-mL) servings.

KID FRIENDLY TIP
Don't add the cayenne until after you've dished out the kids' portions. Then go crazy on yours.

WHAT IS JERK?
Someone who says they'll call and never do. Oh, sorry, that's a jerk. From a foodie's standpoint Jerk is a Jamaican seasoning. The ingredients vary, depending on the cook, but are usually a blend of cinnamon, allspice, cloves, ginger, garlic, thyme, and cayenne. It can be anywhere from mild to extremely spicy. To a real Jamaican, this recipe is for wimps.

ONE SERVING	170 Calories
	4 g Total Fat
	0 g Sat Fat
	0 g Trans Fat
	210 mg Sodium
	25 g CHO
	10 g Fibre
	9 g Protein
UEPC	1 Beans
	½ Fat

Amazing Black Bean Quesadillas

WHERE DO I FIND SOFT WHOLE WHEAT TORTILLAS?
They're usually in the bakery department, but sometimes you can find them in the Mexican food section. My favourite brand in Canada is made by Dempster's. It contains 100% whole wheat and is trans fat free.

The Mexican theme, and teenagers love of it, just keeps popping up. Whether they like it because they think you're serving them fast food, or it's their version of international cuisine, the bottom line is: most kids love Mexican. I say, don't fight it. Go with the flow.

2 tsp (10 mL) **extra virgin olive oil**
1 **onion, diced**
1 **red pepper, diced**
2 **cloves garlic, minced**
½ tsp (2 mL) **cumin**
one 19-oz (540-mL) can **of black beans, drained and rinsed**
1 cup **salsa, mild, medium, or hot**
½ cup + 2 Tbsp (155 mL) **shredded light Monterey Jack cheese**
5 **large whole wheat soft tortillas, trans fat free**

1 Heat a large frying pan over medium heat. Add the oil, onion, and red pepper. Sauté for 3 minutes, or until the veggies are soft.

2 Add the cumin, black beans, and salsa. Stir well. When the beans are heated through, remove from the heat. (This can be made ahead of time and stored in the fridge for up to 3 days.)

3 Preheat the oven to 350°F (180°C). Put a baking sheet in the oven.

4 Heat a medium frying pan over medium heat. Place 1 tortilla in the pan. Spoon ¾ cup (175 mL) of the bean mixture on one half. Sprinkle with 2 Tbsp (30 mL) cheese. Fold the other half over the tortilla over the beans and press down gently with a spatula. Brown the underside and then very carefully flip it over to brown the other side.

5 When the tortilla is cooked, place it in the oven on the baking sheet. Cook remaining quesadillas.

6 When they're all cooked, cut each into 4 triangles. Serve with salsa and low-fat sour cream if desired.

Makes 4 cups (1 L). Makes five ¾-cup (175-mL) servings.

Kid Friendly

ONE SERVING	280 Calories
	6 g Total Fat
	2 g Sat Fat
	0 g Trans Fat
	495 mg Sodium
	45 g CHO
	9 g Fibre
	14 g Protein
UEPC	1 Beans
	1 Fruits & Vegetables
	2 Grains
	¼ Milk

Orange, Avocado, and Black Bean Salsa Salad

Menopause, or as I like to call it, 10 years of forgetting what I was saying right before I got to the good part (and not giving two hoots). Eating complex carbohydrates like those found in black beans, as well as chowing down on lots of fruits and veggies, is supposed to help you make it through the Big M unscathed. I figure even if you do forget why you made this salad, at least you'll still be eating something fabulous. A menopausal win/win situation.

4 **navel oranges**
one 19-oz (540-mL) can **of black beans, drained and rinsed**
½ cup (125 mL) **salsa, mild, medium, or hot**
1 **red pepper, chopped**
1 **small just-ripe avocado, chopped**
½ cup (125 mL) **minced cilantro**
½ cup (125 mL) **diced red onion**
2 Tbsp (30 mL) **fresh lime juice**

1   Cut the top and bottom off the orange. Place on a cutting board and slice off the peel and white stuff (called the pith for all you "Jeopardy" enthusiasts). Cut each orange into 12 pieces. Place in a medium-sized bowl.

2   Add the black beans, salsa, red pepper, avocado, cilantro, red onion, and lime juice. Gently toss. Store in the fridge until serving time. Tastes great for up to 3 days in the fridge.

Makes 6 cups (1.5 L). Makes six 1-cup (250-mL) servings.

I usually buy Haas or California avocados in my grocery store. Store any leftover avocado in the fridge. Cover it with the peel on and the pit intact. This will keep it from turning black. Use within 2 days.

WHAT THE HECK IS A JUST-RIPE AVOCADO?

It's dark green and has a slight give when it's pressed. It's best to buy an unripe avocado and let it ripen at home. They can take up to one week to ripen, so don't run out and buy a rock hard one if you need it in a recipe right away. The best idea is to make them a staple at your house. Liz's suggestions on page 24 are great ways to add them to a sandwich or on a bagel. Buy avocados that are firm and bright green. Bring them home and let them ripen on your counter until they turn a darker green, not black. Black avocados are overripe and squishy. Perfectly ripe avocados slice easily, keep their shape, and have a buttery flavour.

ONE SERVING	215 Calories
	4 g Total Fat
	1 g Sat Fat
	0 g Trans Fat
	360 mg Sodium
	31 g CHO
	7 g Fibre
	8 g Protein
UEPC	1 Beans
	1 Fruits & Vegetables
	1 Fat

New

Nutrition-Packed Curried Lentils with Spinach

SERVING TIP
Serve this with cooked sweet potatoes.

Curry gets its flavour from a blend of spices such as tamarind, coriander, ginger, garlic, chili, pepper, cinnamon, turmeric, cloves, cardamom, cumin, and nutmeg, just to name 12. I'm a big curry fan, especially for its turmeric content, which is one of Liz's all-star healthy spices. This recipe combines all those healthy spices with garlic, lentils, tomatoes, and enough spinach to kick this from super-star to mega-star. This recipe will wow your body and your taste buds all at once.

1 Tbsp + 1 tsp (20 mL) **extra virgin olive oil**
1 **onion, diced**
1 Tbsp (15 mL) **curry powder**
1 tsp (5 mL) **ground cumin**
1 tsp (5 mL) **ground coriander**
¼ tsp (2 mL) **turmeric**
one 19-oz (540-mL) **can lentils, drained and rinsed**
one 28-oz (796-mL) **can diced tomatoes**
4 **cloves garlic, minced**
4 cups (1 L) **baby spinach leaves**

1   Heat a medium saucepan over medium heat. Add the olive oil and onion. Sauté for 2 minutes. Add the curry powder, cumin, coriander, and turmeric. Mix well. Cook for 1 minute, stirring constantly.

2   Add the lentils and diced tomatoes. Stir until well combined.

3   Bring to a boil. Cover and reduce heat. Simmer for 15 minutes, stirring occasionally.

4   Remove lid and turn the heat to medium. Add the garlic and mix well. Add the spinach and stir until it wilts. Serve.

Makes 5 cups (1.25 L). Makes four 1¼-cup (310-mL) servings.

ONE SERVING	
	240 Calories
	5 g Total Fat
	0.5 g Sat Fat
	0 g Trans Fat
	300 mg Sodium
	36 g CHO
	15 g Fibre
	13 g Protein
UEPC	1 Beans
	2½ Fruits & Vegetables
	1 Fat

Hummus Peanut Butter Sandwich Filling

I was a vegetarian in my quasi-hippie period of the early 1970s, right up until I became pregnant in the late '80s. I never missed being a carnivore during those vegetarian days, but I did miss being able to grab a slice of meat and slapping it on a deli-style sandwich. This recipe is my vegetarian answer. No, it doesn't taste like red meat. Are you crazy? But it does give you a wonderful sandwich filling.

My number one combo is two slices of toasted 100% whole grain bread spread with ¼ cup (60 mL) of the filling, then topped with hot pickled peppers, a thin slice of red onion, slivers of sun-dried tomato, and a generous portion of finely chopped cilantro or spinach. Yummy. When's lunch? I'm starving.

1 cup (250 mL) **fresh cilantro**
one 19-oz (540-mL) can **chickpeas, drained and rinsed**
¾ cup (175 mL) **natural peanut butter, smooth or crunchy**
⅓ cup (75 mL) **fresh lemon juice**
2 Tbsp (30 mL) **water**
3 **cloves garlic, chopped**
1 tsp (5 mL) **paprika**
1 tsp (5 mL) **cumin**
pinch **cayenne**

1   Rinse the cilantro. Remove 1 cup (250 mL) of cilantro leaves. Set aside to drain. Store any remaining cilantro in the fridge wrapped in a paper towel.

2   Place the chickpeas, peanut butter, lemon juice, water, chopped garlic, paprika, cumin, and cayenne in a food processor. Pulse until combined. Purée until smooth.

3   Add the cilantro and pulse until combined. Purée until smooth. Yup, it turns sort of greenish, a very cool colour if you're a kid.

4   Store in the fridge for up to 4 days or freeze in ½ to 1 cup (125 to 250 mL) portions for up to 3 months. Thaw overnight in the fridge to make sandwiches the next day.

Makes 3 cups (750 mL). Makes twelve ¼-cup (60-mL) servings.

WHAT KIND OF PEANUT BUTTER DO I USE?

My Vancouver hippy roots are definitely showing when I tell you I use natural peanut butter. No sugar, no salt, just puréed peanuts. The downside is because the peanut butter is just peanuts the oil separates out and you need to stir it once you open the jar to incorporate the oil. I know, it's sort of a mess when you have to mix it together before you store it in the fridge, but for the best flavour, I'm a natural peanut butter kind of girl.

BIG COOKING TIP

The No Swearing Peanut Butter Mixing Method: Store an unopened jar of natural peanut butter upside down for at least 24 hours. Flip right side up, open the jar, and use a metal spatula or a fork to stir the mixture and incorporate the oil. This may take about five minutes. Do a few pliés at the same time—my idea of multitasking. When it has been mixed well, put the lid back on, and store it upright in the fridge to keep it combined.

ONE SERVING	160 Calories
	9 g Total Fat
	1 g Sat Fat
	0 g Trans Fat
	150 mg Sodium
	16 g CHO
	3 g Fibre
	6 g Protein
UEPC	½ Beans
	½ Nuts

Greek Salad with Chickpeas

TIP
English or hothouse cucumbers don't need to be peeled. They aren't waxed and are usually shrink-wrapped in plastic. Just give them a good wash and enjoy the tender peel and added fibre.

FRESH HERBS VS DRIED
Nothing beats the flavour of just picked herbs, and if you have a patch of summer sunshine, you can become an herb botanist. I have pots and pots of fresh herbs on my back deck. I love going to my mini garden in June through October (if I'm lucky and a killer frost hasn't yet hit), and snip fresh oregano, basil, parsley, mint, and thyme. Supermarkets carry fresh herbs all season, but they tend to be pricey in the middle of December. When the prices go up, switch to dried herbs. Substitute 1 tsp (5 mL) dried herbs for 1 Tbsp (15 mL) fresh. You can also try using frozen herbs (a Canadian brand is Toppits).

ONE SERVING	300 Calories
	9 g Total Fat
	2 g Sat Fat
	0 g Trans Fat
	530 mg Sodium
	45 g CHO
	18 g Fibre
	14 g Protein
UEPC	1 Beans
	2½ Fruits & Vegetables
	¾ Fat

The heart healthy Mediterranean diet is loaded with complex carbs, like those found in beans and whole grain pasta. It's also jam-packed with fruits, vegetables, fresh herbs, and olives or olive oil. Dig into this amazing version of a Greek salad and embrace the flavours of Greece. Opa!

1 **English cucumber**
¾ cup (175 mL) **diced red onion**
8 **kalamata olives, pitted and cut in half**
one 19-oz (540-mL) can **chickpeas, drained and rinsed**
2 oz (55 g) or ½ cup (125 mL) **light feta cheese, crumbled**
4 **ripe tomatoes**

Dressing
2 Tbsp (30 mL) **apple cider vinegar**
2 tsp (10 mL) **extra virgin olive oil**
2 **cloves garlic, crushed**
1 Tbsp (15 mL) **diced fresh oregano**
1 Tbsp (15 mL) **diced fresh basil**

1   Wash the cucumber and cut in half lengthwise. Quarter each half. Cut each quarter into ½-inch (1-cm) pieces. Place in a large bowl. Yes, you read that correctly. There's no peeling of the cucumber: the good stuff is in the peel.

2   Add the red onion, olives, chickpeas, and feta. Toss gently.

3   In a separate bowl, whisk together the apple cider vinegar, olive oil, garlic, oregano, and basil. Store the dressing in the fridge. When ready to serve, pour the dressing over the salad and toss gently.

4   Just before serving, wash the tomatoes and cut each tomato into 8 pieces. Gently toss into the salad. This will ensure they stay plump and juicy, not mushy and yucky.

Makes 6 cups (1.5 L). Makes four 1½-cup (375-mL) servings.

BIG COOKING TIP
Don't store tomatoes in the fridge. Cold temperatures interfere with the ripening process and ruin the flavour. Ripen them on the counter and eat as soon as they're ready.

Hummus with Roasted Red Peppers

There's been a real trend in hip chefs creating new hummus's by puréeing every bean known to man. Purist hummus followers know that only a chickpea ends up as a hummus. Everything else is just a bean dip.

one 19-oz (540-mL) can **chickpeas, drained and rinsed**
2 Tbsp (30 mL) **tahini**
2 Tbsp (30 mL) **fresh lemon juice**
2 **cloves garlic (more if you like), chopped**
3 Tbsp (45 mL) **water**
pinch **cayenne (more if you like)**
2 **whole roasted red peppers**

1   In a food processor or blender, purée all the ingredients except the red pepper. Purée until very smooth.

2   Add the red pepper and pulse until well combined. Cover and store in the fridge for up to 1 week.

Makes 2 cups (500 mL). Makes eight ¼-cup (60-mL) servings.

Kid Friendly

WHAT THE HECK IS TAHINI AND WHERE DO I FIND IT?
Tahini is sesame seed paste. You can find it in the ethnic section in your supermarket, or at any health food store. It will last up to 6 months in the fridge. Once you've made this recipe, though, it won't be kicking around the back of your fridge for long.

HOW DO I EAT HUMMUS?
I put hummus into a whole wheat pita and then stuff it with chopped tomato, fresh herbs, hot peppers, and lettuce. You can also serve it as a dip with raw veggies.

BIG COOKING TIP
If you're a wasabi lover, try adding 1 Tbsp (15 mL) wasabi to the recipe. It's a big rush.

ONE SERVING	120 Calories
	3 g Total Fat
	0 g Trans Fat
	180 mg Sodium
	20 g CHO
	4 g Fibre
	5 g Protein
UEPC	½ Beans
	¾ Fat
	½ Fruits & Vegetables

New

Amazing Artichoke and Chickpea Salad

BIG COOKING TIP
All bean salads taste better when they're cold. Store unopened cans of chickpeas and artichokes in the fridge so they're ready to assemble the minute you're ready to make them—sort of like having that prep sous chef guy in your fridge. Okay, not even close.

NUTRITION TIP
Artichokes are an antioxidant hero (see page 21). So make this amazing salad often.

Every time I see a TV cooking show I think how wonderfully easy my life would be if I had a live-in prep sous chef. I like to daydream that I'd roll in from the my extremely busy day and prep sous chef Hugo, and his rippling biceps, would have all the dinner ingredients ready in those cute little bowls. The ingredients just waiting for me to simply toss them about, and bingo, dinner is served. Now some of you are saying, "Forget the prep sous chef guy. I want the chef guy with a killer bod to cook the entire dinner."

Hey, get your own daydream. All I want is the hunky prep sous chef guy. I like the cooking part.

Okay, and maybe the cutie clean-up guy 'cause I really hate doing dishes.

Dressing
1 Tbsp + 1 tsp (20 mL) **extra virgin olive oil**
2 Tbsp (30 mL) **red wine vinegar**
3 **cloves garlic, minced**

Salad
one 14-oz (398-mL) can **artichoke quarters, drained and rinsed**
one 19-oz (540-mL) can **chickpeas, drained and rinsed**
1 **red pepper, diced**
1 cup (250 mL) **loosely packed parsley, minced**
2 **green onions, thinly sliced**
1 Tbsp (15 mL) **minced fresh basil**

1 Whisk together the dressing ingredients in a large bowl.

2 Chop the artichoke quarters into small pieces, about the size of a grape. Add to the bowl.

3 Add the chickpeas, red pepper, parsley, green onions, and basil. Toss until coated with the dressing.

4 Store in the fridge until ready to serve.

Makes 6 cups (1.5 L). Makes six 1-cup (250-mL) servings.

ONE SERVING	
	180 Calories
	4.5 g Total Fat
	0.5 g Sat Fat
	0 g Trans Fat
	280 mg Sodium
	31 g CHO
	8 g Fibre
	7 g Protein
UEPC	¾ Beans
	1 Fat
	1 Fruits & Vegetables

SALMON & SHRIMP

Fish Rules

RULE # 1

How the heck do I know whether or not a fish is fresh?

First of all, if it's smelly, don't buy it.

Remember the rule of thumb: fresh fish should smell like the ocean, clean and fresh. Not smelly and stale like a low tide. Another rule when buying fresh fish: the flesh should be firm to the touch. Ask the fish monger to poke the fish. Ask him nicely. Their finger shouldn't leave an impression in the flesh. If it does, tell him you forgot your keys in the car and walk away. When buying a whole fish, check to see that the eyes are bulging out and clear. Sunken and cloudy? Go with the lost keys story.

RULE # 2

If cooking salmon in the oven, use wet parchment paper to line a pan. Simply crumple up the desired amount under running water, squeeze out the excess water, and mold it into the pan. No big clean up and no added fat to boot.

RULE # 3

How do you know when fish is cooked?

When you prod it with a fork, the flesh should just start to flake or separate. Overcooked fish falls apart easily, and is very dry and chewy. Just done fish is tender, juicy, and melts in your mouth.

Rule of thumb: for each 1 inch (2.5 cm) of thickness, cook for 10 minutes at high heat.

RULE # 4

Why do all the recipes call for 13 oz (370 g) of salmon?

That nasty little thing called shrinkage.

RULE # 5

There are many different varieties of salmon, just like there are many different varieties of apples. A Granny Smith doesn't taste like a Red Delicious, just as wild Sockeye doesn't taste like farmed Atlantic. Explore the world of salmon varieties and enjoy within two days of purchasing.

RULE # 6

We used farmed Atlantic salmon in the nutrient breakdowns; if you decide on a wild variety you'll lower the total fat by 6 grams and drop the calories by an average of 36.

Baked Salmon with Fresh Citrus

How simple can a recipe get? Five ingredients, and a salmon fillet that's ready in 30 minutes or less. Yes, you can make dinner in less time than a pizza delivery.

one 13-oz (370-g) **salmon fillet**
1 **lime**
1 **lemon**
1 **orange**
3 Tbsp (45 mL) **honey**
1 Tbsp (15 mL) **minced fresh ginger**

1 Preheat the oven to 425°F (220°C). Line an 8-inch (20- × 20-cm) square pan with wet parchment paper, or spray with canola oil.

2 Zest the lime, lemon, and orange into one small bowl. Set aside.

3 Juice the lime, lemon, and orange. Mix the juices together. Add the honey and ginger.

4 Lay the salmon in the pan. Pour the citrus/honey/ginger mixture over top. Sprinkle with the zest. Don't be tempted to throw the zest into the juice; it won't have the same zip.

5 Bake for 15 to 20 minutes, or until just done. Remove salmon from the pan and cover. Pour the sauce into a saucepan. Bring to a boil and reduce by half.

6 Serve with brown rice. Spoon the citrus/honey mixture over the salmon and the rice.

Serves 4.

Kid Friendly

KID FRIENDLY TIP:
"WHAT'S THAT FUNNY LOOKING STUFF ON TOP OF THE FISH?"
If you think your child will be zest challenged, leave it off, or scrape it off just before serving.

BIG COOKING TIP
If you want to barbecue this recipe, try marinating it in the citrus/honey/ginger mixture for 15 minutes. Discard the marinade, then grill.

ONE SERVING	220 Calories
	10 g Total Fat
	2 g Sat Fat
	0 g Trans Fat
	55 mg Sodium
	15 g CHO
	0 g Fibre
	19 g Protein
UEPC	1 Fish

Company's Comin' Salmon

BIG COOKING TIP

If the parchment paper or tin foil won't keep its shape around the fish, lightly crinkle up a piece of parchment paper or tin foil into a ball and place it between the pouch and the side of the pan.

As I've mentioned before, the trick to really good salmon is really fresh salmon. It should smell clean like the ocean, without any hint of a fishy odour. If you walk into a fish store and the odour makes you want to faint, make sure the door doesn't hit you on the behind as you're leaving.

13 oz (370 g) **salmon fillet, skinned**

Poaching Liquid
½ cup (125 mL) **dry white wine**
¼ cup (60 mL) **frozen orange juice concentrate, thawed**
2 tsp (10 mL) **fresh lime juice**
2 Tbsp (30 mL) **diced shallots**
1 tsp (5 mL) **mixed peppercorns**

1   Preheat the oven to 425°F (220°C). Line an 8-inch (20- × 20-cm) square pan with wet parchment paper or tin foil.

2   Cut the salmon fillet into 4 equal pieces. Place the fillets in the pan, leaving ½ inch (1 cm) between the pieces.

3   In a small bowl, mix together the white wine, orange juice concentrate, lime juice, shallots, and peppercorns.

4   Pour the poaching liquid over top of the fillets. Pull up the sides of the parchment paper or foil to make sure the poaching liquid stays close to the salmon.

5   Bake for 15 to 20 minutes, or until just done.

Serves 4.

ONE SERVING	175 Calories
	10 g Total Fat
	2 g Sat Fat
	0 g Trans Fat
	55 mg Sodium
	2 g CHO
	0 g Fibre
	18 g Protein
UEPC	1 Fish

Garlic Lovers Lemon Shrimp

Garlic lovers will be shocked that all this garlic doesn't hit them over the head or kill them. It does have a definite garlic hit, but not as strong as you'd think 10 cloves would have. The good news is that you'll be safe from random vampire attacks for at least 13 days.

one 1-lb (454-g) bag **peeled, de-veined, thawed, and uncooked shrimp (about 31 to 40 shrimp)**
10 **cloves garlic, minced**
2 tsp (10 mL) **canola oil**
zest of 2 **lemons**
⅔ cup (150 mL) **fresh lemon juice**

1   Mix together the garlic and canola oil in a medium resealable plastic bag.

2   Add the shrimp and toss until coated. Refrigerate for 1½ hours.

3   Remove the shrimp from the refrigerator and add lemon zest and juice. Make sure the shrimp is coated with the marinade. Pop back into the fridge. Marinate up to 30 minutes.

4   Remove the shrimp from the bag and discard the marinade. Heat a medium frying pan over medium heat. Add 1 tsp (5 mL) canola oil and the shrimp. Stir fry until the shrimp are cooked. They'll turn a wonderful pink. Serve with lemon wedges.

Serves 4.

ONE SERVING	140 Calories
	3 g Total Fat
	0 Sat Fat
	0 g Trans Fat
	170 mg Sodium
	1 g CHO
	0 g Fibre
	23 g Protein
UEPC	1 Fish

New

Grilled Salmon with Raspberries

This is a fabulous way to get some omega-3 fatty acids, a hit of antioxidants, and feel like you just ate a treat. Salmon and raspberries are an awesome combo.

one 13-oz (370-g) **salmon fillet**

Marinade/Dressing
½ cup (125 mL) **Ribena blackcurrant concentrate (see page 146)**
½ cup (125 mL) **chopped fresh cilantro**
¼ cup (60 mL) **grainy Dijon mustard**
¼ cup (60 mL) **fresh lime juice**

1 **head dark green leaf lettuce**
4 cups (1 L) **frozen raspberries, thawed**

1 Whisk together the dressing/marinade. Reserve ½ cup (125 mL). Pour the remaining 1 cup (250 mL) into a resealable plastic bag. Add the salmon. Seal the bag and place it in the refrigerator. Marinate up to 30 minutes.

2 Wash and dry the lettuce. Set aside.

3 Preheat an indoor grill or outside barbecue. Remove the salmon from the plastic bag and discard the marinade. Grill the salmon on medium heat for 5 to 10 minutes, or until cooked through, turning once.

4 Mix together the reserved dressing with ½ of the thawed raspberries. Set aside.

5 Chop the lettuce and divide equally between 4 plates, about 1½ cups (375 mL) per plate.

6 Divide the cooked salmon into 4 equal pieces and place each piece on top of the lettuce. Spoon a quarter of the raspberry mixture over the salmon. Garnish with the extra raspberries. Serve to raves.

Serves 4.

Kid Friendly

HISTORY LESSON
The Fraser Valley in British Columbia grows more than 80% of Canada's red raspberries, making Clearbrook, BC, the Raspberry Capital of Canada. If you happen to be in Hopkins, Minnesota, in the beginning of July, you're in for a treat. America's Raspberry Capital celebrates raspberry season with the Hopkins Raspberry Festival. They have tent dances, loads of sporting events, a raspberry cooking contest, a gigantic arts & crafts fair, and a parade.

CAN I USE FRESH RASPBERRIES?
Sure, gently mash ½ of them, add to the dressing, and toss.

WHY CAN'T I MARINATE THE SALMON FOR LONGER THAN 30 MINUTES?
The acid from the lime juice will start to cook the protein in the fish. This process is called a seviche, but for this recipe we want the barbecue to cook the fish, not the lime juice.

ONE SERVING	270 Calories
	10 g Total Fat
	2 g Sat Fat
	0 g Trans Fat
	128 mg sodium
	24 g CHO
	9 g Fibre
	20 g Protein
UEPC	1 Fish
	2 Fruits & Vegetables

Poached Salmon with Mairlyn's World-Famous Lime Mayo

Most novice cooks overcook fish. The trick is to *just* cook it, and poaching is a sensational way to accomplish this culinary feat. The liquid should be slightly bubbling. You aren't boiling it. You're gently cooking those tender protein chains so they remain delicate and brimming with flavour.

2 cups (500 mL) **orange juice, fresh or from concentrate**
one 13-oz (370-g) **salmon fillet, cut into 4 equal pieces**

World-Famous Lime Mayo
2 Tbsp + 2 tsp (40 mL) **low-fat mayonnaise**
2 Tbsp (30 mL) **fresh lime juice**
zest of 1 **lime (optional)**

1   Unless you own a fish poacher, bring the orange juice to a boil in a covered frying pan.

2   When the juice begins to boil, add the salmon. The juice should just cover the fillets. Cover with lid.

3   Gently poach for 5 to 10 minutes.

4   While poaching, mix together the mayonnaise, lime juice, and lime zest (if using). Set aside.

5   When the salmon is cooked, use a slotted spoon to remove from the pan. Serve with the sauce.

Serves 4.

Kid Friendlly

**BIG COOKING TIP:
COLD POACHED SALMON**
Poach individual portions, preferably wrapped loosely in cheesecloth. Once cooked, carefully lift the salmon out of the poaching liquid onto a plate. Let it cool. Remove the cheesecloth. Cover and store in the refrigerator for up to 24 hours. At serving time, drizzle with my World-Famous Lime Mayo and garnish with slices of lime.

WORLD-FAMOUS SAUCE
I did a fair amount of catering back in the '70s and '80s, mostly for family and friends. I'd have tons of gorgeous foods out and always a salmon with my World-Famous Lime Mayo. Well, dollars to donuts, someone would always ask me for my sauce recipe after the event. I never gave it away, not because it was such a big secret, but because I didn't want anyone to know how simple it was.

ONE SERVING	210 Calories
	13 g Total Fat
	2.5 g Sat Fat
	0 g Trans Fat
	54 mg Sodium
	2 g CHO
	0 g Fibre
	19 g Protein
UEPC	½ Fat
	1 Fish

Classic Favourite
Really Great Salmon

KID FRIENDLY TIP: FILLET OR STEAK?

I always buy fillets. I find that without the hassle of bone excavation, my son will eat a fillet in a minute. Even though they're more money, you only need 3 oz (85 g) for 1 serving. And a fillet gets completely eaten. A salmon steak on the over hand, has a fair amount of waste. Then there's the care of checking for bones, and the whole skin thing. When Andrew was little he wouldn't even have the skin on his plate, let alone touching anything else—and he isn't a picky eater. So when I weigh out the pros and cons, I always end up buying the fillets.

SERVING TIP
Goes great with brown rice and steamed broccoli.

Every time I serve this, people say, "Hey, this is really great salmon." So I thought, what the heck, it may not be the most creative name for a recipe, but it's really great salmon.

one 13-oz (370-g) **salmon fillet**
2 Tbsp (30 mL) **low-sodium soy sauce**
1 tsp (5 mL) **Worcestershire sauce**
¼ tsp (1 mL) **dry mustard**
¼ tsp (1 mL) **fresh cracked black pepper**
1 **clove garlic, minced**

1 Preheat the oven to 425°F (220°C). Line an 8-inch (20- × 20-cm) square pan with wet parchment paper or spray with canola oil.

2 Place the salmon in the pan.

3 Mix together the soy sauce, Worcestershire, dry mustard, pepper, and minced garlic. Pour over the salmon fillet.

4 Bake for 15 to 20 minutes or until just done. Spoon the really great sauce that's in the pan over the salmon.

Serves 4.

ONE SERVING	180 Calories
	10 g Total Fat
	2 g Sat Fat
	0 g Trans Fat
	370 mg Sodium
	1 g CHO
	0 g Fibre
	19 g Protein
UEPC	1 Fish

Sensational Salmon with Mango Salsa

This recipe has become a classic among Ultimate Healthy Eating Plan fans. The salsa takes the grilled salmon to another level, which is chef-speak for "feel the love."

KID FRIENDLY TIP
Omit the salsa. Serve the fish with some slices of mango and red pepper on the side.

Salsa
1 **large ripe mango, diced**
½ **red pepper, diced**
2 Tbsp (30 mL) **fresh lime juice**
2 Tbsp (30 mL) **finely chopped fresh chives**
¼ tsp (1 mL) **red pepper flakes**

one 13-oz (370-g) salmon fillet

1   Mix together the mango, red pepper, lime juice, chives, and red pepper flakes in a bowl.

2   Cover and set aside in the refrigerator for up to 1 day in advance. You can leave it covered on the counter for up to 30 minutes.

3   Heat indoor grill or outdoor barbecue on high.

4   Cut the fillet into 4 equal pieces.

5   Place the salmon on the grill, reduce the heat to medium, and close the lid. Grill the salmon until just cooked. Avoid cooking the living daylights out of it. Most people don't like fish because they had a bad overcooked fillet experience at one time. In 5 to 10 minutes per side, the fish should start to flake easily.

6   Serve with the mango salsa on the top of each fillet.

Serves 4.

Kid Friendly

ONE SERVING	210 Calories
	10 g Total Fat
	2 g Sat Fat
	0 g Trans Fat
	55 mg Sodium
	11 g CHO
	1 g Fibre
	19 g Protein
UEPC	1 Fish
	½ Fruits & Vegetables

Classic Favourite

Terrific Salmon Teriyaki

This recipe is my West Coast specialty. I've always professed that most fish abstainers have just never eaten really fantastically fresh fish cooked to perfection. Case in point: I served this on a long weekend up at my friend Michale's cottage, and Susan, a long-time salmon slagger, had seconds. Another salmon miracle.

one 13-oz (370-g) **salmon fillet**
2 Tbsp (30 mL) **low-sodium soy sauce**
2 Tbsp (30 mL) **rice vinegar**
2 Tbsp (30 mL) **brown sugar**
2 tsp (10 mL) **minced fresh ginger**

1   Preheat the oven to 425°F (220°C). Line an 8-inch (20- × 20-cm) square pan with wet parchment paper or spray with canola oil.

2   Place the salmon in the pan.

3   Mix together the soy sauce, rice vinegar, brown sugar, and fresh ginger. Pour over the fish.

4   Bake for 15 to 20 minutes or until the fish is just done. Serve with brown rice and spoon the sauce over top.

Serves 4.

Kid Friendly

ONE SERVING	200 Calories
	10 g Total Fat
	2 g Sat Fat
	0 g Trans Fat
	360 mg Sodium
	7 g CHO
	0 g Fibre
	19 g Protein
UEPC	1 Fish

Spicy Salmon Cakes

My oldest and dearest friend Michale and her husband Lutz have a cottage in Muskoka. Most summer weekends you can find us on the dock discussing the ins and outs of child rearing, the annoying habits of our loved ones, how perfect we are, what we're going to eat next, and what the best ever martini recipe is—not necessarily in that order (see page 275 for the best martini recipe!). I'd been working on this salmon cake recipe for a while, and it was ready for an official taste test. I was making eight different dishes that night at the cottage, so Michale suggested we make the salmon cakes appetizer size. We did, and they were most excellent. I like them best as a main course, but they're also great as an appetizer.

1½ cups (375 mL) **Post Cereal Spoon Size Shredded Wheat
   + Bran**
two 7.5-oz (213-g) cans **sockeye salmon, well drained**
2 Tbsp (30 mL) **low-fat mayonnaise**
2 Tbsp (30 mL) **low-fat plain probiotic yogurt**
1 Tbsp (15 mL) **Dijon mustard**
½ tsp (2 mL) **Worcestershire sauce**
2 tsp (10 mL) **garlic chili sauce**
½ **medium onion, minced**
½ **red pepper, minced**
¼ cup (60 mL) **finely chopped fresh cilantro**
1 Tbsp (15 mL) **fresh lime juice**

ONE SERVING	280 Calories
	13 g Total Fat
	2 g Sat Fat
	0 g Trans Fat
	265 mg Sodium
	20 g CHO
	3 g Fibre
	21 g Protein
UEPC	½ Fat
	1 Fish
	½ Grains

1   Preheat the oven to 425°F (220°C).

2   In a food processor, pulse the cereal until fine. Measure out ½ cup (125 mL) and set aside to use for the coating.

3   Put the salmon (bones and all) into the food processor and pulse several times.

4   Add the mayonnaise, yogurt, Worcestershire, garlic chili sauce, onion, and red pepper. Pulse until well combined.

5   Add the cilantro and lime juice and pulse until combined.

6   Using a ¼ cup (60 mL) ice cream scoop with a release button, scoop out 8 salmon scoops and place into the reserved crumbs.

7   Press the salmon gently into the crumbs and make sure both sides are well coated. Flatten to ¾ inch (2 cm) thickness.

8   Place them on a cookie sheet lined with parchment paper. Bake for 20 minutes. Serve.

Makes eight 3-inch (8-cm) cakes. Makes four 2-cake servings.

The Ultimate Salmon Sandwich Filling

My mom packed me salmon sandwiches every time I stayed at school for lunch. I'd open my Barbie lunchbox and no one would say, "What the heck did your mom pack you?" Their moms had packed them the same thing. When I moved to Ontario many years ago and packed my salmon sandwiches for work, I got so many comments I was almost tempted to stop bringing them. But then I thought, "Who cares what people think. I love these sandwiches." Moral of the story: Don't let people ruin your lunch. If it's heart healthy and you love it, pack it and enjoy.

one 7.5-oz (213-g) can **Sockeye salmon**
¼ cup (60 mL) **diced celery (about 1 stalk)**
¼ cup (60 mL) **sweet green pickle relish**
3 Tbsp (45 mL) **minced red onion**
1 Tbsp (15 mL) **low-fat mayonnaise**
**Adult Version: add ⅛–¼ tsp (1 mL) wasabi paste for every
⅓ cup (75 mL) filling**

1   Drain the salmon well. Transfer to a medium bowl. Gently mash salmon, including the skin and bones. Yes, mash it all up. Make sure the bones are well mashed— most people don't like crunchy salmon.

2   Gently mix in the celery, relish, red onion, and mayonnaise. Mix until well combined.

3   If you're adding wasabi, measure out the correct amount and mix it in well.

4   Measure out ⅓ cup (75 mL) per sandwich and start building your sandwich. See page 237.

Makes 1⅓ cups (325 mL). Makes four ⅓-cup (75-mL) servings.

Kid Friendly

ONE SERVING	300 Calories
	7 g Total Fat
	1.5 g Sat Fat
	0 g Trans Fat
	240 mg Sodium
	56 g CHO
	2 g Fibre
	10 g Protein
UEPC	½ Fish

Build Your Own Sandwich

PACKING A SANDWICH FOR SCHOOL OR THE OFFICE?
To cut down on added fat, line both halves of the bread or bun with lettuce, spinach, or a green of your choice rather than a lining of non-hydrogenated margarine. Cover the greens with the salmon filling and any other add-ons. Top with the other half of the bread or bun. Wrap tightly and pack next to something cold. I freeze a Tetra Pak of either 100% juice or milk the night before. The frozen drink, which doesn't explode because it's in a Tetra Pak, keeps the lunch cold and will be thawed for the ride home from school or work.

WHERE THE HECK DO I BUY WASABI PASTE?
Most grocery stores carry the increasingly popular wasabi paste in the Asian section, or in a bunker with the sushi ingredients. Once opened, store it in the refrigerator for up to 6 months.

Bread
100% whole wheat or whole grain bread
100% whole wheat English muffin
100% whole wheat tortilla
100% whole wheat hamburger bun
100% whole wheat pita

Veggies
Sun-dried tomatoes
Sliced tomato
Spinach
Diced herbs—basil, cilantro, dill, or parsley are all great
Sliced pickles
Sliced avocado
Romaine lettuce, shredded

My Favourite Combo

I add wasabi paste to The Ultimate Salmon Sandwich Filling, then put it in a toasted whole wheat English muffin. I add just one skinny slice of avocado, chopped spinach, diced cilantro, and a sliced pickle. It's amazing.

Totally Kid Friendly Salmon Cakes

You've read Liz's chapter on fish and now you're panicking trying to find a recipe your picky kids will even look at. Read no further. This is the one. Not as adventurous as the Spicy Salmon Cakes, these are definitely kid friendly.

1½ cups (375 mL) **Post Cereal Spoon Size Shredded Wheat + Bran**
two 7.5-oz (213-g) cans **Sockeye salmon, well drained**
1 **small onion, quartered**
2 **cloves garlic**
2 Tbsp (30 mL) **sweet green pickle relish**
2 Tbsp (30 mL) **low-fat creamy caesar salad dressing**

1   Preheat the oven to 425°F (220°C).

2   In a food processor, pulse the cereal until fine. Measure out ½ cup (125 mL) and set aside to use as the coating.

3   Add the onion and garlic into the food processor and pulse until chunky.

4   Add the salmon (bones and all) and pulse several times. Add the pickle relish and caesar salad dressing. Pulse until well combined.

5   Using a ¼-cup (60-mL) ice cream scoop with a release button, scoop out 8 salmon scoops and place into the reserved crumbs.

6   Press the salmon gently into the crumbs, making sure both sides are well coated. Flatten balls to ¾ inch (2 cm) thickness.

7   Place on a cookie sheet lined with parchment paper. Bake for 20 minutes. Serve.

Makes eight 3-inch (8-cm) cakes. Makes four 2-cake servings.

Kid Friendly

ONE SERVING	275 Calories
	13 g Total Fat
	2.5 g Sat Fat
	0 g Trans Fat
	290 mg Sodium
	18 g CHO
	3 g Fibre
	20 g Protein
UEPC	½ Fat
	½ Grains
	1 Fish

Classic Favourite

Wasabi Salmon

WHAT THE HECK IS WASABI?

Wasabi is a green horseradish that's used in Japanese cooking, especially in sushi. It has a very hot effect, different from regular spicy food. Wasabi goes right up to the top of your head, clearing your sinuses on its way. It's very distinctive, and once you've tried it, you're either hooked, or not. Personally, I'm hooked.

SERVING TIP

Serve with short-grain brown rice and cooked sweet potato.

WHY SHORT-GRAIN BROWN RICE?

Short-grain gives you stickier rice than long-grain and is more like traditional sticky Japanese rice.

I'd always thought that a wasabi salmon dish would be terrific. I could imagine the flavours in my head. The first time I made it, you couldn't even taste the wasabi. My friend Michale thought that reserving some of the wasabi sauce to drizzle over the fish would do the trick. For once, I went along with her, and you know, she was right. Write it in the record books: I was wrong. Again. Reserve some for the final drizzle.

one 13-oz (370-g) **salmon fillet**
1 Tbsp (15 mL) **dark brown sugar**
2 tsp (10 mL) **wasabi paste**
2 tsp (10 mL) **low-sodium soy sauce**
2 tsp (10 mL) **rice vinegar**
2 tsp (10 mL) **minced fresh ginger**

1 Preheat the oven to 425°F (220°C). Line an 8-inch (20- × 20-cm) square pan with wet parchment paper or spray with canola oil.

2 Place salmon in the pan.

3 In a small bowl, mix together the brown sugar, wasabi paste, soy sauce, rice vinegar, and ginger.

4 Reserve 2 tsp (10 mL) of this sauce and pour the remaining sauce over the fish.

5 Bake the fish for 15 to 20 minutes or until just done.

6 Once cooked, pour the reserved wasabi sauce over the fish.

Serves 4.

ONE SERVING	185 Calories
	10 g Total Fat
	2 g Sat Fat
	0 g Trans Fat
	160 mg sodium
	4 g CHO
	0 g Fibre
	19 g Protein
UEPC	1 Fish

West Coast Salmon Chowder

I love soups and chowders. Not only are they a complete meal in a bowl, but you eat all the nutrients in the broth. Add a 100% whole wheat bun, and you have all the food groups present and accounted for. Who says eating well has to be hard when you can make a meal like this in 30 minutes?

3 cups (750 mL) **lower-sodium chicken broth**
1 **medium onion, diced**
3 **cloves garlic, minced**
3 **large carrots, chopped**
2 **stalks celery, chopped**
1 **red pepper, chopped**
1 **small potato, diced (peel on)**
1 cup (250 mL) **corn kernels, fresh, cooked or frozen**
13 oz (370 g) **salmon fillet**
1 cup (250 mL) **fat-free evaporated milk**

1   In a large pot with a tight fitting lid, add the chicken broth, onion, garlic, and carrots. Bring to a boil.

2   Add the celery, red pepper, potato, and corn. Stir well.

3   Bring back to a boil and reduce the heat to simmer. Cover and simmer for 10 minutes, or until the veggies are cooked.

4   Cut the salmon into 1-inch (2.5-cm) cubes. Add the salmon and simmer covered for 5 minutes or until the salmon is just cooked.

5   Add the fat-free evaporated milk. Stir until combined. Add pepper to taste. Serve.

Makes 8 Cups. Makes four 2-cup (500-mL) servings.

Kid Friendly

QUICK TIP

The next time salmon is on sale, buy an extra 13-oz (370-g) fillet. Cut it into 1-inch (2.5-cm) cubes and freeze in a freezer bag. Making the chowder for dinner? Take the bag out of the freezer and drop it into a sink full of cold water; it will be thawed in about 20 minutes. Or take the frozen salmon cubes out of the bag, microwave to defrost, and add to the pot.

ONE SERVING	340 Calories
	11 g Total Fat
	2.5 g Sat Fat
	0 g Trans Fat
	400 mg Sodium
	36 g CHO
	5 g Fibre
	29 g Protein

UEPC	1 Fish
	3 Fruits & Vegetables
	½ Milk

POULTRY

Poultry Rules

All raw meat needs to be handled carefully, or you could be running to the loo for a couple of days—or worse. Food-borne illnesses are preventable if you follow some simple rules.

RULE # 1

Always wash your hands before handling food, especially raw meat, beef, pork, or poultry.

RULE # 2

Don't wash raw chicken. The water will splatter all over the sink, faucets, etc. If desired, pat the meat dry with a paper towel. Just make sure to discard the paper towel immediately.

RULE # 3

Store raw poultry in the refrigerator for up to three days, or until the day on the "best before" label.

RULE # 4

Thaw frozen chicken pieces in the refrigerator for 10 hours per kilogram (5 hours per pound).

RULE # 5

Rapid method: thaw poultry in a sink full of cold water. Two hours per kilogram (one hour per pound). Change the water frequently. Once the chicken is thawed, remove it from sink, wash the sink with a mild bleach solution (mild bleach solution formula: 1 tsp/5 mL of bleach to every 3 cups/750 mL of water).

RULE # 6

Use a special cutting board that you use exclusively for raw meat. Wash the used board with the mild bleach solution listed above, rinse with clean water, and let it air dry.

RULE # 7

Wash the counters, faucets, and all other surfaces that may have come in contact with the raw meat with the mild bleach solution.

RULE # 8

The best way to know if your chicken is cooked is by testing the internal temperature. A meat thermometer should read 165°F (74°C) on a skinless, boneless breast or thigh.

RULE # 9

Don't forget to sanitize the thermometer after each use.

Chicken with Dried Cranberries and Orange

In the poultry world, nothing is worse than dried out, rubbery chicken. Follow the cooking instructions below and your chicken should end up tender and moist every time you make this recipe. It's all about having the proper technique and equipment, something any carpenter knows.

14 oz (400 g) **skinless boneless chicken breasts, cut into
   4 equal pieces**

Sauce
2 Tbsp (30 mL) **orange marmalade**
2 Tbsp (30 mL) **hot pepper jelly**
2 Tbsp (30 mL) **frozen orange juice concentrate, thawed**
1 Tbsp (15 mL) **balsamic vinegar**
½ cup (125 mL) **dried cranberries**
¼ tsp (1 mL) **hot pepper flakes**

1 Preheat the oven to 450°F (230°C). Line an 8-inch (2-L) square metal baking pan with wet parchment paper (see page 260) or spray with canola oil. Lay the chicken on top.

2 In a medium bowl, mix together the marmalade, hot pepper jelly, orange juice concentrate, and balsamic vinegar.

3 Stir in the dried cranberries. Pour the sauce over the chicken. Sprinkle with hot pepper flakes.

4 Bake for 20 to 25 minutes, or until the chicken has reached an internal temperature of 165°F (74°C)

5 Pour the liquid into a frying pan. Leave the chicken in the baking pan on top of the stove and cover. Bring the liquid to a boil and leave it to reduce for about 5 minutes, or until slightly thickened. Pour it over the chicken. Serve.

Serves 4.

ONE SERVING	250 Calories
	2 g Total Fat
	0.5 g Sat Fat
	0 g Trans Fat
	65 mg Sodium
	28 g CHO
	1 g Fibre
	28 g Protein
UEPC	1 Meat
	½ Fruits & Vegetables

New

Chicken with Lime, Garlic, and Cashews

Today's average skinless, boneless chicken breast is 7 oz (200 g), which means that for this particular recipe one little 'ole chicken breast is going to serve four people. What? Yes, you read that correctly: four people. The cashews you're going to add are a meat alternative. If you want more chicken and no cashews, feel free to add one more chicken breast.

one 7-oz (200-g) **skinless, boneless chicken breast**

Marinade
4 **cloves garlic, minced**
2 Tbsp (30 mL) **low-sodium soy sauce**
2 Tbsp (30 mL) **garlic chili sauce**
2 tsp (10 mL) **canola oil**
2 tsp (10 mL) **fresh lime juice**

Stir-Fry
2 **large red peppers, thinly sliced**
1 cup (250 mL) **snap or snow peas**
6 **green onions, chopped into 4-inch (10-cm) pieces**
¼ cup (60 mL) **unsalted cashews, chopped coarsely**

1   Slice the chicken into ¼-inch (5-mm) slices. If this is hard to do, place the chicken in the freezer for 20 minutes to firm for easier slicing.

2   In a resealable plastic bag, mix together the garlic, soy sauce, chili sauce, 1 tsp (5 mL) of the canola oil, and lime juice. Add the sliced chicken. Marinate in the refrigerator from 20 minutes to 12 hours.

3   When the chicken is marinated, heat a medium-sized frying pan over medium heat. Add 1 tsp (5 mL) canola oil and the red peppers. Sauté for 1 minute. Remove the peppers from the pan and set aside on a plate.

4   Remove the chicken from the marinade and add to the frying pan. Discard marinade. Stir-fry the chicken for 4 minutes. Return the red peppers to the pan and continue cooking for 1 minute. Add the green onion and cook for 2 minutes. Sprinkle with cashews and stir-fry for 1 minute. Serve.

Serves 4.

**BIG COOKING TIP:
FREEZER METHOD**
You can freeze the chicken while it's marinating, just follow steps 1 and 2, then pop the chicken in its resealable bag into the freezer for up to 2 months. The night before you're ready to use, remove from the freezer and thaw in the refrigerator. It will be thawed and marinated by the time you cook it the next evening.

TIP
If you're garlic challenged reduce the garlic to 2 cloves.

ONE SERVING	175 Calories
	5 g Total Fat
	1 g Sat Fat
	0 g Trans Fat
	102 mg Sodium
	15 g CHO
	4 g Fibre
	18 g Protein
UEPC	¼ Fat
	½ Meat
	2 Fruits & Vegetables
	½ Nut

Chicken with Mango and Apricots

WHAT THE HECK IS FROZEN ORANGE JUICE CONCENTRATE AND WHERE DO I FIND IT?

It's the frozen juice that you find in the frozen juice aisle. You knew that.

WHAT THE HECK DOES A REALLY RIPE MANGO LOOK LIKE?

Mangoes are in season from May to September. Look for heavy ones that have a golden yellow skin with red mottling. This will be a deliciously ripe mango loaded with flavour and nutrition. Keep a ripe mango in the refrigerator for up to 4 days. To ripen a green mango, store it in a paper bag on the counter until the skin turns that golden yellow colour.

SERVING TIP

Tastes great with Quinoa 101 on page 189.

ONE SERVING	300 Calories
	2 g Total Fat
	0.5 Sat Fat
	0 g Trans Fat
	300 mg Sodium
	38 g CHO
	3 g Fibre
	30 g Protein
UEPC	1 Fruits & Vegetables
	1 Meat

This is my co-author's all time favourite recipe in the book. She makes this at least twice a month. It's a winner—easy, quick, delicious, and Liz approved.

14 oz (400 g) **boneless skinless chicken breasts, cut into 4 equal pieces**

Sauce
one 14-oz (398-mL) **can apricots in light syrup**
3 Tbsp (45 mL) **frozen orange juice concentrate, thawed**
⅓ cup (75 mL) **mango chutney**
1 Tbsp (15 mL) **low-sodium soy sauce**
1 **large, really ripe mango**

1   Preheat the oven to 425°F (220°C). Line an 8-inch square (2-L) metal baking pan with wet parchment paper (see page 260) or spray with canola oil. Lay the chicken in the pan.

2   Drain the apricots. Reserve ⅓ cup (75 mL) of the liquid. Set the apricots aside.

3   Mix the reserved liquid with the orange juice concentrate, mango chutney, and soy sauce. Pour over the chicken.

4   Bake for 20 to 25 minutes, or until the chicken reaches an internal temperature of 165°F (74°C).

5   While it's cooking, cut and peel the mango. Cut it into 1-inch (2-cm) slices. Set aside.

6   When the chicken is cooked, remove from the oven and pour the liquid into a frying pan. Leave the chicken in the baking pan on top of the stove and cover. Turn the heat onto high and add the apricots and mango to the frying pan. Bring to a boil and leave it to reduce for about 5 minutes, or until slightly thickened. Pour the sauce over the chicken. Serve.

Serves 4.

Kid Friendly

CAN'T FIND CANNED APRICOTS?

Use fresh or dried ones and add ⅓ cup (75 mL) apricot nectar, which you can find in the juice aisle. Most brands of apricot nectar are sold in Tetra Paks and are usually found with the drink boxes.

Polynesian-Style Slow Cooker Chicken

My church has an annual dinner theatre to raise money for our much depleted coffers. *Murder at the Family Reunion*, the 2006 show, was set in a Tiki Bar, and I crazily volunteered to create a menu to feed the masses. Note: If you ever get the opportunity to cook for 92 people, think long and hard and make sure you'll be working alongside fun, calm people. My partner in the kitchen, Judi, was all that and more. We had a blast, a few mini breakdowns, and many great laughs. Moral of the story: volunteering is very good for the soul.

¼ cup (60 mL) **whole wheat flour**

1 tsp (5 mL) **paprika**

1 tsp (5 mL) **curry powder**

8 **skinless boneless chicken thighs**

1 **medium onion, diced**

¼ tsp (1 mL) **black pepper**

3 Tbsp (45 mL) **low-sodium soy sauce (see sidebar)**

1 Tbsp (15 mL) **dark brown sugar**

one 19-oz (540-mL) **can pineapple chunks in pineapple juice**

2 **large red peppers, sliced into thin strips (culinary term: julienne)**

1   In a plastic bag, mix together the flour, paprika, and curry powder. Place the chicken in the bag, close it, and then give it a good shake.

2   Dump or, as they say in culinary terms, gently place the chicken and any of the remaining flour into the slow cooker.

3   Sprinkle with the onion and pepper.

4   Mix together the soy sauce and brown sugar. Pour over chicken. Pour the can of pineapple and its juices over top.

5   Place the lid on the slow cooker and cook on low for 4 to 5 hours, or until the chicken is cooked.

6   Remove the lid and add peppers. Replace the lid and continue cooking for 30 to 45 minutes, or until peppers are soft.

Serves 4.

Kid and Church Dinner Friendly

LOW-SODIUM OR LIGHT SOY SAUCE

Using low-sodium or light soy sauce is a great way to reduce your sodium intake. I use Kikkoman because it's made with real soybeans, has no artificial flavours, and tastes fantastic.

SERVING TIP

Goes great with short-grain brown rice.

BIG COOKING TIP

If you decide to double this recipe, add 1 to 3 more hours of cooking time. Serve half the recipe (four servings) on day one. Two days later, reheat the leftovers in a medium pot over medium heat, add 2 cups (500 mL) cooked brown rice and 2 cups (500 mL) frozen peas. Heat through. Add one 14-oz (385-mL) can of fat-free evaporated milk. Stir well and voila! Polynesian Chicken Chowder. Serves 4.

ONE SERVING	300 Calories
	6 g Total Fat
	1.5 g Sat Fat
	0 g Trans Fat
	590 mg Sodium
	37 g CHO
	4 g Fibre
	25 g Protein
UEPC	1 Meat
	2 Fruits & Vegetables

New

Grilled Herb Chicken

BIG COOKING TIP
Use dried herbs if you're going to make this recipe for the Freezer Method (page 244). The fresh herbs will discolour and get a tad slimy when frozen.

Insanely easy and absolutely delicious. Create a different flavour every time you make it by mixing up the fresh herbs. Try using one herb, or a combo of basil, oregano, and rosemary. My son's friend, Andrew D, a confessed picky eater, loves this—in itself a ringing endorsement.

14 oz (400 g) **skinless, boneless chicken breasts or thighs**

Marinade
1 Tbsp (15 mL) **canola oil**
⅓ cup (75 mL) **fresh lemon juice**
2 **cloves garlic, minced**
¼ cup (60 mL) **diced fresh herbs (I use a combo of basil, oregano, and rosemary)**

1   Place all the marinade ingredients in a resealable plastic bag. Add the chicken and marinate in the refrigerator from 1 to 12 hours.

2   Preheat the indoor grill or outdoor barbecue on high.

3   Remove the chicken from the refrigerator and let it sit for 15 minutes.

4   Remove the chicken from the marinade and place on the hot grill. If using a barbecue, close the lid and reduce the heat to medium. Discard marinade.

5   Cook chicken on direct medium heat until it's no longer pink inside, or until the internal temperature reaches 165°F (74°C), about 6 to 12 minutes per side, depending on the thickness of the chicken.

6   Remove from the grill and place on a clean plate. Let it sit covered for 5 minutes.

7   Divide the chicken evenly between four plates. Goes great with new potatoes and the Grilled Veggie Salad on page 168.

Serves 4.

Kid Friendly

ONE SERVING	150 Calories
	2.6 g Total Fat
	0.5 g Sat Fat
	0 g Trans Fat
	65 mg Sodium
	0 g CHO
	0 g Fibre
	28 g Protein
UEPC	1 Meat

Honey Mustard Chicken Your Honey Will Love

I like to marinate chicken overnight. While I whip up dinner the night before, I multitask and mix up the marinade in a resealable plastic bag, drop in the chicken, and pop the whole thing in the refrigerator until the next evening. If you want to make a quick dinner the next day, it's all about mixin', droppin', and poppin'.

14 oz (400 g) skinless, boneless chicken breasts

Marinade
2 Tbsp (30 mL) **Dijon mustard**
2 Tbsp (30 mL) **honey**
2 Tbsp (30 mL) **fresh lime juice**
1 tsp (5 mL) **canola oil**

1   Mix all the marinade ingredients in a medium resealable plastic bag.

2   Drop in the chicken and let it marinate in the refrigerator for 12 to 24 hours. You can freeze it for up to 2 months. Just thaw it in the refrigerator the night before.

3   Take the chicken out of the refrigerator 15 minutes before grilling.

4   Preheat indoor grill or outdoor barbecue on high.

5   Remove the chicken from the marinade and place on the hot grill. If using a barbecue, close the lid and reduce the heat to medium. Discard marinade.

6   Cook the chicken on direct medium heat until it's no longer pink inside, or until the internal temperature reaches 165°F (74°C), about 6 to 12 minutes per side, depending on the size of the chicken.

7   Remove the chicken from the grill and place it on a clean plate. Let sit covered for 5 minutes, then transfer to 4 plates and serve.

Serves 4.

Kid Friendly

ONE SERVING	150 Calories
	2 g Total Fat
	0.5 g Sat Fat
	0 g Trans Fat
	81 mg Sodium
	1 g CHO
	0 g Fibre
	28 g Protein
UEPC	1 Meat

New

Tex Mex Turkey Skillet Dinner

FYI
I got the original idea for this recipe off butterball.ca.

You cooked a 28-lb (13-kg) turkey and now have enough leftovers to feed 47 of your closest friends. Aside from the usual turkey sandwiches, turkey pot pies, and turkey surprises, you could whip up this amazing dinner in about 20 minutes to raves, or you could freeze those leftovers and make it three weeks later to cheers. Your pick. Just remember, if you want applause from your family, make this dinner. You'll be buying turkeys all the time for the leftovers and the cheers.

1 Tbsp (15 mL) **canola oil**
1 **medium onion, diced**
2 cups (500 mL) **frozen whole kernel corn, thawed (see page 183)**
2 cups (500 mL) **chopped cooked turkey**
1 cup (250 mL) **salsa, mild, medium, or hot**
8 cups (2 L) **baby spinach leaves**

1   Heat a large skillet over medium heat. Add the oil and onion and sauté for 2 minutes.

2   Add the corn, turkey, and salsa. Heat about 5 minutes or until it bubbles.

3   Add the spinach and stir until wilted. Serve.

Makes 6 cups (1.5 L). Makes four 1½-cup (375-mL) servings.

Kid Friendly

ONE SERVING	
	270 Calories
	8 g Total Fat
	1 g Sat Fat
	0 g Trans Fat
	420 mg Sodium
	33 g CHO
	5 g Fibre
	21 g Protein

UEPC	
	¾ Fat
	3½ Fruits & Vegetables
	1 Meat

BEEF & PORK

Beef Bourguignonne

BIG COOKING TIP

If you're a rosemary lover, mince the fresh rosemary and add it to the stew when you add the other herbs. Adding the sprig and then removing it is for the non-rosemary lovers in the crowd.

WHAT THE HECK IS A DUTCH OVEN?

It's a large pot with a lid that can be used either in the oven or on top of the stove.

There's something homey about the fall and making a big pot of hearty stew. For me, stew is a comfort food that evokes memories of my mom and Sunday night dinner, her regular oven fire, and my dad running around with the fire extinguisher.

2 lb (1 kg) **lean stewing beef**
2 **medium onions, chopped into quarters**
3 cups **chopped carrots (approx 6)**
2 cups (500 mL) **cubed rutabaga 1 × 2 inch (2.5 × 5 cm)**
4 **cloves garlic, minced**
1 tsp (5 mL) **thyme**
1 tsp (5 mL) **summer savory**
½ tsp (2 mL) **cracked pepper**
½ tsp (2 mL) **tarragon leaves**
¼ cup (50 mL) **whole wheat flour**
one 10-oz (284-mL) can **lower-sodium beef broth, undiluted**
1 cup (250 mL) **crushed canned tomatoes**
1 cup (250 mL) **red wine, Merlot or Burgundy**
½ cup (125 mL) **water**
1 Tbsp (15 mL) **Worcestershire sauce**
2 **sprigs fresh rosemary (see sidebar)**

1 Preheat the oven to 350°F (180°C).

2 Place the beef, onions, carrots, rutabaga, and garlic in a large Dutch oven.

3 Sprinkle with thyme, summer savory, pepper, tarragon, summer savory, and flour. Toss to coat.

4 Add the beef broth, crushed tomatoes, red wine, and Worcestershire sauce. Stir. Place rosemary sprigs on top.

5 Cover and cook for 2½ to 3 hours. You don't even need to stir this while it's cooking (what a recipe!). Remove from the oven. Remove rosemary, stir, let sit for 15 minutes, and serve. Store leftovers in the fridge for up to 3 days.

Makes 8 cups (2 L). Makes eight 1-cup (250-mL) servings.

Kid Friendly

ONE SERVING	
	280 Calories
	8 g Total Fat
	3 g Sat Fat
	0 g Trans Fat
	230 g Sodium
	19 g CHO
	4 g Fibre
	28 g Protein
UEPC	1 Meat
	2 Vegetables and Fruit

Garlic Pork with Stir-Fried Peppers

Google "garlic" and you'll get 44,300,000 hits in 0.35 seconds for the lovely stinking rose. With over 400 varieties, make sure the bulb you choose is perfect. It should be dry, with plenty of paper covering. If you see any green shoots, the garlic is either old, or wasn't dried properly.

According to folklore, garlic was used for everything from a mosquito repellent to a cure for the Plague. You win some, you lose some. Aside from its amazing addition to most savory dishes, it also reduces the formation of carcinogens when cooking at a high heat. Yup, good things really do come in small packages.

1 lb (500 g) **pork tenderloin**

Marinade
3 **garlic cloves, minced**
2 Tbsp (30 mL) **low-sodium soy sauce**
1 tsp (5 mL) **honey**
½ tsp (2 mL) **cracked black pepper**

Sauce
½ cup (125 mL) **lower-sodium chicken broth**
¼ cup (60 mL) **low-sodium soy sauce**
4 **cloves garlic, minced**
2 tsp (10 mL) **rice vinegar**
½ tsp (2 mL) **red pepper flakes**
½ tsp (2 mL) **honey**
1 Tbsp (15 mL) **cornstarch**

Stir-fry
2 tsp (10 mL) **canola oil**
2 **red peppers, julienned (sliced into thin strips)**
2 **green onions, finely chopped**

ONE SERVING	230 Calories
	4.5 Total Fat
	1.5 Sat Fat
	0 g Trans
	680 mg Sodium
	12 g CHO
	2 g Fibre
	29 g Protein
UEPC	1 Meat
	1 Fruits & Vegetables
	¼ Fat

BIG COOKING TIP
Having trouble slicing the pork
tenderloin into ⅛-inch (3-mm)
slices? Semi-frozen pork is
easier to slice. Place pork in
the freezer for 15 minutes and
then slice.

1 Slice the pork tenderloin thinly, about ⅛ inch (3 mm)
   thick.

2 In a medium bowl, whisk together the garlic, soy sauce,
   honey, and pepper. Add the pork and marinate for 15 to
   20 minutes.

3 In a medium bowl, whisk together the chicken broth,
   soy sauce, minced garlic, rice vinegar, red pepper flakes,
   honey, and cornstarch. Set aside.

4 Remove pork from the marinade. Drain well.

5 Heat a large frying pan over medium heat. Add canola oil
   and stir-fry pork until cooked. Set aside.

6 Add red peppers and onions. Stir-fry for 1 minute.

7 Return the pork to the pan. Pour the sauce mixture over
   top and cook until the sauce bubbles. Serve.

Serves 4.

Kid Friendly

Jamaican Spiced Marinade for Beef and Pork

Anytime you blacken a food containing protein—on a stove, in the oven, indoor grill, or barbecue—you're producing carcinogens. Novice grillers tend to cook on high heat, ending up with blackened pieces of meat that are overcooked on the outside and raw in the middle, or just plain burnt. This is a one-way ticket to carbon overload.

How the heck can we cut down on those nasty carcinogens? Marinate. Specifically, marinate with anti-oxidant-high ingredients like pomegranate juice, lemon juice, green tea, garlic, and herbs. This Jamaican Spiced Marinade is slightly sweet, and has a wonderfully light spicy flavour. Experiment by adding diced fresh basil, oregano, or rosemary.

Always preheat your grill on high. Place the meat on grill, reduce heat to medium, and close the lid. Let it sear for two minutes, then flip the meat frequently until cooked. Yes, this is probably the exact opposite of what you might presently be doing, but it's the safest and best way to grill.

Marinade
1 cup (250 mL) **pomegranate juice**
2 Tbsp (30 mL) **dark brown sugar**
4 **cloves garlic, minced**
1½ tsp (7 mL) **ground ginger**
1 tsp (5 mL) **thyme**
1 tsp (5 mL) **ground allspice**
1 tsp (5 mL) **cinnamon**
1 tsp (5 mL) **extra virgin olive oil**
1 tsp (5 mL) **low-sodium soy sauce**
½ tsp (2 mL) **cracked pepper**

1 lb (500 g) **boneless grilling steak or butterflied pork tenderloin (see sidebar, page 255)**

ONE SERVING	155 Calories
	4.5 g Total Fat
	1.5 g Sat Fat
	0 g Trans Fat
	65 mg Sodium
	1 g CHO
	0 g Fibre
	26 g Protein
UEPC	1 Meat

HOW THE HECK DO I BUTTERFLY THE PORK?

A great way to make sure that the marinade will touch as much of the pork as possible is to butterfly it. Simply slice the pork tenderloin lengthwise, cutting to, but not through, the other side. When you open it, it's supposed to look like a butterfly. You may have to use your imagination on this one.

WHY DO I DISCARD THE MARINADE IN THE PLASTIC BAG AND BOIL THE RESERVED MARINADE?

Basically, if you don't, you could die! The marinade that was used to tenderize and add flavour to the meat is now full of bacteria. That's why you reserved ⅔ cup (150 mL) of the marinade at the beginning to use as a sauce. It needs to be boiled just so it can thicken.

1   In a 2-cup (500-mL) measuring cup, whisk together the marinade ingredients. Reserve ⅔ cup (150 mL) of the marinade and pour the remaining into a resealable bag.

2   Add the meat to the bag and reseal. Make sure the meat is fully covered with the marinade. Place the bag in the fridge and marinate for 20 minutes to 24 hours.

3   Once marinated, remove the meat from the fridge and let it sit at room temperature for 15 minutes. Preheat the grill to high. Remove the meat from the bag and discard the bagged marinade.

4   Place the meat on the grill, and reduce heat to medium. Grill the meat until the internal temperature reaches 160°F (71°C).

5   Once cooked, remove the meat from the grill, cover, and let it sit for 10 minutes.

6   While the meat is resting, pour the reserved marinade into a small saucepan and bring to a boil. Reduce the marinade to ⅓ cup (75 mL); this will take about 5 minutes. Set aside.

7   Divide the meat into 4 equal portions. Pour the cooked marinade over top and serve.

Serves 4.

Kid Friendly

EGGS

New

Breakfast Burrito

A power breakfast to rival all those fast food joints. Teach your family how to whip these up and you may even get breakfast in bed one day. Note: if you have teenagers, don't hold your breath.

1 **omega-3 egg**
½ tsp (2 mL) **canola oil**
1 small (6-inch/15-cm) **100% whole wheat soft tortilla, trans fat free**
1 Tbsp (15 mL) **salsa, mild, medium, or hot**
1 Tbsp (15 mL) **diced red pepper**
1 Tbsp (15 mL) **shredded light aged cheddar cheese**

1   In a small bowl, beat the egg until fluffy.

2   Heat a small frying pan over medium heat. Add the oil, then scramble the egg until cooked through.

3   Warm the tortilla in the microwave at medium-high (60%) for 10 seconds. Remove from the microwave and add the egg. Top with the salsa, red pepper, and cheese. Roll and enjoy.

Makes 1 serving. Recipe can be doubled, quadrupled, or even sextupled.

Kid Friendly

ONE SERVING	190 Calories
	8 g Total Fat
	2 g Sat Fat
	0 g Trans Fat
	330 mg Sodium
	22 g CHO
	2 g Fibre
	11 g Protein
UEPC	½ Fat
	1 Egg
	1 Grain

Greek Pizza Frittata

Frittatas are for the omelet challenged. No stirring, jiggling, or flipping needed. Just heat a frying pan, pour in the eggs, add the bells and whistles, and presto! You've got dinner. If only finding a bathing suit was that easy.

1 tsp (5 mL) **extra virgin olive oil**
4 **omega-3 eggs**
¾ tsp (4 mL) **dried oregano**
1 Tbsp (15 mL) **diced fresh basil**
1 tsp (5 mL) **Dijon mustard**
½ tsp (2 mL) **cracked black pepper**
2 cups (500 mL) **chopped baby spinach**
4 **kalamata olives, pitted and diced**
2 oz (55 g) **or** ½ cup (125 mL) **crumbled light feta cheese**
¼ cup (60 mL) **salsa, mild, medium, or hot**
2 **green onions, chopped**

1   In a medium bowl, beat the eggs until fluffy. Beat in the oregano, basil, Dijon, and pepper.

2   Heat an 11-inch (28-cm) frying pan over medium heat. Add the oil, then pour in the egg mixture. Let it cook for 2 minutes, or until partially set.

3   Sprinkle the spinach, olives, feta cheese, salsa, and green onions over the top.

4   Cover the pan with a lid and reduce the heat to low. Cook for 3 to 4 minutes, or until the eggs are cooked through and the cheese has melted.

Makes one 12-inch (30-cm) frittata. Serves four.

Kid Friendly

ONE SERVING	140 Calories
	9 g Total Fat
	3 g Sat Fat
	0 g Trans Fat
	400 mg Sodium
	5 g CHO
	1 g Fibre
	10 g Protein
UEPC	¼ Fat
	1 Fruit and Vegetables
	¼ Milk

FRUIT

Best Ever Berry Crisp

I love to serve this warm crisp as a breakfast treat. Note: if you want this crisp for breakfast, make it the night before. Scott, my partner in crime, can't understand the concept of making something that smells amazing and then not demolishing it immediately. So if you live with someone like this, hide the crisp after it comes out of the oven and nowhere near the remote control. Warm the crisp the next morning before serving.

Topping
1½ cup (375 mL) **large flake rolled oats**
½ cup (125 mL) **whole wheat flour**
½ cup (125 mL) **dark brown sugar**
1 Tbsp (15 mL) **cinnamon**
½ cup (125 mL) **canola oil**

Berries
6 cups (1.5 L) **mixed berries, fresh or frozen. Use raspberries, blueberries, and blackberries—or any combo you love.**
1 Tbsp (15 mL) **quick cooking tapioca**
1 tsp (5 mL) **cinnamon**

1   Preheat the oven to 350°F (180°C). Line an 8-inch (2-L) square baking pan with wet parchment paper. Set aside.

2   In a medium bowl, stir together the oats, flour, brown sugar, and cinnamon. Mix in the canola oil using a large spoon. The mixture should be well combined and look wet.

3   Place the berries into the prepared pan. Sprinkle with the tapioca and cinnamon.

4   Pour topping over the berries. Press down lightly.

5   Bake for 45 to 50 minutes, or until it bubbles. If you use frozen berries, cook for 15 to 20 minutes longer.

6   Serve warm or cold. Will keep up to 2 days in the fridge, covered.

Makes 5 cups (1.25 L). Makes eight ⅔-cup (150-mL) servings.

Kid Friendly

BIG COOKING TIP: WET PARCHMENT PAPER? ARE YOU KIDDING?

No. When you're baking or roasting something in the oven, thoroughly wetting a piece of parchment paper will help with clean up. Squeeze out excess water and line your pan with it. You'll never have to scrub a casserole pan or baking dish again. Most excellent.

WHY ARE THERE SO MANY CALORIES IN YOUR CRISP?

To make a crispy topping I used ½ cup (125 mL) of heart-healthy canola oil. You can do one of two things: make this with ¼ cup (60 mL) canola oil to reduce the grams of fat by half, or leave it as is and enjoy the crisp on a day where you've eaten low-fat elsewhere. Remember that heart-healthy fats eaten in moderation are a good thing.

ONE SERVING	310 Calories
	16 g Total Fat
	1 g Sat Fat
	0 g Trans Fat
	10 mg Sodium
	46 g CHO
	7 g Fibre
	4 g Protein
UEPC	1½ Fruits and Vegetables
	3 Fat
	½ Grains

Dried Fruit Compote

TIP
If you love dried cherries, substitute them for the dried cranberries.

I know you're looking at this and thinking, old people food.

Fruit compote, albeit an extremely popular nursing home food, is not just for aging boomers who aren't getting enough fibre. No one is getting enough fibre. Try this on for size and, who knows, you may become a dried fruit convert long before you hit retirement.

2 cups (500 mL) **orange juice**
20 **prunes**
20 **dried apricots**
½ cup (125 mL) **dried cranberries**
4 **cinnamon sticks**

1   In a medium saucepan, combine the orange juice, prunes, apricots, and cranberries. Submerge the cinnamon sticks.

2   Bring to a boil. Cover and reduce the heat to low. Simmer for 10 minutes. Remove from the heat and let sit for 20 minutes.

3   Cover and store in the fridge for up to 1 week.

Makes 3 cups (750 mL) dried fruit and 1 cup (250 mL) juice.
Makes six ½-cup (125-mL) servings.

ONE SERVING	190 Calories
	0 g Total Fat
	0 g Sat Fat
	0 g Trans Fat
	0 g Sodium
	48 g CHO
	4 g Fibre
	2 g Protein
UEPC	2½ Fruits & Vegetables

Revised

Fantastic Frozen Yogurt Times Four

My mom, dad, sister, brother, and myself (in short, the whole famdamily) are ice cream fanatics. We all love that cold creamy texture. Unfortunately, none of us love the fat. Okay, I don't love the fat. The rest of the family couldn't give a hoot or a holler, even though the good Lord knows I've tried to convince them otherwise. Oh, how I've tried.

You can buy low-fat frozen yogurts, but I'm not a huge fan of the bells and whistles they add to improve the flavour, texture, and what we call in the biz, mouth feel. I make my own. All you need is yogurt, frozen fruit, and a food processor.

Basic Fantastic Frozen Yogurt

2 cups (500 mL) **frozen fruit or berries, unsweetened (see sidebar)**
1 cup (250 mL) **low-fat French probiotic vanilla yogurt**

1 Blend the frozen fruit or berries and the yogurt in the food processor. Pulse occasionally and blend until smooth. It's going to be noisy, but it's totally worth it.

2 Serve immediately. Too cinchy.

Makes 2 cups (500 mL). Makes four ½-cup (125-mL) servings.

Kid Friendly

BIG EATING TIP
You have to eat this right away. It doesn't do well in the freezer.

FLAVOUR IDEAS
Frozen Mango Yogurt—
2 cups (500 mL) frozen unsweetened mango chunks

Frozen Raspberry Yogurt—
2 cups (500 mL) frozen unsweetened raspberries

Frozen Blueberry Yogurt—
2 cups (500 mL) frozen unsweetened wild blueberries

Frozen Mixed Berry Yogurt—
2 cups (500 mL) frozen unsweetened mixed berries

ONE SERVING	90 Calories
	1 g Total Fat
	0.5 g Sat Fat
	0 g Trans Fat
	45 mg Sodium
	19 g CHO
	2 g Fibre
	3 g Protein
UEPC	1 Fruits & Vegetables
	¼ Milk

New

My Very Own Fast Food Berry Parfait

This is one of my all-time favourite packable treats. I've been making this parfait for the past 10 years. I put frozen berries in the bottom of a plastic container, add the yogurt, then pack it in a thermal bag. At lunch time, I add my homemade granola. Voila, my very own personal fast food treat.

1 cup (250 mL) **fresh or frozen berries**
½ cup (125 mL) **low-fat probiotic French vanilla yogurt or unsweetened plain probiotic yogurt**
¼ cup (60 mL) **granola (recipe follows on next page)**

1 Place the berries in a bowl, and top with yogurt and granola. Eat. You didn't need instructions for this one, did you?

Makes 1¾ cups (425 mL). Makes one 1¾-cup (425-mL) serving.

Kid Friendly

ONE SERVING with granola	320 Calories
	7 g Total Fat
	1 g Sat Fat
	0 g Trans Fat
	90 mg Sodium
	58 g CHO
	6 g Fibre
	10 g Protein
UEPC	2 Fruit and Vegetables
	¾ Fat
	½ Grains
	¾ Milk
ONE SERVING without granola	190 Calories
	2 g Total Fat
	1 g Sat Fat
	0 g Trans Fat
	90 mg Sodium
	37 g CHO
	4 g Fibre
	7 g Protein
UEPC	2 Fruits & Vegetables
	¾ Milk

Crunchy Cinnamon Granola

In the late '60s, my family took a trip to San Francisco where we had our very first hippy sighting. My parents thought these long-haired, granola-eating kids were just a bunch of tree huggers who wanted nothing more than to run naked and have wild sex. Sounded pretty darned exciting to me. Whoa baby!

1½ cup (375 mL) **large flake rolled oats**
¼ cup (60 mL) **wheat germ**
2 Tbsp (30 mL) **canola oil**
2 Tbsp (30 mL) **honey**
2 Tbsp (30 mL) **brown sugar**
1 Tbsp (15 mL) **cinnamon**
1 tsp (5 mL) **pure vanilla extract**

1   Preheat the oven to 325°F (180°C). Line a 9- × 13-inch (3.5-L) metal baking pan with parchment paper.

2   In a medium bowl, mix the oats and wheat germ.

3   In a small microwaveable bowl, mix together the canola oil, honey, brown sugar, cinnamon, and vanilla extract. Heat at medium-high (60%) in the microwave for 15 seconds. Pour over the oat mixture. Toss well.

4   Pour the mixture into the lined baking pan and bake in the oven for 15 minutes.

5   Remove from the oven and stir. Return to the oven and continue baking for 10 minutes.

6   Remove from the oven and let it cool completely. Store in an airtight container for up to 2 months.

Makes 2 cups (500 mL). Makes eight ¼-cup (50-mL) servings.

Kid Friendly

NUTRITION TIP
Granola isn't a low-fat cereal. Just because it's made with healthy ingredients doesn't give you carte blanche to eat the whole thing. Stick to ¼ cup (60 mL) per serving.

ONE SERVING	130 Calories
	5 g Total Fat
	0 g Sat Fat
	0 g Trans Fat
	0 mg Sodium
	21 g CHO
	2 g Fibre
	3 g Protein
UEPC	½ Grains
	¾ Fat

BEVERAGES

Super Quick Blender Shakes

Using frozen fruit in a smoothie turns it into the consistency of a milkshake—a big hit with kids. They may even think you've lost your mind by giving them a milkshake for breakfast or snack. It's okay, let them think that. It'll keep them on their toes.

HOW THE HECK DO I FREEZE A BANANA?
Peel and cut overripe bananas into 2-inch (5-cm) chunks and freeze them in plastic bags. When the urge for a blended drink hits you, break off 6 to 8 chunks and, voila, you now have one frozen banana.

Revised
Super Banana Chocolate Shake
Get your soy and chocolate fix all at the same time. Most chocolate soy milk products have different amounts of fat, and therefore calories. Try choosing a low-fat one. I use So Nice or Silk.

1 cup (250 mL) **chocolate soy milk**
1 **frozen banana, in chunks**
1 Tbsp (15 mL) **natural cocoa powder**

1   Whirl everything in a blender. Drink.

Serves 1.

ONE SERVING	280 Calories
	4 g Total Fat
	0.5 g Sat Fat
	0 g Trans Fat
	111 mg Sodium
	54 g CHO
	6 g Fibre
	8 g Protein
UEPC	2 Fruits & Vegetables
	1 Beans

Classic Favourite
Super Soy Strawberry Smoothie
You can find strawberry soy milk in Tetra Paks at most grocery stores beside the canned milk.

1 cup (250 mL) **strawberry soy milk**
½ cup (125 mL) **frozen strawberries or any frozen berry**

1   Whirl everything together in the blender. Drink.

Serves 1.

FROZEN BERRIES
In berry season, I freeze my own. Gently wash, dry on paper towels, and freeze on trays. Once frozen, pack them into containers. In the off season, you can buy unsweetened frozen berries in the freezer section at your local grocery store. Either way, they're great.

ONE SERVING	175 Calories
	6 g Total Fat
	0.5 g Sat Fat
	125 mg Sodium
	22 g CHO
	4 g Fibre
	8 g Protein
UEPC	1 Fruits & Vegetables
	1 Beans

TIP
You can buy frozen mango and pineapple in the freezer section, or freeze your own.

HOW THE HECK DO I GET THE FISH OIL OUT OF THAT TABLET?
Very carefully. Through trial and error I discovered the best way is to pierce the tablet in the middle with the sharp point of a small knife. Hold the tablet over the blender and gently squeeze both sides in a downward motion. Hopefully, the oil will go into the blender and not all over you. Make sure the kids aren't watching. In this case, what they don't know won't hurt them.

Or you can do what I do. I use Nutra Sea, a fish oil product from Norway, made by Ascenta. I use the original formula, lemon zest flavour. You can buy it at most health food stores. It comes in a bottle that you keep in the fridge once opened. Measure out 1 tsp (5 mL) for this recipe and omit the lemon juice.

ONE SERVING	110 Calories
	1 g Total Fat
	0 g Sat Fat
	0 g Trans Fat
	25 mg Sodium
	25 g CHO
	1 g Fibre
	3 g Protein
UEPC	1½ Fruits & Vegetables
	½ Milk

New
Omega-3 Tropical Smoothie

My grandma always said that fish was brain food—she wasn't that far off. We need to be eating those omega-3s in fish form at least twice a week. What's a harried working person, with kids, a spouse, and a dog to do? Well, you could give everyone a fish oil tablet and a glass of water, but that sounds pretty darn gross. Help is on the way! Try making this smoothie, so chock full of tropical flavours that it camouflages the added fish oil. I've served this shake to the pickiest eaters I know. No one ever said, "Boy, does that ever taste like salmon." Nope. It was, "Great!" Every time.

½ cup (125 mL) **orange juice, with pulp**
¼ cup (60 mL) **frozen mango chunks**
¼ cup (60 mL) **frozen pineapple chunks**
½ **banana**
one 100-g container **of probiotic French vanilla yogurt**
1 Tbsp (15 mL) **fresh lemon juice**
1 **fish oil tablet**

1   Don't just throw the whole fish oil pill in the blender. Remove the oil from tablet (see sidebar).

2   Whirl everything in a blender until smooth. Divide between 2 glasses. Serve.

Makes 1½ cups (375 mL). Makes two ¾-cup (175-mL) servings.

WHERE THE HECK DO I FIND PROBIOTIC YOGURT?
There are many companies out there selling probiotic yogurts: Activia, Astro, and Bio K. Pick the one you love and buy it often. I used Activia's French vanilla for this recipe.

New

Purple Pomegranate Smoothie

An excellent purple colour, this antioxidant superstar smoothie is a mini meal in a glass. Loaded with berries, cinnamon, and pomegranate, one sip feels like a party in your mouth. Warning: this stuff stains like crazy. Drink sitting down, or invest in one of those portable stain removers if you're on the go. You want to drink the purple power, not wear it.

½ cup (125 mL) **pomegranate juice**
1 cup (250 mL) **frozen mixed berries**
¼ cup (60 mL) **probiotic French vanilla yogurt**
½ tsp (2 mL) **cinnamon**

1   Whirl everything in a blender. Drink.

Serves 1.

ONE SERVING	210 Calories
	1 g Total Fat
	0 g Sat Fat
	0 g Trans Fat
	75 mg Sodium
	47 g CHO
	6 g Fibre
	6 g Protein
UEPC	3 Fruits & Vegetables
	½ Milk

New

Two Incredible Cocoa Creations

NOT SWEET ENOUGH?
**Add an extra tablespoon
(15 mL) of granulated sugar.**

My son plays hockey, which means I've dragged myself out of bed at the crack of 5:00 a.m. I've cheered him on through thick and thin, and have consumed a lot of really terrible hockey rink cocoa. For whatever reason, some rinks call the thin brown liquid hot chocolate, and others call it cocoa. They could call it the Elixir of the Gods. It still tastes like dishwater.

For all you hot chocolate or cocoa lovers, here's my basic cocoa recipe, along with a variation for the sweet tooth in the family. Plus there's a summer version that's a staple at my house during those hot, humid days.

Basic Cocoa

An adult version that's not too sweet. Buy a mini whisk, sometimes called a cocoa whisk, to make sure your cocoa is lump free. (See Must-Have Kitchen Toys.)

1 cup (250 mL) **low-fat soy milk or skim milk**
2 Tbsp (30 mL) **natural cocoa powder**
1 Tbsp (15 mL) **granulated sugar**

1   Make a paste with the cocoa powder, sugar, and 3 Tbsp (45 mL) of the milk or soy milk.

2   Heat the rest of the milk or soy milk in the microwave or on top of the stove, until steaming.

3   Whisk the hot milk or soy milk into the cocoa paste until frothy. Drink.

Serves 1.

ONE SERVING made with skim milk	
	180 Calories
	2 g Total Fat
	0 g Sat Fat
	0 g Trans Fat
	120 mg Sodium
	31 g CHO
	2 g Fibre
	11 g Protein
UEPC	1 Milk

ONE SERVING made with soy milk	
	175 Calories
	4.6 g Total Fat
	0.8 g Sat Fat
	0 Trans Fat
	130 mg Sodium
	25 g CHO
	3 g Fibre
	8 g Protein
UEPC	1 Milk

Frozen Cocoa

Hormones are a powerful thing. Out of the blue, they'll scream in your ear, "Must have chocolate!" Now, I've never been one to argue with my hormones, so the last time I heard the chocolate voice I remembered I had seen a recipe for frozen hot chocolate on Oprah. The way she danced around, I just knew I had to try some. I googled frozen hot chocolate, and no wonder Ms Winfrey had gone mental: it was loaded with tons of high end chocolate, whipping cream, and full-fat milk. By now you know I don't do the full-fat thing, so I came up with a lower fat, heart healthy version. It packs a cocoa punch that'll have you drinking and dancing all summer long.

1 cup (250 mL) **skim milk**
2 Tbsp (30 mL) **natural cocoa powder**
1 Tbsp (15 mL) **granulated sugar (see sidebar)**
1 tsp (5 mL) **pure vanilla extract (see sidebar)**
2 Tbsp (30 mL) **skim milk powder**
2 cups **ice cubes**

1   Put all the ingredients into a blender. Whirl until smooth. This can be noisy, but well worth it. Divide into 2 equal servings and share. Viva la cocoa!

Makes 3 cups (750 mL). Makes two 1½-cup (375-mL) servings.

The first time my most blessed assistant Tracey tried the Frozen Cocoa, she said she'd sign a waiver if she could have the recipe before the book came out. Tracey is a pastry chef and a weight watcher, so I'm taking this as a ringing endorsement.

BIG COOKING TIP
Feel free to double, triple, quadruple, whatever. Who knew math would end up being so important?

SWEET TOOTH?
This isn't a sweet drink. If you need more sweetness go ahead and add an extra 1 tablespoon (15 mL) of granulated sugar. Just one. You must use pure vanilla extract. Nothing else comes close.

MUST-HAVE KITCHEN TOYS
A cocoa whisk or a mini whisk. You're going to be drinking a lot of cocoa, so you might as well splurge for a $1 mini whisk. They're absolutely a must-have in the cocoa department.

WHERE THE HECK DO I FIND SKIM MILK POWDER?
It's in the same aisle as the canned milk, usually on the bottom shelf. Loaded with protein and calcium, it can really bump up the nutrition and the creaminess of a blender drink.

ONE SERVING	145 Calories
	2 g Total Fat
	0 g Sat Fat
	0 g Trans Fat
	90 mg Sodium
	18 g CHO
	1 g Fibre
	9 g Protein
UEPC	1 Milk

The Perfect Cup of Tea

I was raised in an English/Irish/Scottish home. One of the things my grandmother and my great aunt taught me was how to make a great pot of tea.

My Grannie and Great Aunt Nellie's Tea Making Rules

1 Always use a clean teapot. That whole nonsense about never washing out your teapot is just another culinary myth. The old tannins that stick to the inside of your pot affect your next pot's flavour. And not in a good way.

2 Use fresh cold water. Don't boil anything but fresh cold water. Believe it or not, some people use hot water from the tap. No. Bad. Don't even think about it. That cold tap water has oxygen in it, which really affects the flavour of the tea. Bet you didn't know that bit of tea trivia.

3 Hot the pot. Translation: preheat the teapot by using some of the boiling water from the kettle, swirl it around for 10 seconds, then dump it out.

4 Measure out the correct amount of tea. One teaspoon (5 mL) per 6-oz (175-mL) cup. Most of us think a cup is 8 oz (250 mL), but to the tea world, a cup is 6 oz (175 mL). I use 1 teaspoon (5 mL) per serving, and because my Great Aunt Nellie made tea that could dissolve a spoon, I do throw in that extra teaspoon (5 mL) for the pot. If you don't like strong tea, forget it. If you're using tea bags to make a pot, use 1 bag per cup (unless it's a 2-cup tea bag).

5 Most new teapots have built in strainers, an excellent idea if you use loose tea. If you can, run out and buy one immediately. The wire mesh balls aren't as good, but in a pinch they'll do. Tea bags are okay, but I'm a loose tea kinda girl.

6 Add the tea and pour in the boiling water. It's really important not to overboil the water. This will get rid of the much needed oxygen that's in the just boiled water, which as I mentioned before really affects the flavour of the tea.

7 Let the tea steep for the required time. Black teas usually take from 3 to 5 minutes.

8 Remove the tea leaves or bag, unless you want your fortune told (google "tea-leaf readers").

9 Pour into a china cup—okay, whatever you like.

10 Serve with milk, sweetener, or leave it clear.

The Perfect Cup of Green Tea

The rules are different for green tea. If you've been brewing green tea the same way you brew black tea and wondering why it tastes so bitter, read on—these rules are for you.

Green Tea Rules

1   Always use a clean teapot.

2   Bring fresh cold water to a boil.

3   The correct temperature to brew green tea is just below the boiling point. How do you know when that is? After the water has boiled, pour it into the pot and let it sit for 1 to 2 minutes. Alternately, use a thermometer to gage when the water is between 160°F and 175°F (70°C and 80°C).

4   Add the tea bags, or measure out the tea leaves, 1 teaspoon (5 mL) per cup. For loose leaves, put them in a wire mesh ball or wire basket. Brew for 3 to 5 minutes, unless your tea merchant or the label states otherwise.

5   Remove the leaves after the recommended time and drink clear.

New

Iced Tea

TIP
If you drink really weak tea, this recipe may be too strong. Add extra cold water to your liking.

On a hot summer day there's nothing like a glass of iced tea. Commercial iced teas are loaded with sugar, sugar, and more sugar. Plus the valuable antioxidants are destroyed in the processing.

This recipe let's you use those antioxidants as well as create your desired sweetness level.

Old-Fashioned Iced Black Tea

Although most people think of iced tea as regular old black tea cooled down, be a bit creative. Brew a pot of Earl Grey, Irish Breakfast, or your favourite blended tea. Then ice and enjoy.

½ cup (125 mL) **loose tea or eight 2-cup tea bags**
4 cups (1 L) **boiling water**
4 cups (1 L) **cold water**

1   Hot your clean, 4-cup (1-L) tea pot. See page 271.

2   Add the loose tea or tea bags. Pour boiling water into the pot and let the tea steep for 4 to 6 minutes.

3   Fill a 10-cup (2.5-L) jug with 4 cups (1 L) of cold water.

4   Stir the hot tea. Gently squeeze the tea bags into the tea and then discard them. If you want sweet iced tea, add the desired amount of granulated sugar (2 to 3 Tbsp/ 30 to 45 mL should do it) to the hot tea, then stir to dissolve. Pour the tea into the jug of cold water. If you're using loose leaves, pour the tea into the cold water through a strainer to catch the loose leaves. Refrigerate until cold.

5   If desired, add lemon to serve. Pour into glasses filled with ice.

Makes 9 cups.

Iced Spiced Black Tea

Add 4 cinnamon sticks and 4 cloves to the pot before you add the tea. Follow the directions for Old-Fashioned Iced Black Tea.

Iced Blackcurrant Tea

Add 1 Tbsp (15 mL) blackcurrant syrup (can be bought under the brand name of Ribena) to 1 cup (250 mL) unsweetened iced tea.

Iced Green Tea

Brew green tea normally. Refrigerate. Add sweetener if desired.

Iced Cinnamon Mint Green Tea

In a 4-cup (1-L) tea pot, brew green tea, 3 mint herbal tea bags, and 3 cinnamon sticks. Remove green tea bags after 3 to 5 minutes. Remove mint tea bags and cinnamon sticks after 8 to 10 minutes. Cool. Serve unsweetened, with ice.

Liz's Spiced Green Tea

In a 4-cup (1-L) tea pot, brew 3 green tea bags, 3 cinnamon sticks, and 5 whole cloves. Remove the green tea bags after 3 to 5 minutes. Remove the cinnamon sticks and cloves after 8 to 10 minutes. Cool. Serve unsweetened, with ice.

TIP

Used tea leaves make wonderful food for your garden. Those antioxidants just don't stop. Sprinkle loose leaves, or the contents from tea bags, around your plants. You and your posies will be healthier.

New

Pomegranate Martini

WHAT KIND OF POMEGRANATE JUICE SHOULD I BUY?
I've tried several different brands of pomegranate juice, but I keep going back to POM. You can find it in most grocery stores in the chilled produce section. For me it has the perfect blend of tart and sweet.

BIG BIG TIP
Ever wonder why you might be gaining weight? Check the calories on this one. 240 big ones is nothing to sneeze at. Just another reason to have only one little old martini.

May the trend of martinis live a long and happy life. This purple drink has become my favourite summer, fall, winter, and spring drink. Not only am I getting the HDL raising ethanol from the vodka, I'm also packing in the antioxidants from the pomegranate juice. I feel incredibly virtuous when I have one of these. But remember, one martini is all we girls get. And that's only if we've made sure to have our 7 to 10 servings of fruits and veggies. Guys, feel free to have two. What's with that testosterone, anyway?

1½ oz **Vodka**
juice of ½ **a lime**
1 cup (250 mL) **pomegranate juice (I recommend POM)**

1   Shake all the ingredients in a cocktail shaker filled with ice until well chilled. Strain into a martini glass. Drink slowly.

Or for a cocktail

1   In a tall glass, mix together all the ingredients. Fill the glass with ice and enjoy.

Serves 1.

Pomegranate Mocktini

Mix together ½ cup (125 mL) pomegranate juice with an equal amount of mineral water. Add a little squeeze of lime and serve over ice.

ONE SERVING	240 Calories
	0 g Total Fat
	0 g Sat Fat
	0 g Trans Fat
	30 mg Sodium
	36 g CHO
	0 g Fibre
	1 g Protein
UEPC	2 Fruits & Vegetables

MUFFINS, PANCAKES, & FRENCH TOAST

Whole Wheat Muffins 101

Never made a 100% Whole Wheat Mairlyn Muffin before? Follow these rules.

RULE # 1
Measure carefully. Spoon all dry ingredients into dry ingredient measuring cups. They are usually the metal or plastic ones. The glass ones are for liquid measures. Once you've spooned the dry ingredients into the measuring cups, level them off with a straight edge. A metal spatula or the back of a knife both work, as long as they're flat.

RULE # 2
You can't overmix a whole wheat muffin. The old rule about mixing until just combined is out the window. There isn't enough gluten—the protein that causes baked goods to toughen—in whole wheat, so stir away. Better yet, get your kids to help. They can't wreck them.

RULE # 3
Use paper cup liners for your muffin pans. There will be less clean-up.

   When you start filling the muffin cups, you'll think: "Hey, hold the phone. There's a ton of batter here. I'm going to make 16 muffins instead of the 12 Miss Home Ec Teacher Smarty Pants said." Don't. Back away from the batter. Whole wheat muffins don't rise to the same height as muffins made with white flour. So fill those muffin cups equally so that they're almost ¾ full and bake them as instructed. You'll have 12 gorgeous muffins begging to be consumed.

RULE # 4
How do you get your homemade muffins to look uniform?

   You need to buy one of my Must-Have Kitchen Tools—a ¼-cup (60-mL) ice cream scoop with a release button. Simply scoop out the muffin batter, squeeze the release button, and voila! Perfect muffins every time.

RULE # 5
Bake up a double batch. Leave a couple out for eating and freeze the rest. All the muffins in this chapter freeze well. The best way is to freeze the muffins individually in plastic bags. Take one out of the freezer and pop it in your purse, briefcase, or backpack. It will be thawed in about two hours.

RULE # 6
Some, but not all, whole wheat flour is 100% whole grain. In some cases the germ portion of the grain has been removed. To ensure that the muffins you make are 100% whole grain, consider adding 2 Tbsp (30 mL) wheat germ to each recipe when you add the dry ingredients.

Banana Chocolate Chip Muffins

These muffins are my family's favourite. My son can eat them for breakfast, lunch, snacks, or even for dessert, but not for every meal in the same day. These deliciously moist muffins are loaded with fibre and flavour.

Warning: each muffin contains 6 grams of fibre, which is about 6 times more than a commercial muffin, so don't go pigging out and eat a half dozen. To put it mildly, you'll be in for a big surprise about 12 hours later.

Dry Ingredients
1 cup (250 mL) **whole wheat flour**
¾ cup (175 mL) **wheat bran**
¾ cup (175 mL) **ground flaxseed**
¼ cup (60 mL) **chopped dark chocolate, M&M's baking bits, or mini chocolate chips**
1½ tsp (7 mL) **baking powder**
1 tsp (5 mL) **baking soda**
2 Tbsp (30 mL) **cinnamon**

Wet Ingredients
1½ cups (375 mL) **mashed banana, about 4 really ripe bananas**
¾ cup (175 mL) **dark brown sugar**
¾ cup (175 mL) **buttermilk**
1 **omega-3 egg**

BIG COOKING TIP
For a moist muffin, make sure the bananas are really ripe. You want them to look almost all black and be fairly squishy. You can either let your bananas hit this state of ripeness on your counter (attracting fruit flies) or look in the markdown produce section for some ripe ones, then let them sit on your counter to get even riper. Freeze any that you won't be using right away. When it's time to make these muffins, pull out 4 or 5 of the blackened bananas. Freezing really turns them black. Thaw, cut off the tops and squish them into a measuring cup; discard the slimy peel into your composter. Voila! Perfect, intensely-flavoured mushy banana, albeit slightly gross looking.

ONE SERVING	180 Calories
	5 g Total Fat
	1 g Sat Fat
	0 Trans Fat
	170 mg Sodium
	36 g CHO
	6 g Fibre
	5 g Protein
UEPC	1 Flax
	½ Fruits & Vegetables
	1½ Grains

WHAT THE HECK IS FLAXSEED AND WHY IS IT IN SO MANY OF YOUR RECIPES?

I'm guessing you didn't read Liz's section on flaxseed. Go to page 86 for a tutorial. To learn how to cook with flaxseed, read on.

GROUND FLAXSEED

I like to buy flaxseed whole and then grind it up in my coffee bean mill. That way I grind up only what I'll be using in the next week. Don't become overzealous and grind them into flour. Just keep pulsing until they look like coarse sand. Once the flaxseeds have been ground, store them in a covered container in the fridge. They'll stay fresh for up to 90 days. A coffee bean mill is the only thing that grinds up the seeds well enough. Trust me: I've tried blenders, food processors, an old fashioned coffee bean grinder, and a hammer. The coffee bean mill works the best. Considering you're going to be eating 1 to 2 tablespoons (15 to 30 mL) of ground flaxseed every day for the rest of your life, it's worth the purchase. I used whole flaxseed, which I ground myself for all the recipes in this book.

1 Preheat the oven to 400°F (200°C). Line a muffin pan with paper cup liners.

2 In a large bowl, using a fork or a wire whisk, mix together all the dry ingredients: whole wheat flour, wheat bran, flaxseed, chocolate, baking powder, baking soda, and cinnamon.

3 In a medium bowl, beat together all the wet ingredients: mashed banana, brown sugar, buttermilk, and egg. The mashed banana needs to be mixed in well.

4 Pour the wet ingredients into the dry ingredients and mix until combined.

5 Scoop into muffin cups. Bake for 20 to 25 minutes or until done.

Makes 12 servings.

Kid Friendly

Wild Blueberry Muffins

When I signed up for parenthood I was vaguely aware that I needed to be a shift worker in top physical condition, with first aid and psychology training under my belt. A sense of humor was required, catering skills a must, and managerial and organizational skills were advantageous. I had no idea that baking muffins every week would be one of the most important skills I had. Goes to show you that cooking is love.

BIG COOKING TIP
Try using non-stick baking cups. In Canada my favourite brand is Chef's Select.

Topping
1 Tbsp (15 mL) **granulated sugar**
1½ Tbsp (17 mL) **lemon zest, about one lemon**

Wet Ingredients
1 **omega-3 egg**
3 Tbsp (45 mL) **canola oil**
¾ cup (175 mL) **buttermilk**
1½ cups (375 mL) **oat bran**
¾ cup (175 mL) **honey**
2 Tbsp (30 mL) **fresh lemon juice**

Dry Ingredients
1 cup (250 mL) **whole wheat flour**
1½ tsp (7 mL) **baking powder**
1 tsp (5 mL) **baking soda**
2 Tbsp (30 mL) **cinnamon**
2 cups (500 mL) **wild blueberries, fresh or frozen**

ONE SERVING	190 Calories
	5 g Total Fat
	0.5 g Sat Fat
	0 g Trans Fat
	160 mg Sodium
	39 g CHO
	4 g Fibre
	5 g Protein
UEPC	¾ Fat
	¼ Fruits & Vegetables
	1½ Grains

SHOULD I USE FROZEN OR FRESH BLUEBERRIES?

It doesn't really matter what you choose. I use fresh wild blueberries when they're in season and frozen ones when they aren't. I freeze the fresh wild ones in August so that I'm stocked up for the winter. I'd have made a great pioneer. Wait, I just remembered the outhouse thing. I may need to rethink the whole homesteader option.

Wild blueberries are smaller than cultivated commercial ones, and I think they bake up better. If you go with frozen berries, don't worry about the thick batter it creates. The berries are freezing it. The batter will bake just the same. Make sure that you test for doneness. And that would be? Using a toothpick to pierce the muffin and see if it comes out clean. If it isn't all gummy with raw batter, the muffins are done.

1 Preheat the oven to 400°F (200°C). Line a muffin pan with paper cup liners.

2 Mix sugar and lemon zest in a small bowl. Set aside.

3 In a large bowl, mix together all the wet ingredients. Set aside while you measure the dry ingredients. This is a really important step. It allows the oat bran to act like a sponge and absorb most of the liquid. Skipping it will leave you with soggy muffins instead of moist ones. When you're expecting a delectable blueberry muffin and you bite into a smooshie mess, that's a bad thing.

4 In a small bowl, using a fork or a wire whisk, mix together all the dry ingredients. Pour the dry ingredients into the wet ingredients and mix with a large spoon or spatula until combined.

5 Gently fold in the blueberries using a rubber spatula. Don't overmix or you'll end up with purple muffins, although, if you have small children, baking something purple can be a very cool thing.

6 Scoop into muffin cups. Sprinkle each muffin with some of the sugar/lemon zest mixture. Bake for 20 to 25 minutes or until done.

Makes 12 servings.

Kid Friendly

Super Nutritious Bran Muffins, a.k.a the BM Bullets

These muffins are loaded with powerfully nutritious ingredients like whole grains, ground flaxseed, dates, prunes, buttermilk, and dark chocolate. They honestly taste too good to be healthy for you, but they are— somebody pinch me.

Dry Ingredients

1¼ cups (310 mL) **whole wheat flour**

1 cup (250 mL) **wheat bran**

¾ cup (175 mL) **ground flaxseed**

½ cup (125 mL) **chopped dates**

¼ cup (60 mL) **chopped dark chocolate, M&M's baking bits, or mini chocolate chips**

2 Tbsp (30 mL) **cinnamon**

1 tsp (5 mL) **baking powder**

1 tsp (5 mL) **baking soda**

Wet Ingredients

1¼ cups (310 mL) **buttermilk**

1 **omega-3 egg**

one 4.5-oz (128-mL) **jar baby food strained prunes, no added sugar or starch**

¾ cup (175 mL) **dark brown sugar**

¼ cup (60 mL) **molasses**

1   Preheat the oven to 400°F (200°C.) Line a muffin pan with paper cup liners.

2   In a large bowl, using a fork or a wire whisk, mix together all the dry ingredients.

3   In a medium bowl, beat together all the wet ingredients.

4   Pour the wet ingredients into the dry ingredients and mix until combined.

5   Scoop into muffin cups. Bake for 20 to 25 minutes or until done.

Makes 12 servings.

DO YOU REMEMBER THE MUFFIN METHOD FROM GRADE 8 HOME EC?
Mix all the dry ingredients in one bowl. Mix all the wet ingredients in another bowl. Add the wet to the dry and stir until just mixed. So you're probably thinking, "Brown sugar isn't a wet ingredient." Well, you'd be correct. Your Home Ec teacher would be proud. But when brown sugar is dissolved with the wet ingredients, it combines for a better muffin. Just call this the Mairlyn Muffin Method.

WHERE THE HECK DO I FIND A JAR OF BABY FOOD STRAINED PRUNES, NO ADDED SUGAR OR STARCH?
Haven't had a baby? Never want a baby? Too old to remember your kids as babies? Go to the baby food section of your local supermarket. Look at all those tiny jars and make sure you buy the jar that has no sugar or starch added.

ONE SERVING	220 Calories
	5 g Total Fat
	1 g Sat Fat
	0 g Trans Fat
	170 mg Sodium
	45 g CHO
	7 g Fibre
	6 g Protein
UEPC	1 Flax
	1½ Grains

Double Chocolate Muffins

BIG COOKING TIP
Pure pumpkin purée and canned pumpkin pie filling are two totally different things. Make sure you buy the pure pumpkin purée and not the pie filling, which is loaded with sugar.

WHAT THE HECK DO I DO WITH THE REST OF THE PUMPKIN FROM THE HUGE CAN I JUST OPENED?
Go to the Soup chapter and make the Jamaican Black Bean Pumpkin Soup on page 158. Or freeze the leftover pumpkin in 1 cup (250 mL) portions for the next time you want to make these chocolatey muffins.

Don't let the pumpkin in the recipe mislead you. These muffins don't have the faintest hint of pumpkin flavour. They're chocolate all the way. These have become one of Liz's daughters favourite in the book. She says it's like packing a chocolate cupcake for lunch.

Wet Ingredients
1 cup (250 mL) **buttermilk**
1 cup (250 mL) **pure pumpkin purée**
1 cup (250 mL) **dark brown sugar**
½ cup (125 mL) **oat bran**
1 **omega-3 egg**

Dry Ingredients
1 cup (250 mL) **whole wheat flour**
¾ cup (175 mL) **ground flaxseed**
½ cup (125 mL) **natural cocoa powder**
2 Tbsp (30 mL) **cinnamon**
1½ tsp (7 mL) **baking powder**
1 tsp (5 mL) **baking soda**
¼ cup (60 mL) **chopped dark chocolate, M&M's baking bits, or mini chocolate chips**

1   Preheat the oven to 400°F (200°C.) Line a muffin pan with paper cup liners.

2   In a medium bowl, beat together all the wet ingredients. Set aside.

3   In a large bowl, using a fork or a wire whisk, mix together all the dry ingredients.

4   Pour the wet ingredients into the dry ingredients and mix until combined.

5   Scoop into muffin cups. Bake for 20 to 25 minutes or until done.

Makes 12 servings.

Kid Friendly

ONE SERVING	200 Calories
	5 g Total Fat
	1 g Sat Fat
	0 g Trans Fat
	180 mg Sodium
	38 g CHO
	5 g Fibre
	6 g Protein
UEPC	1 Flax
	1 Grain

Banana Walnut Bread Muffins

Looking back on my childhood, aside from fruit, rice pudding, and the odd date square, my mom didn't make desserts very often. She was into loaves and breads. There was the date loaf, walnut loaf, lemon loaf, and my favourite, banana bread—always wondered why it wasn't a loaf. Mom was raised during the depression and didn't squander food, so banana bread was a great way to get rid of those overripe, black bananas, which are perfect for this recipe. Take a trip down memory lane and enjoy.

Wet Ingredients
¾ cup (175 mL) **skim milk**
1 Tbsp (15 mL) **fresh lemon juice**
¾ cup (175 mL) **dark brown sugar**
¼ cup (60 mL) **oat bran**
¼ cup (60 mL) **Kellogg's All-Bran Buds (see page 286)**
¼ cup (60 mL) **wheat bran**
1 **omega-3 egg**
1½ cups (375 mL) **mashed ripe banana (about 4 bananas)**

Dry Ingredients
1 cup (250 mL) **whole wheat flour**
¾ cup (175 mL) **ground flaxseed**
¼ cup (60 mL) **walnuts, finely chopped**
2 Tbsp (30 mL) **cinnamon**
1½ tsp (7 mL) **baking powder**
1 tsp (5 mL) **baking soda**

1   Preheat the oven to 400°F (200°C). Line a muffin pan with paper cup liners.

2   In a large bowl, mix together the skim milk, lemon juice, brown sugar, oat bran, All-Bran Buds, and wheat bran. Let sit for 5 minutes. Beat in the egg and mashed bananas.

3   In a medium bowl, using a fork or wire whisk, mix together all the dry ingredients.

4   Pour the dry ingredients into the wet ingredients and mix until well combined.

5   Scoop into muffin cups. Bake for 20 to 25 minutes or until done.

Makes 12 servings.

Kid Friendly

ONE SERVING	
	200 Calories
	6 g Total Fat
	0 g Sat Fat
	0 g Trans Fat
	160 mg Sodium
	37 g CHO
	6 g Fibre
	6 g Protein

UEPC	
	1 Flax
	½ Fruits & Vegetables
	1½ Grains

Revised

Cranberry Orange Muffins

WHAT THE HECK DO I DO WITH THE LEFTOVER ORANGE?
Eat it. If it was a large orange, count it as two fruit servings. It all adds up.

WHERE DO I FIND DRIED CRANBERRIES?
Dried fruit, especially dried cranberries, are becoming more and more popular. Dried fruit is found in the fresh fruit produce section. I guess it makes sense, but I've always thought they should be in the baking section.

KID FRIENDLY TIP
Make the Banana Chocolate Chip Muffins. You eat the Cranberry Orange; they eat the Banana Chocolate Chip. It's a win-win situation. Or better yet, teach them how to make the Banana Chocolate Chip Muffins.

ONE SERVING	230 Calories
	6 g Total Fat
	0.5 g Sat Fat
	0 g Trans Fat
	170 mg Sodium
	45 g CHO
	6 g Fibre
	6 g Protein
UEPC	1 Flax
	½ Fruits & Vegetables
	1½ Grains

Food has the sensory power to conjure up memories. Cranberries are one of those foods for me. My dear friend, confidante, and pseudo mother, Nina Roberts, made me cranberry walnut tarts every Christmas. There would be a knock on my front door, and there she'd be with my Christmas treat.

Nina passed away in 2006 at 91 and I'll miss her forever. But every time I have cranberries, I think of her spirit of laughter, sense of fun, and how lucky I was to have my personal fairy godmother.

Wet Ingredients
1 cup (250 mL) **oat bran**
1 **omega-3 egg**
1¼ cups (310 mL) **buttermilk**
1 cup (250 mL) **dark brown sugar**

Dry Ingredients
1 cup (250 mL) **whole wheat flour**
¾ cup (175 mL) **ground flaxseed**
¼ cup (60 mL) **walnuts, coarsely chopped**
1 tsp (5 mL) **baking powder**
1 tsp (5 mL) **baking soda**
2 Tbsp (30 mL) **cinnamon**
1 cup (250 mL) **dried cranberries**
1 cup (250 mL) **fresh or frozen whole cranberries**
zest of 1 **large orange**

1   Preheat the oven to 400°F (200°C.) Line a muffin pan with paper cup liners.

2   In a large bowl, mix together all the wet ingredients.

3   In a medium bowl, using a wire whisk or fork, mix together all the whole wheat flour, ground flaxseed, walnuts, baking powder, baking soda, and cinnamon. Add the dried cranberries, whole cranberries, and the orange zest.

4   Add the dry ingredients to the wet ingredients and mix until combined.

5   Scoop into muffin cups. Bake for 20 to 25 minutes or until done.

Makes 12 servings.

Kid Friendly

Pumpkin Chocolate Chip Muffins

Pumpkin and chocolate? You've got to be kidding. Nope, it isn't a misprint. Chocolate can make just about anything taste better, except mixed with garlic. Pumpkin is one of those foods we need to eat more often, so here's another muffin recipe that uses this nutritious ingredient. This time you can actually taste the pumpkin, as opposed to the Double Chocolate Muffins on page 283.

BIG COOKING TIP
All-Bran Buds is a cereal made by Kellogg's. It's made with psyllium fibre and has 19.5 grams of fibre per ½ cup (125 mL). Don't substitute. Nothing else works—trust me.

Wet Ingredients
1 cup (250 mL) **buttermilk**
1 cup (250 mL) **pure pumpkin purée**
1 cup (250 mL) **dark brown sugar**
1 **omega-3 egg**
½ cup (125 mL) **Kellogg's All-Bran Buds cereal (see sidebar)**

Dry Ingredients
1¼ cups (310 mL) **whole wheat flour**
½ cup (125 mL) **wheat bran**
¾ cup (175 mL) **ground flaxseed**
2 Tbsp (30 mL) **wheat germ**
2 Tbsp (30 mL) **cinnamon**
1½ tsp (7 mL) **baking powder**
1 tsp (5 mL) **baking soda**
¼ cup (60 mL) **chopped dark chocolate, M&M's baking bits, or mini chocolate chips**

1 Preheat the oven to 400°F (200°C). Line a muffin pan with paper cup liners.

2 In a large bowl, mix together all of the wet ingredients. Let sit for 5 minutes.

3 In a medium bowl, using a wire whisk or fork, mix together all of the dry ingredients.

4 Add the wet ingredients to the dry ingredients and mix until combined.

5 Scoop into muffin cups. Bake for 20 to 25 minutes or until done.

Makes 12 servings.

Kid Friendly

ONE SERVING	200 Calories
	6 g Total Fat
	1 g Sat Fat
	0 g Trans Fat
	200 mg Sodium
	41 g CHO
	8 g Fibre
	6 g Protein
UEPC	1 Flax
	1½ Grains

Classic Favourite

Whole Wheat Blueberry Buttermilk Pancakes

When my son was in primary school, I'd go in and make pancakes for the kids on Shrove Tuesday, or as some people call it, Pancake Tuesday. Every kid ate them with great enthusiasm. Some kids even asked for the recipe to bring home to their parents. My son is in high school now and would die a million deaths if I showed up to make pancakes for his homeroom. But he'll eat them everyday for breakfast if I make them.

Dry Ingredients
1 cup (250 mL) **whole wheat flour**
½ cup (125 mL) **wheat germ**
1 Tbsp (15 mL) **granulated sugar**
1 tsp (5 mL) **baking soda**
1 tsp (5 mL) **baking powder**
1 Tbsp (15 mL) **cinnamon**

Wet Ingredients
1 **omega-3 egg**
1 Tbsp + 1 tsp (20 mL) **canola oil**
1½ cups (375 mL) **buttermilk**
1 cup (250 mL) **wild blueberries, fresh or frozen**

1 Preheat the oven to warm at 200°F (95°C).

2 In a large bowl, using a wire whisk or fork, mix together all of the dry ingredients.

3 In a medium bowl, mix together all of the wet ingredients.

4 Pour the wet ingredients into the dry ingredients and stir until just mixed. Add the blueberries and combine gently.

5 Heat a large skillet over medium heat. Lightly spray the skillet with canola oil, or add ¼ tsp (1 mL) canola oil to the pan and wipe with a paper towel. If the skillet looks dry while cooking, wipe it again with the same paper towel.

6 Drop pancake batter onto the pan and cook until the underside is golden brown. Flip and cook until done. Place cooked pancakes on an ovenproof dish and put in the pre-warmed oven. Cook remaining pancakes.

7 Serve with real or light maple syrup.

Makes 16 medium pancakes. Serves 4.

Kid Friendly

ONE SERVING	300 Calories
	9 g Total Fat
	1.5 g Sat Fat
	0 g Trans Fat
	500 mg Sodium
	45 g CHO
	7 g Fibre
	13 g Protein
UEPC	1 Fat
	½ Fruits & Vegetables
	3 Grains

Mairlyn's Pancake Mix

Instead of measuring all the ingredients every time you have a pancake attack, make this dry mix once and have enough for six recipes.

Following the Pancake Mix recipe are three pancake recipes. They taste great, are easy to make, and are healthier than anything out there. I'm going to have to put a patent on this one.

3½ cups (875 mL) **whole wheat flour**
2½ cups (625 mL) **ground flaxseed**
1½ cup (375 mL) **quick cooking oats**
1 cup (250 mL) **skim milk powder**
½ cup (125 mL) **ground cinnamon**
2 Tbsp (30 mL) **baking powder**
1 tsp (5 mL) **baking soda**

1   In a large bowl, using a wire whisk or a fork, mix together all the ingredients until well combined. Store in the fridge or freezer in a 12-cup (3-L) covered container, or in a resealable plastic bag. Keeps up to 1 month in the fridge and up to 3 months in the freezer.

Makes 9 cups, enough for 6 pancake recipes.

Kid Friendly

WHAT THE HECK AM I GOING TO DO WITH THE LEFTOVER SKIM MILK POWDER?
Check out the Frozen Cocoa recipe on page 270.

BIG COOKING TIP
This recipe is great to take to the cottage or cabin. Pre-measure Mairlyn's Pancake Mix into small resealable plastic bags. Add the egg, milk, and oil when you make them.

CAMPING TRIP?
Pack the pre-measured dry mix and just add 1¼ cups (310 mL) water to make a batter.

Recipes Using Mairlyn's Pancake Mix

Banana Pancakes

1 **omega-3 egg**
1 cup (250 mL) **skim milk**
1 Tbsp (15 mL) **canola oil**
1 **ripe mashed banana**
1½ cups (375 mL) **Mairlyn's Pancake Mix**
2 Tbsp (30 mL) **chopped dark chocolate or mini chocolate chips (optional)**

1   Preheat the oven to warm at 200°F (95°C).

2   In a medium bowl, beat together the egg, milk, and oil. Add the mashed banana.

3   Shake or whisk the pancake mix. Measure out and add to the banana mixture. Add chocolate (if using) and stir until well combined.

4   Heat a medium frying pan over medium heat. Lightly spray with canola oil, or add ¼ tsp (1 mL) canola oil to the pan and wipe with a paper towel. If the pan looks dry while cooking, wipe it again with the same paper towel.

5   Drop pancake batter onto the frying pan and cook until the underside is golden brown. Flip and cook until done. Place cooked pancakes on an ovenproof dish and put in the pre-warmed oven. Cook remaining pancakes.

6   Serve with real or light maple syrup.

Makes 12 medium pancakes. Serves 4.

Kid Friendly

ONE SERVING without chocolate	250 Calories
	11 g Total Fat
	0.5 g Sat Fat
	0 g Trans Fat
	200 mg Sodium
	35 g CHO
	7 g Fibre
	12 g Protein
UEPC	¾ Fat
	1 Grains
	1 Flax

Recipes Using Mairlyn's Pancake Mix (cont'd)

Blueberry Pancakes

1 omega-3 egg
1 cup (250 mL) **skim milk**
1 Tbsp (15 mL) **canola oil**
1½ cups (375 mL) **Mairlyn's Pancake Mix**
1 cup (250 mL) **wild blueberries, fresh or frozen**

1 Preheat the oven to warm at 200°F (95°C).

2 In a medium bowl, beat together the egg, milk, and oil.

3 Shake or whisk the pancake mix. Measure out and add to the milk/egg mixture. Stir until well combined. Lightly fold in the blueberries.

4 Heat a medium frying pan over medium heat. Lightly spray with canola oil, or add ¼ tsp (1 mL) canola oil to the pan and wipe with a paper towel. If the pan looks dry while cooking, wipe it again with the same paper towel.

5 Drop pancake batter onto the frying pan and cook until the underside is golden brown. Flip and cook until done. Place the cooked pancakes on an ovenproof dish and put in the pre-warmed oven. Cook remaining pancakes.

6 Serve with real or light maple syrup.

Makes 12 medium pancakes. Serves 4.

Kid Friendly

ONE SERVING	250 Calories
	11 g Total Fat
	0.5 g Sat Fat
	0 g Trans Fat
	200 mg Sodium
	33 g CHO
	7 g Fibre
	12 g Protein

UEPC	¾ Fat
	¼ Fruits & Vegetables
	1 Grains
	1 Flax

Apple Pancakes

1 **omega-3 egg**
1 cup (250 mL) **skim milk**
1 Tbsp (15 mL) **canola oil**
1 **large apple, grated (peel on)**
1½ cups (375 mL) **Mairlyn's Pancake Mix**

1   Preheat the oven to warm at 200°F (95°C).

2   In a medium bowl, beat together the egg, milk, and oil. Add the grated apple or grate the apple right into the bowl.

3   Shake or whisk the pre-made pancake mix. Measure out and add to the apple mixture. Stir until well combined.

4   Heat a medium frying pan over medium heat. Lightly spray with canola oil, or add ¼ tsp (1 mL) canola oil to the pan and wipe with a paper towel. If the pan looks dry while cooking, wipe it again with the same paper towel.

5   Drop pancake batter onto the frying pan and cook until the underside is golden brown. Flip and cook until done. Place cooked pancakes on an ovenproof dish and put in the pre-warmed oven. Cook remaining pancakes.

6   Serve with real or light maple syrup. Tastes great with applesauce as well.

Makes 12 medium pancakes. Serves 4.

Kid Friendly

ONE SERVING	260 Calories
	11 g Total Fat
	0.5 g Sat Fat
	0 g Trans Fat
	200 mg Sodium
	36 g CHO
	8 g Fibre
	12 g Protein
UEPC	¾ Fat
	1 Grains
	1 Flax

Overnight Oats

When my brother and I were kids, my mom made us oatmeal for breakfast in the winter. She'd serve it in wide soup bowls. My brother John would create a river system in his bowl, complete with tributaries. He'd pour the milk on top and use brown sugar as dams. Big surprise that he taught high school geography for years. You never know where playing with your food can lead.

4 cups (1 L) water
1 cup (250 mL) Steel Cut Oats, sometimes called either Irish Oats or 8 grain cereal

1 Pour water into a medium pot. Turn heat to high.

2 When the water boils, sprinkle in the oats and stir. Cover and remove from the heat. Let cool for 1 hour and then pour into a container. Cover and place in the fridge overnight.

3 The next morning remove from the fridge, pour into a pot over medium-high heat, and bring back to a boil. Cover and reduce heat to medium. Simmer for 5 to 8 minutes, stirring occasionally, until heated through.

4 Want some pizzazz? See Build a Better Bowl, page 293.

Makes 4 cups (1 L). Serves 4.

ONE SERVING	150 Calories
	3 g Total Fat
	0 g Sat Fat
	0 g Trans Fat
	0 mg Sodium
	27 g CHO
	4 g Fibre
	5 g Protein
UEPC	1¼ Grains

Build a Better Bowl

WANT YOUR DRIED FRUIT TO BE JUICIER?

Add your favourite dried fruit to the pot in the morning before you bring the Overnight Oats to a boil.

OTHER TOPPING IDEAS

» Sprinkle 2 Tbsp (30 mL) ground or chopped walnuts over the top and add a splash of maple syrup.
» 1 chopped banana with ¼ tsp (1 mL) cinnamon
» ¼ cup (60 mL) unsweetened applesauce and ¼ tsp (1 mL) cinnamon
» Grate one apple, peel on, and sprinkle with ¼ tsp (1 mL) cinnamon.

These toppings are for 1 bowl.

1 Add ¼ cup (60 mL) dried fruit, such as cranberries, currants, raisins, mango, apricots, or blueberries. Go wild and add a combo of your favourite. See the sidebar.

2 Add ½ to 1 cup (125 to 250 mL) skim milk or low-fat soy milk.

3 Sprinkle with 1 to 2 Tbsp (15 to 30 mL) ground flaxseed.

4 Sprinkle with ¼ to ½ tsp (1 to 2 mL) cinnamon.

5 If you need a little sweetness, add 1 tsp (5 mL) brown sugar or maple syrup.

Classic Favourite

French Toast

This was one of the first things I taught my son to cook. It requires him to follow directions, measure, beat, cook over heat, and use the oven. Once a Home Ec teacher, always a Home Ec teacher.

Aside from Andrew gaining confidence in the kitchen, I've also guaranteed myself a great breakfast in bed on Mother's Day and my birthday. One year I even got scrambled eggs. The woman Andrew decides to spend his life with is going to be one lucky lady.

4 **omega-3 eggs**
1 cup (250 mL) **skim or soy milk**
2 tsp (10 mL) **cinnamon**
1 tsp (5 mL) **pure vanilla extract**
8 **slices 100% whole wheat bread**

1   Warm the oven at 200°F (95°C).

2   In a shallow dish, beat together the eggs, milk, cinnamon, and vanilla.

3   Heat a large frying pan over medium heat.

4   Soak the bread in the egg mixture, one slice at a time. Lightly spray the pan with canola oil. Cook each slice of bread over medium heat until done on both sides. Keep the cooked ones in the pre-warmed oven until all the slices are cooked.

5   Serve with light or regular maple syrup.

Makes 4 servings.

Kid Friendly

DO I USE SKIM MILK OR SOY MILK?
The choice is yours. This recipe is great if you're trying to add soy to your diet. You won't be able to tell the difference between French toast made with regular milk or soy milk. My son's best friend, who is a very picky eater, couldn't tell. And if Andrew D. can't tell, no one can.

100% WHOLE WHEAT BREAD
Is your family whole wheat challenged? This recipe is a great way to introduce a new ingredient. Aside from being one of the wonderful whole grain foods Liz talks about in the grain chapter, whole wheat bread has more flavour than white bread. Even my son's whole wheat challenged friend—yes, Andrew D.— gobbles it up when I serve it.

PURE VANILLA EXTRACT
If you don't have the pure stuff, don't even think of using the artificial. Back away from the cupboard. Write a note to buy some of the genuine stuff the next time you're out shopping. Note to self: throw that fake stuff out. It just doesn't taste like the real thing.

ONE SERVING	240 Calories
	7 g Total Fat
	1.5 g Sat Fat
	0 g Trans Fat
	220 mg Sodium
	33 g CHO
	4 g Fibre
	14 g Protein
UEPC	1 Egg
	2 Grains
	¼ Milk

COOKIES & TREATS

Cookie Rules

RULE #1

Baking is a science, so you need to measure accurately. Don't go guessing how much flour or baking powder to add. Measure it out. Measure whole wheat flour by spooning the flour into a dry measuring cup (those are the ones you can't see through, either made of metal or plastic). Then level it off with a metal spatula or the flat edge of a knife. The same levelling technique applies to baking powder and baking soda.

RULE #2

The kind of fat you use really makes a difference.

I love unsalted, non-hydrogenated margarine for baking—and I think you'll enjoy it if you're an unsalted butter lover. All of the cookie recipes in this book can be made with salted or unsalted non-hydrogenated margarine.

RULE #3

Granulated sugar means white sugar, not icing sugar

RULE #4

Must-Have Kitchen Toys
Take a tip from the pros and use a mini ice cream scoop with a release button when measuring out cookie dough. They're one of my best kitchen toys. It makes cookies and mini muffins the same size and the same calories. The scoops come in different sizes. It's best to have a 1 teaspoon (5 mL) size, which is perfect for all the cookies in this book, except the Big Breakfast Cookie, which uses a ¼-cup (60-mL) scoop.

RULE #5

All cookie sheets aren't the same. Some are insulated, some aren't. I baked all the cookies in this chapter on insulated cookie sheets. If you don't have an insulated cookie sheet, don't panic. Use what you have and reduce the baking time: your cookies will bake faster. Decrease time by 3 to 7 minutes.

RULE #6

I don't like to wash dishes, so I use parchment paper on my cookie sheets. It's slippery, so be careful when you throw those cookie sheets into the oven. A warning from a person who's been there, done that: the cookies will slide off if you aren't careful. And cookies don't taste great after you've scraped them off the bottom of an oven. Been there, done that.

RULE #7

Cool them on the cookie sheet before putting them on a cooling rack. They're a lot easier to remove once they've set.

RULE #8

Store cookies in an airtight container for up to 1 week, or freeze them for up to 3 months.

New

Cocoa Crisps

Theobroma cacao, or chocolate as we mere mortals refer to the Food of the Gods, originated in the Amazon basin, revered by the Mayans. They used the beans from the chocolate trees as currency. According to a 16th-century Spanish chronicle, a rabbit was worth 10 cocoa beans and a mule cost 50 beans. I'd say that your typical run-of-the-mill rabbit is probably worth about a wheelbarrow of cocoa beans in today's inflated market. Makes you wonder how much a car would be.

¼ cup + 2 Tbsp (90 mL) **canola oil**
¾ cup (175 mL) **dark brown sugar**
¼ cup (60 mL) **granulated sugar**
1 **omega-3 egg**
1 tsp (5 mL) **pure vanilla extract**
1 cup (250 mL) **whole wheat flour**
¼ tsp (1 mL) **baking soda**
½ cup (125 mL) **natural cocoa powder**

1   Preheat the oven to 375°F (190°C). Line a cookie sheet with parchment paper.

2   In a medium mixing bowl, beat together the canola oil, brown sugar, granulated sugar, eggs, and vanilla for 3 minutes.

3   In a medium bowl, stir the flour, baking soda, and cocoa together with a whisk. Add to the canola oil mixture. Blend for 1 minute or until well incorporated.

4   Drop by teaspoonfull onto the lined cookie sheet, or use that 1 tsp (5 mL) mini scoop. Press down gently on the cookies. Bake for 13 to 15 minutes or until the outside looks crunchy. See Cookie Rules on page 296 Rule #5. Remove from the oven. Let them cool for 3 minutes, then remove from the cookie sheet. Let them cool the rest of the way on a wire rack.

Makes 44 cookies. 1 serving = 2 cookies.

Kid Friendly

ONE SERVING	
	100 Calories
	6 g Total Fat
	0 g Sat Fat
	0 g Trans Fat
	20 mg Sodium
	15 g CHO
	1 g Fibre
	1 g Protein
UEPC	1 Fat

Chewy Chocolate Chip Cookies

For 99.9% of women worldwide, chocolate can be the difference between losing your mind and just losing your cool. Yes, on a really bad day there's nothing like that hit of decadent dark chocolate. In a pinch, even not so decadent chocolate will do. I've been known on occasion to wolf down a handful of chocolate chips while standing in front of the open pantry. A girl's gotta do what a girl's gotta do.

½ cup (125 mL) **unsalted non-hydrogenated margarine**
½ cup (125 mL) **dark brown sugar**
¼ cup (60 mL) **granulated sugar**
1 **omega-3 egg**
1 tsp (5 mL) **pure vanilla extract**
1¼ cups (310 mL) **whole wheat flour**
½ tsp (2 mL) **baking soda**
¼ cup (60 mL) **chopped dark bittersweet chocolate or M&M's baking bits**

1   Preheat the oven to 375°F (190°C). Line a cookie sheet with parchment paper.

2   In a medium bowl, cream the margarine. Beat in the brown and granulated sugars until fluffy.

3   Add the egg and vanilla. Beat until fluffy.

4   Stir in the whole wheat flour, baking soda, and chocolate.

5   Drop by rounded teaspoonful onto the cookie sheet, or use that 1 tsp (5 mL) mini scoop.

6   Bake for 10 to 12 minutes. See Cookie Rules on page 296 Rule #5. Cool slightly before removing from the cookie sheet.

Makes 40 cookies. 1 serving = 2 cookies.

Kid Friendly

BIG COOKING TIP
If you want crispy and sweet cookies, add another ¼ cup (60 mL) each of granulated sugar and whole wheat flour.

ONE SERVING	110 Calories
	6 g Total Fat
	0.6 g Sat Fat
	35 mg Sodium
	15 g CHO
	1 g Fibre
	1 g Protein
UEPC	1 Fat

Peanut Butter Cookies

If it wasn't for George Washington Carver, an African-American educator, botanist, and scientist from Alabama's Tuskegee Institute, we'd never munch on peanut butter cookies. The cotton crops in the southern United States had been attacked by the boll weevil, and Carver promoted peanuts as an alternative crop. Once again, you just never know when something good comes from something not so good. Thanks, you nasty old boll weevil you.

½ cup (125 mL) **unsalted non-hydrogenated margarine**
½ cup (125 mL) **smooth or crunchy natural peanut butter**
1 cup (250 mL) **dark brown sugar**
1 **omega-3 egg**
½ tsp (2 mL) **pure vanilla extract**
1 Tbsp (15 mL) **water**
1¼ cup (310 mL) **whole wheat flour**
½ tsp (2 ml) **baking soda**
½ tsp (2 mL) **cinnamon** ·
¼ cup (60 mL) **M&M's baking bits or chopped bittersweet chocolate (optional)**

1 Preheat the oven to 350°F (180°C). Line a baking sheet with parchment paper.

2 In a medium bowl, cream together the non-hydrogenated margarine and the peanut butter. Beat in the brown sugar.

3 Add the egg, vanilla, and water. Beat until creamy.

4 Stir together the whole wheat flour, baking soda, and cinnamon. Stir into the peanut butter mixture. Stir in M&M's or chocolate chunks, if you're using them.

5 Drop onto the lined cookie sheet by teaspoonfuls, or use that 1 tsp (5 mL) mini scoop.

6 Bake for 10 to 12 minutes. See Cookie Rules on page 296 Rule #5. Cool slightly before removing from the cookie sheet. Let them cool the rest of the way on a wire rack.

Makes 48 cookies. 1 serving = 2 cookies.

Kid Friendly

ONE SERVING without chocolate	135 Calories
	7.5 g Total Fat
	1 g Sat Fat
	0 g Trans Fat
	35 mg Sodium
	16 g CHO
	1 g Fibre
	2 g Protein
UEPC	1 Fat

Oatmeal Raisin Cookies

This will make 50 cookies, if and only if you use no more than 1 teaspoonful (5 mL) of batter per cookie. Just another great reason to buy that mini scoop I keep harping about. See page 296. Remember that no matter what they say, size does matter. Always has, always will.

½ cup (125 mL) **unsalted non-hydrogenated margarine**
½ cup (125 mL) **dark brown sugar**
¼ cup (60 mL) **granulated sugar**
1 **omega-3 egg**
2 Tbsp (30 mL) **water**
½ tsp (2 mL) **pure vanilla extract**
1¼ cups (310 mL) **whole wheat flour**
1¼ cups (310 mL) **rolled oats, old fashioned or large flake**
2 tsp (10 mL) **cinnamon**
½ tsp (2 mL) **baking soda**
¾ cup (175 mL) **raisins**

1   Preheat the oven to 375°F (190°C). Line a cookie sheet with parchment paper.

2   In a medium bowl, cream the margarine. Beat in the white and brown sugars until fluffy.

3   Add the egg, water, and vanilla. Beat until creamy.

4   Add the whole wheat flour, rolled oats, baking soda, and cinnamon. Mix until combined. Stir in the raisins.

5   Drop by rounded teaspoonful (5 mL) onto the cookie sheet or use that 1 tsp (5 mL) mini scoop.

6   Bake for 12 to 14 minutes. See Cookie Rules on page 296 Rule #5. Cool slightly before removing them from the cookie sheet. Let them cool the rest of the way on a wire rack, if you can wait that long.

Makes 50 cookies. 1 serving = 2 cookies.

Kid Friendly

ROLLED OATS

When you wander through the cereal aisle looking for oats, make sure you buy the kind your recipe calls for. Oats come in many different forms. There are instant, quick-cooking, and rolled oats. The rolled oats are sometimes called old fashioned oats or large flake oats. If that isn't confusing enough, there are also different varieties such as Irish oats or steel cut oats and Scotch oats. So don't grab the first package you see. These cookies use the old fashioned or large flake type. I always say, do your homework. Read the label and buy the right one.

ONE SERVING	115 Calories
	4.5 g Total Fat
	0 g Sat Fat
	0 g Trans Fat
	30 mg Sodium
	18 g CHO
	1 g Fibre
	2 g Protein
UEPC	1 Fat

New

Snappy Gingersnaps

CHOCOLATE LOVERS
Go ahead and add ¼ cup
(60 mL) chopped dark
bittersweet chocolate, M&M's
baking bits, or mini chocolate
chips at the same time you add
the flour.

I've always baked gingersnaps for Christmas. Several years ago when my dad had open-heart surgery, I changed his favourite gingersnap recipe into one made with a heart healthy fat. If you're a real ginger lover, try adding ¼ cup (60 mL) diced candied ginger.

½ cup (125 mL) **canola oil**
1¼ cup (310 mL) **granulated sugar**
¼ cup (60 mL) **molasses**
1 **omega-3 egg**
1¾ cup (425 mL) **whole wheat flour**
1 tsp (5 mL) **baking soda**
1 tsp (5 mL) **baking powder**
2 tsp (10 mL) **ground ginger**
1 Tbsp (15 mL) **ground cinnamon**

1 Preheat the oven to 375°F (190°C). Line a cookie sheet with parchment paper.

2 In a large mixing bowl, beat together the oil and 1 cup (250 mL) of the sugar. Reserve ¼ cup (60 mL).

3 Add the molasses and egg. Beat until fluffy.

4 Stir in the flour, baking soda, baking powder, ginger, and cinnamon until the dough becomes stiff.

5 Scoop out teaspoonfuls and roll in the reserved sugar. Press down lightly on the cookies to flatten them slightly.

6 Bake for 12 to 15 minutes or until golden brown. See Cookie Rules on page 296 Rule #5. Let them cool on the cookie sheet for 1 minute, then remove and let them cool the rest of the way on a wire rack.

Makes 36 cookies. 1 serving = 2 cookies.

Kid Friendly

ONE SERVING	160 Calories
	7 g Total Fat
	0.5 g Sat Fat
	0 g Trans Fat
	90 mg Sodium
	25 g CHO
	1 g Fibre
	2 g Protein
UEPC	1 Fat

Big Breakfast Cookies
A Snack'n Powerhouse

My fabulous friend Jann and I meet at Starbucks several times a month to solve the world's problems. We do this over non-fat decaf lattes and huge soft cookies. I have no idea what the Starbuck's recipe is, but after many attempts, I've created a big, healthy, delicious cookie that Starbuck's would kill for. Calorie watchers—better sit down for this one—Starbuck's big fat cookie is over 500 calories. Mine is only 160 calories. And to make things even better, my cookies have 4 g of fibre each.

2 cups (500 mL) **large flake rolled oats**
2 cups (500 mL) **whole wheat flour**
½ cup (125 mL) **oat bran**
½ cup (125 mL) **ground flaxseed**
2 cups (500 mL) **dried cranberries**
2 Tbsp (30 mL) **cinnamon**
1 tsp (5 mL) **baking soda**
½ cup (125 mL) **dark brown sugar**
2 **omega-3 eggs**
¼ cup (60 mL) **canola oil**
one 4.5-oz (128-mL) **jar baby food strained prunes**
2 tsp (10 mL) **pure vanilla extract**

ONE SERVING	160 Calories
	4.5 g Total Fat
	0 g Sat Fat
	0 g Trans Fat
	60 mg Sodium
	29 g CHO
	4 g Fibre
	4 g Protein
UEPC	½ Fat
	1 Grain

TIP

These cookies are great as a snack or breakfast on the run. Pack milk and a handful of nuts, and you're good to go.

1 Preheat the oven to 375°F (190°C). Line a cookie sheet with parchment paper.

2 In a large bowl, mix together the oats, flour, oat bran, flaxseed, dried cranberries, cinnamon, and baking soda.

3 In a medium bowl, whisk together the brown sugar, eggs, canola oil, prunes, and vanilla extract.

4 Add this to the dry ingredients and stir until well combined. You can use a stand mixer if you like, but all those muscles working to mix the batter burns calories. Who says baking can't be good for you?

5 Drop the batter onto the cookie sheet using either a ¼ cup (60 mL) measuring cup or ¼ cup (60 mL) ice cream scoop. Gently press down on the cookies so they're ⅛ inch (3 mm) thick. If it's too sticky, lightly dampen your hands, then press down.

6 Bake for 15 to 18 minutes. See Cookie Rules on page 296 Rule #5. Remove the cookies from the oven. Let them sit on the cookie sheet for 5 minutes to set. Gently move the cookies to a cooling rack. Let them cool completely and then store in an airtight container for up to 1 week. Or separate, bag, and freeze them for up to 3 months. They'll be ready to pop into your briefcase or purse on the way out the door.

Makes 24 really big cookies. 1 serving = 1 really big cookie.

Super Snackers

If you loved those white rice marshmallow squares your mom made when you were seven, you're going to take one look at these and say, "What the heck are all those healthy nuts, dried fruit, and whole grains doing in there?"

Well, big surprise. I upped the ante. You can treat yourself to these babies and know you're getting a whole lot of goodness. It's a grand slam super snacker that tastes spectacular.

2 Tbsp (30 mL) **unsalted non-hydrogenated margarine**
40 **large marshmallows**
4 cups (1 L) **whole grain bran flakes**
⅔ cup (150 mL) **Kellogg's All-Bran Buds**
½ cup (125 mL) **chopped almonds**
½ cup (125 mL) **unsalted peanuts**
½ cup (125 mL) **chopped dried apricots**
¼ cup (60 mL) **chopped dark bittersweet chocolate**

1   Line an 8-inch (2-L) pan with parchment paper. Set aside.

2   In a large pot, stir the margarine and the marshmallows over low heat until melted. Remove from heat.

3   Add the bran flakes, All-Bran Buds, almonds, peanuts, and dried apricots. Stir until combined.

4   Stir in the chocolate quickly (you don't want it to melt).

5   Spoon the mixture into the pan. Dampen hands and press the mixture into the pan. Let it cool completely before cutting. If you're in a hurry, pop the pan into the fridge for 30 minutes.

6   Cut into 16 bars. Cover and store at room temperature for up to 4 days.

Makes 16 bars.

Kid Friendly

CHOPPING DRIED APRICOTS
It's a sticky mess at the best of times. Use kitchen scissors. They make the job go fast, and it's a great way to get your kids involved. "Hey kids, let's snip the apricots!" Boy, do I know how to entertain kids or what?

PEANUT AWARENESS
Lots of schools are now peanut-free zones. My son's school is, so I never pack these in his lunch, although we do eat them after school. If you or your child has an allergy to nuts, substitute ½ cup (125 mL) raisins for the peanuts and add an extra ½ cup (125 mL) of chopped dried apricots instead of the almonds.

MICROWAVE METHOD
Put the margarine and marshmallows into a large microwaveable bowl. Heat on medium-high (60%) for 1½ minutes. Remove from the microwave and stir until melted. If it isn't completely melted, heat and stir in 10-second increments. Add all the remaining ingredients, except the chocolate. Stir to combine, then add the chocolate. Follow the rest of the recipe method from step #5.

ONE SERVING	185 Calories
	6 g Total Fat
	1.2 g Sat Fat
	0 g Trans Fat
	115 mg Sodium
	32 g CHO
	5 g Fibre
	4 g Protein
UEPC	¼ Fat
	¼ Grains
	¼ Nuts

Revised

Old-Fashioned Date Squares

My mother raised my brother, sister, and I on power foods. We just didn't know it. As a matter of fact, neither did my mom.

Dates are a powerhouse of antioxidants and a must-have in this version of mom's 1950s date squares.

One ¾ lb (375 g) package **pitted dates, or 2 cups (500 mL) chopped dates**
1 cup (250 mL) **water**
zest of 1 **orange**
¼ cup (60 mL) **freshly squeezed orange juice**
1½ cups (375 mL) **whole wheat flour**
1½ cups (375 mL) **large flake rolled oats**
¾ cup (175 mL) **dark brown sugar**
1 Tbsp (15 mL) **ground cinnamon**
⅓ cup (75 mL) **canola oil**
½ cup (125 mL) **frozen orange juice concentrate, thawed**

1 In a medium saucepan, bring the dates and the water to a boil. Reduce the heat to low and stir until it becomes a thick paste. Remove from the heat.

2 Stir in the orange zest and the freshly squeezed orange juice. Set aside to cool.

3 Preheat the oven to 350°F (180°C). Line an 8-inch (2-L) metal pan with parchment paper.

4 In a medium bowl, mix together the flour, oats, brown sugar, and cinnamon.

5 In a small bowl, mix together the oil and the orange juice concentrate. Pour this into the flour mixture. Blend until the flour mixture looks wet. Pat half of this mixture into the bottom of the pan. Spread the date mixture on top. Spoon the rest of the flour mixture over the date mixture. Lightly press down.

6 Bake for 30 minutes. Cool completely before cutting it into 16 pieces.

Makes sixteen 2- × 2-inch (5- × 5-cm) pieces.

Kid Friendly

ONE SERVING	230 Calories
	6 g Total Fat
	0 g Sat Fat
	0 g Trans Fat
	5 mg Sodium
	46 g CHO
	4 g Fibre
	4 g Protein
UEPC	1 Fat
	½ Fruits & Vegetables
	½ Grains

Decadent Brownies

Way back in the late 1990s I came up with The Best Brownie Recipe ever. I even had the gall to call them Better Than Sex Brownies. I boasted that I'd rather eat a small piece of a fat-laden, artery cloggin' brownie than a large piece of a low-fat, tasteless brownie facsimile. Man oh man was I bold.

Now most decadent brownies get their decadence from chocolate. Lots of it.

I've come up with a decadent brownie that's lower in fat, uses whole wheat flour, and is made with (are you sitting down?) cocoa. Yes, high flavanol cocoa. This is an excellent time to review Liz's chapter Don't Forget the Chocolate. And here's the best part: it doesn't taste like a low-fat brownie made with whole wheat flour and cocoa. It tastes like a high-fat, artery cloggin' decadent brownie. Success is sweet.

⅓ cup (75 mL) **canola oil**
2 **omega-3 eggs**
1 cup (250 mL) **granulated sugar**
1 tsp (5 ml) **pure vanilla extract**
½ cup + 2 Tbsp (155 mL) **natural cocoa powder**
½ cup (125 mL) **whole wheat flour**
1 tsp (5 mL) **baking powder**

ONE SERVING	120 Calories
	8 g Total Fat
	0.5 g Sat Fat
	0 g Trans Fat
	25 mg Sodium
	17 g CHO
	1 g Fibre
	2 g Protein
UEPC	1 Fat

1 Preheat the oven to 325°F (160°C). Line an 8-inch (2-L) metal pan with parchment paper. Make sure to use enough parchment paper so that it hangs over the edges of your pan. You can thank me for this tip later when you lift the brownies out of the pan unscathed.

2 Beat together the oil and eggs. Add the sugar and beat until slightly thickened.

3 Add the vanilla and cocoa powder. Slowly beat in.

4 Stir in the whole wheat flour and baking powder. The batter will be fairly thick.

5 Spoon the batter into the prepared pan and gently spread.

6 Bake for 25 minutes. Let it cool in the pan for 10 minutes. Pick up the parchment paper at the sides and lift the brownie out. Finish cooling on a wire rack.

7 Cut into 16 equal pieces, not "here's a really big one for me and a teeny one for you." Store the leftovers in an airtight container for up to 2 days. Like they're going to last that long.

Makes sixteen 2- × 2-inch (5- × 5-cm) pieces. Serves 1 chocoholic and anyone with whom they choose to share.

Kid Friendly

The Ultimate Healthy Chocolate Treat

You know, sometimes you just luck out with a creation. This treat is really the ultimate as far as chocolate is concerned, and it tastes as good on the plate as it did in my imagination. These are so excellent, you may not be able to share. Not only are you getting the benefits of bittersweet chocolate, you're also getting a ton of fibre. Warning: since these have a ton of fibre in them—something not usually found in a treat—you may want to reconsider having more than one a day. You may not make it into work, although depending where you work, this may not be such a bad thing.

WHAT KIND OF WHOLE GRAIN CEREAL SHOULD I PICK?
Any whole grain flake will do. Or you can try Cheerios, Kellogg's All Bran Flakes, or Nature's Path Flax Plus Flakes.

½ lb (250 g) **dark bittersweet chocolate, chopped into ½-inch (1-cm) chunks**
1½ cups (375 mL) **whole grain cereal**
2 cups (500 mL) **Kellogg's All Bran Buds**

1 Line a 9- × 13-inch (3.5-L) pan with parchment paper. Set aside.

2 Melt the chocolate in a metal bowl over gently simmering water. Remove from the heat just as it starts to melt. Continue to stir until completely melted and cool to the touch.

3 Mix the cereals in a large bowl. Pour in the melted chocolate. Stir gently until combined.

4 Spread evenly into the pan. Let it sit for 20 minutes or until set.

5 Cut into 16 pieces. This is a tad tricky. Good luck. Store in an airtight container for up to 1 week.

Makes 16 pieces. 1 piece per serving.

Kid Friendly

ONE SERVING	130 Calories
	6 g Total Fat
	3 g Sat Fat
	0 g Trans Fat
	75 mg Sodium
	21 g CHO
	7 g Fibre
	2 g Protein
UEPC	½ Grain

New

Creamy Rice Pudding

BIG COOKING TIP
BIG COOKING TIP
You can find short-grain brown rice in any health food store or in most large grocery stores in the health food section. Don't substitute long-grain brown rice. Short-grain tends to be stickier, which makes this rice pudding very creamy.

My Irish, Scottish, and English roots are showing with this recipe. Here's a healthy spin on me dear old mom's classic.

4 cups (1 L) **soy milk**
¾ cup (175 mL) **short-grain brown rice**
⅓ cup (75 mL) **dark brown sugar**
¼ cup (60 mL) **raisins**
¼ cup (60 mL) **dried cranberries**
1 tsp (5 mL) **cinnamon**

1 In a medium saucepan, stir together the soy milk and the rice. Bring the mixture to a boil and cover. Reduce the heat to medium-low and simmer. Stir occasionally. Cook until the rice is tender, approximately 60 minutes.

2 Once the rice is tender, remove from the heat and stir in the brown sugar, raisins, dried cranberries, and cinnamon. Stir until it becomes creamy. Cover and let it sit for 15 minutes.

3 Don't be tempted to skip the 15-minute time-out. This adds the creamy texture to the pudding. Stir once more and serve warm.

Makes 4 cups (1 L). Makes eight ½-cup (125-mL) servings.

ONE SERVING	170 Calories
	1.5 g Total Fat
	0 g Sat Fat
	0 g Trans Fat
	50 mg Sodium
	37 g CHO
	2 g Fibre
	4 g Protein
UEPC	½ Milk
	¼ Fruits & Vegetables

Revised

Don't Forget to Leave Room for Chocolate Cake

If this cake had been around when Marie Antoinette shrieked her famous, "Let them eat cake!" chances are the French Revolution would have been rewritten, depriving future musical theatre lovers of the *Les Miserables* experience.

1 cup (250 mL) **whole wheat flour**
⅔ cup (150 mL) **all-purpose flour**
1½ cups (375 mL) **granulated sugar**
⅔ cups (150 mL) **natural cocoa powder**
1½ tsp (7 mL) **baking soda**
¼ cup (60 mL) **canola oil**
1 cup (250 mL) **chocolate soy milk**
2 tsp (10 mL) **fresh lemon juice**
1 **omega-3 egg**
one 4.5-oz (128-mL) jar **baby food strained prunes, no added sugar or starch**
1 Tbsp (15 mL) **pure vanilla extract**

Icing
2 Tbsp (30 mL) **unsalted non-hydrogenated margarine**
1 oz (30 g) **unsweetened chocolate**
6 Tbsp (90 mL) **chocolate soy milk**
2½ cups (625 mL) **icing sugar**
⅓ cup (75 mL) **natural cocoa powder**

ONE SERVING	150 Calories
	4 g Total Fat
	0.5 g Sat Fat
	0 g Trans Fat
	75 mg Sodium
	29 g CHO
	1 g Fibre
	2 g Protein
UEPC	1 Fat

1. Preheat the oven to 350°F (180°C). Line a 9- × 13-inch (3.5-L) metal cake pan with parchment paper, or lightly spray with a canola oil cooking spray.

2. In a large bowl, mix together the whole wheat flour, all-purpose flour, granulated sugar, cocoa powder, and baking soda.

3. Add the oil, chocolate, soy milk, lemon juice, egg, prunes, and vanilla.

4. Blend the ingredients together for 1 minute using a hand-held mixer or wire whisk. Scrape the bowl often.

5. Turn the speed up to medium, or whisk like your life depends on it, and mix for another 2 minutes.

6. Pour into the prepared pan and bake for 30 to 35 minutes, or until a toothpick comes out clean.

7. Cool the pan on a wire rack for 10 minutes. Remove the cake from the pan and continue cooling on the rack.

8. Prepare icing. Put the margarine, unsweetened chocolate, and chocolate soy milk in a microwaveable dish. Heat on medium-low for 1 minute. Stir. Repeat until almost melted. Remove from the microwave and stir until completely melted. Alternately, melt the ingredients over the stove. The key is to under-do it. Scorched chocolate is ruined chocolate. In some countries this is considered a sin.

9. Pour this melted chocolate mixture into a medium bowl. Don't lick this yet—it's unsweetened. Add the icing sugar and cocoa powder. Beat until smooth. If it's too thick, add a little bit of chocolate soy milk until you reach your desired spreading consistency. Now you can lick the beaters.

10. Spread the icing on the cooled cake. Lick the bowl. The cake can be served immediately or the next day. Remember that tomorrow it will taste better. Your choice.

Serves 30. 1 Serving = one 2- × 2-inch (5- × 5-cm) square.

Kid Friendly

APPENDIX

Healthy Weight, Blood Pressure, and Blood Cholesterol Levels

How healthy are you? Use the guidelines below to see how well you rate. If you haven't had your blood pressure or blood cholesterol checked lately, do so the next time you visit your family doctor.

Healthy Blood Cholesterol Levels

LDL cholesterol
Less than 100 mg/dL (2.6 mmol/L)

Total cholesterol
Less than 200 mg/dL (5.2 mmol/L)

HDL cholesterol
Greater than 45 mg/dL (1.17 mmol) is acceptable. Equal to or greater than 60 mg/dL is optimal (1.56 mmol/L).

Triglyceride Levels
Less than 150 mg/dL (2.3 mmol/L) is normal.

Healthy Blood Pressure
Less than 120/80 mmHg is optimal.

High blood pressure is greater than or equal to 140/90 mmHg.

Waist Circumference
If you carry excess weight in your abdominal area, you're at higher risk of developing disease like diabetes and heart disease.

High risk for men is a waist greater than 40 inches (102 cm) around.

High risk for women is waist greater than 35 inches (88 cm) around.

Healthy Weight Guidelines

Early diagnosis of an unhealthy weight (also referred to as body mass index) can aid in the prevention of disease and provide advanced warning of health problems.

HEIGHT	HEALTHY WEIGHT	CAUTION ZONE	HEALTH RISK ZONE
4'11" (150 cm)	99–123 pounds	124–133 pounds	over 133 pounds
5' (153 cm)	102–127 pounds	128–138 pounds	over 138 pounds
5'1" (155 cm)	106–131 pounds	132–143 pounds	over 143 pounds
5'2" (158 cm)	109–135 pounds	136–147 pounds	over 147 pounds
5'3" (160 cm)	113–140 pounds	141–152 pounds	over 152 pounds
5'4" (163 cm)	116–144 pounds	145–157 pounds	over 157 pounds
5'5" (165 cm)	120–149 pounds	150–162 pounds	over 162 pounds
5'6" (168 cm)	124–154 pounds	155–167 pounds	over 167 pounds
5'7" (170 cm)	127–158 pounds	159–172 pounds	over 172 pounds
5'8" (173 cm)	131–163 pounds	164–177 pounds	over 177 pounds
5'9" (175 cm)	135–168 pounds	169–182 pounds	over 182 pounds
5'10" (178 cm)	139–173 pounds	174–188 pounds	over 188 pounds
5'11" (180 cm)	143–178 pounds	179–193 pounds	over 193 pounds
6' (183 cm)	147–183 pounds	184–199 pounds	over 199 pounds
6'1" (185 cm)	151–188 pounds	189–204 pounds	over 204 pounds
6'2" (188 cm)	155–193 pounds	194–210 pounds	over 210 pounds
6'3" (190 cm)	160–199 pounds	200–216 pounds	over 216 pounds

Note: To convert pounds to kilograms divide by 2.2.

This chart shouldn't be used to evaluate the weight of children, the frail elderly, serious bodybuilders, or pregnant or breast-feeding women. If your extra weight comes from muscle, not fat, you may have a high body mass index even though you're healthy.

BIBLIOGRAPHY

Good Fats, Bad Fats

Albert, C., et al. "Dietary alpha-linolenic acid intake and risk of sudden cardiac death and coronary heart disease." *Circulation* 112 (2005): 3232-3238

Ascherio, A., et al. "Dietary fat and risk of coronary heart disease in men: cohort follow up study in the United States." *British Medical Journal* 313 (1996): 84-90.

Asher, M., et al. "Intake of trans fatty acids and prevalence of childhood asthma and allergies in Europe. ISAAC Steering Committee." *Lancet* 353 (1999): 2040-2041.

Brown, M., et al. "Carotenoid bioavailability is higher from salads ingested with full-fat than with fat-reduced salad dressings as measured with electrochemical detection." *American Journal of Clinical Nutrition* 80 (2004): 396-403.

Colditz, G., et al. "The Nurses' Health Study: 20-Year Contribution to the Understanding of Health Among Women." *Journal of Women's Health* 6 (1997): 49-62.

Denke, M., et al. "Individual Cholesterol Variation in Response to a Margarine or Butter Based Diet." *Journal of the American Medical Association* 284 (2000): 2740-2747.

DeFilippis, A., and L. Sperling. "Understanding omega-3's." *American Heart Journal* 151 (2006): 564-570.

Hashim, Y., et al. "Components of olive oil and chemoprevention." *Nutrition Reviews* 63 (2005): 374-386.

Hu, F., et al. "Dietary intake of alpha-linolenic acid and risk of fatal ischemic heart disease among women." *American Journal of Clinical Nutrition* 69 (1999): 890-897.

Kaklamani, L., et al. "Dietary factors in relation to rheumatoid arthritis: a role for olive oil and cooked vegetables?" *American Journal of Clinical Nutrition* 71 (2000): 1010.

Lorgeril, M., et al. "Mediterranean alpha-linolenic acid-rich diet in secondary prevention of coronary heart disease." *Lancet* 343 (1994): 1454-1459.

Lorgeril, M., and P. Salen. "Alpha-linolenic acid and coronary heart disease." *Nutrition, Metabolism and Cardiovascular Diseases* 3 (2004): 162-169.

Lorgeril, M., et al. "Mediterranean Diet, Traditional Risk Factors, and the Rate of Cardiovascular Complications after Myocardial Infarction." *Circulation* 99 (1999): 779-785.

Mozaffarian, D. "Does alpha-linolenic acid intake reduce the risk of coronary heart disease? A review of the evidence." *Alternative Therapies in Health and Medicine* 11 (2005): 24-30.

Perona, J., et al. "The role of virgin olive oil components in the modulation of endothelial function." *Journal of Nutritional Biochemistry* 12 (2005): epub.

Ruano, J., et al. "Phenolic Content of Virgin Olive Oil Improves Ischemic Reactive Hyperemia in Hypercholesterolemic Patients." *Journal of the American College of Cardiology* 46 (2005): 1864-1868.

Stampfer, M., et al. "Primary Prevention of Coronary Heart Disease in Women Through Diet and Lifestyle." *New England Journal of Medicine* 343 (2000): 16-22.

Stender, S., and J. Dyerberg. "Influence of trans fatty acids on health." *Annals of Nutrition and Metabolism* 48 (2004): 61-66.

Williams, C., and G. Burdge. "Long-chain n-3 PUFA: plant v. marine sources." *The Proceedings of the Nutrition Society* 65 (2006): 42-50.

Woodside, J., and D. Kromhout. "Fatty acids and CHD." *The Proceedings of the Nutrition Society* 64 (2005): 554-564.

Phenomenal Fruits & Vegetables

Andres-Lacueva, C., et al. "Anthocyanins in aged blueberry-fed rats are found centrally and may enhance memory." *Nutritional Neuroscience* 8 (2005): 111-120.

Ard, J., et al. "One-year follow-up study of blood pressure and dietary patterns in dietary approaches to stop hypertension (DASH)-sodium participants." *American Journal of Hypertension* 17 (2004): 1156-1162.

Aviram, M., et al. "Pomegranate juice consumption for 3 years by patients with carotid artery stenosis reduces common carotid intima-media thickness, blood pressure and LDL oxidation." *Clinical Nutrition* 23 (2004): 423-433.

Dauchet, L., et al. "Fruit and vegetable consumption and risk of stroke: a meta-analysis of cohort studies." *Neurology* 65 (2005): 1193-1997.

Djousse, L., et al. "Fruit and vegetable consumption and LDL cholesterol: the National Heart, Lung, and Blood Institute Family Heart Study." *American Journal of Clinical Nutrition* 79 (2004): 213-217.

Giovannucci, E., et al. "A prospective study of tomato products, lycopene, and prostate cancer risk." *Journal of the National Cancer Institute* 94 (2002): 391-398.

Joseph, J., et al. "Blueberry supplementation enhances signaling and prevents behavioral deficits in an Alzheimer disease model." *Nutritional Neuroscience* 6 (2003): 153-162.

Key, T., "Diet, nutrition and the prevention of cancer." *Public Health Nutrition* (2004): 187-200.

Lau, F., et al. "The beneficial effects of fruit polyphenols on brain aging." *Neurobiology of Aging* 26 (2005): 128-132.

Liu, R., et al. "Apples prevent mammary tumors in rats." *Journal of Agriculture and Food Chemistry* 53 (2005): 2341-2343.

Loren, D., et al. "Maternal dietary supplementation with pomegranate juice is neuroprotective in an animal model of neonatal hypoxic-ischemic brain injury." *Pediatric Research* 57 (2005): 858-864.

Magkos, F., et al. "Organic food: buying more safety or just peace of mind? A critical review of the literature." *Critical Reviews in Food Science & Nutrition* 46 (2006): 23-56.

Malik, A., et al. "Pomegranate fruit juice for chemoprevention and chemotherapy of prostate cancer." *Proceedings of the National Academy of Science* 102 (2005): 14813-14818.

Neuhouser, M. "Dietary flavonoids and cancer risk: evidence from human population studies." *Nutrition & Cancer* 50 (2004): 1-7.

Nishino, H., et al. "Cancer prevention by phytochemicals." *Oncology* 69 (2005): S38-S40.

Piao, X., et al. "Protective effects of broccoli (Brassica oleracea) and its active components against radical-induced oxidative damage." *Journal of Nutritional Science and Vitaminology* 51 (2005): 142-147.

Rolls, B., et al. "What can intervention studies tell us about the relationship between fruit and vegetable consumption and weight management?" *Nutrition Reviews* 62 (2004): 1-17.

Sacks, F., et al. "A Dietary Approach to Prevent Hypertension: A Review of the Dietary Approaches to Stop Hypertension (DASH) Study." *Clinical Cardiology* 22 (1999): 6S-10S.

Sesso, H., et al. "Dietary Lycopene, Tomato-Based Food Products and Cardiovascular Disease in Women." *Journal of Nutrition* 133 (2003): 2336-2341.

Song, Y., et al. "Associations of dietary flavonoids with risk of type 2 diabetes, and markers of insulin resistance and systemic inflammation in women: a prospective study and cross-sectional analysis." *Journal of the American College of Nutrition* 24 (2005): 376-84.

Wang, Y., et al. "Dietary supplementation with blueberries, spinach, or spirulina reduces ischemic brain damage." *Experimental Neurology* 193 (2005): 75-84.

Wu, X., et al. "Lipophilic and hydrophilic antioxidant capacities of common foods in the United States." *Journal of Agriculture and Food Chemistry* 52 (2004): 4026-4037.

Zhang, Y., et al. "Vegetable-derived isothiocyanates: anti-proliferative activity and mechanism of action." *The Proceedings of the Nutrition Society* 65 (2006): 68-75.

Spice Up Your Life

Bengmark, S. "Curcumin, an atoxic antioxidant and natural NFkappaB, cyclooxygenase-2, lipooxygenase, and inducible nitric oxide synthase inhibitor: a shield against acute and chronic disease." *Journal of Parenteral and Enteral Nutrition* 30 (2006): 45-51.

Bray, G., et al. "A further subgroup analysis of the effects of the DASH diet and three dietary sodium levels on blood pressure: results of the DASH-Sodium Trial." *American Journal of Cardiology* 94 (2004): 222-227.

Campbell, F., and G. Collett. "Chemopreventive properties of curcumin." *Future Oncology* 1 (2005): 405-414.

Chu, Y., et al. "Antioxidant and antiproliferative activities of common vegetables." *Journal of Agriculture and Food Chemistry* 50 (2002): 6910-6916.

Dickinson, H., et al. "Lifestyle interventions to reduce raised blood pressure: a systematic review of randomized controlled trials." *Journal of Hypertension* 24 (2006): 215-233.

Dragland, S., et al. "Several culinary and medicinal herbs are important sources of dietary antioxidants." *Journal of Nutrition* 133 (2003): 1286-1290.

El-Bayoumy, K., et al. "Cancer chemoprevention by garlic and garlic-containing sulfur and selenium compounds." *Journal of Nutrition* 136 (2006): 864S-869S.

Herman-Antosiewicz, A., and S. Singh. "Signal transduction pathways leading to cell cycle arrest and apoptosis induction in cancer cells by Allium vegetable-derived organosulfur compounds: a review." *Mutation Research* 555 (2004): 121-131.

Khanum, F., et al. "Anticarcinogenic properties of garlic: a review." *Critical Reviews in Food Science and Nutrition* 44 (2004): 479-488.

Khan, A., et al. "Cinnamon Improves Glucose and Lipids of People with Type 2 Diabetes." *Diabetes Care* 26 (2003): 3215-3218.

Lai P., and Roy, J. "Antimicrobial and chemopreventive properties of herbs and spices." *Current Medicinal Chemistry* 11 (2004): 1451-1460.

Maheshwari, R. "Multiple biological activities of curcumin: a short review." *Life Sciences* 78 (2006): 2081-2087.

Mang, B., et al. "Effects of a cinnamon extract on plasma glucose, HbA, and serum lipids in diabetes mellitus type 2." *European Journal of Clinical Investigation* 36 (2006): 340-344.

Milner, J. "Preclinical perspectives on garlic and cancer." *Journal of Nutrition* 136 (2006): 827S-831S.

Ninfali, P., et al. "Antioxidant capacity of vegetables, spices and dressings relevant to nutrition." *British Journal of Nutrition* 93 (2005): 257-266.

Rahman, K., and G. Lowe. "Garlic and cardiovascular disease: a critical review." *Journal of Nutrition* 136 (2006): 736S-740S.

Ringman, J. "A potential role of the curry spice curcumin in Alzheimer's disease." *Current Alzheimer Research* 2 (2005): 131-136.

Sengupta A., et al. "Allium vegetables in cancer prevention: an overview." *Asian Pacific Journal of Cancer Prevention* 5 (2004): 237-245.

Shan, B., et al. "Antioxidant capacity of 26 spice extracts and characterization of their phenolic constituents." *Journal of Agriculture and Food Chemistry* 53 (2005): 7749-7759.

Yang, J., et al. "Varietal differences in phenolic content and antioxidant and antiproliferative activities of onions." *Journal of Agriculture and Food Chemistry* 52 (2004): 6787-6793.

A "Whole" Lot More with Whole Grains

Adom, K., et al. "Phytochemicals and antioxidant activity of milled fractions of different wheat varieties." *Journal of Agriculture and Food Chemistry* 53 (2005): 2297-2306.

Bazzano, L., et al. "Dietary Intake of Whole and Refined Grain Breakfast Cereals and Weight Gain in Men." *Obesity Research* 13 (2005): 1952-1960.

Jacobs, D., et al. "Is Whole Grain Intake Associated with Reduced Total and Cause-Specific Death Rates in Older Women? The Iowa Women's Health Study." *American Journal of Public Health* 89 (1999): 322-329.

Jacobs, D., and D. Gallaher. "Whole grain intake and cardio-vascular disease: a review." *Current Atheroscler Reports* 6 (2004): 415-423.

Jensen, M., et al. "Intakes of whole grains, bran, and germ and the risk of coronary heart disease in men." *American Journal of Clinical Nutrition* 80 (2004): 1492-1499.

Larsson, S., et al. "Whole grain consumption and risk of colourectal cancer: a population-based cohort of 60,000 women." *British Journal of Cancer* 92 (2005): 1803-1807.

Lui, S., et al. "A prospective study of dietary glycemic load, carbohydrate intake and risk of coronary heart disease in US women." *American Journal of Clinical Nutrition* 71 (2000): 1455-1461.

Lui, S., et al. "A Prospective Study of Whole-Grain Intake and Risk of Type 2 Diabetes mellitus in US Women." *American Journal of Public Health* 90 (2000): 1409-1415.

Liu, S., et al. "Relation between changes in intakes of dietary fibre and grain products and changes in weight and development of obesity among middle-aged women." *American Journal of Clinical Nutrition* 78 (2003): 920-927.

Lui, S., et al. "Whole-grain consumption and risk of coronary heart disease: results from the Nurses' Health Study." *American Journal of Clinical Nutrition* 70 (1999): 412–419.

Lui, S., et al. "Whole Grain Consumption and Risk of Ischemic Stroke in Women." *Journal of the American Medical Association* 284 (2000): 1534–1540.

McKeown, N., et al. "Carbohydrate Nutrition, Insulin Resistance, and the Prevalence of the Metabolic Syndrome in the Framingham Offspring Cohort." *Diabetes Care* 27 (2004): 538-546.

Miller, H., et al. "Antioxidant Content of Whole Grain Breakfast Cereals, Fruits and Vegetables." *Journal of the American College of Nutrition* 19 (2000): 312S-319S.

Rampersaud, G., et al. "Breakfast habits, nutritional status, body weight, and academic performance in children and adolescents." *Journal of the American Dietetic Association* 105 (2005): 743-760.

Sahyoun, N., et al. "Whole-grain intake is inversely associated with the metabolic syndrome and mortality in older adults." *American Journal of Clinical Nutrition* 83 (2006): 124-131.

Slavin, J. "Dietary fibre and body weight." *Nutrition* 21 (2005): 411-488.

Slavin, J. "Whole Grains and Human Health." *Nutrition Research Reviews* 17 (2004): 1-12.

Seal, C. "Whole grains and CVD risk." *The Proceedings of the Nutrition Society* 65 (2006): 24-34.

Low-Fat Milk Makes Sense

Boonen S., et al. "Addressing the musculoskeletal components of fracture risk with calcium and vitamin D: a review of the evidence." *Calcification Tissue International* 78 (2006): 257-270.

Chapuy, M., et al. "Vitamin D3 and calcium to prevent hip fractures in the elderly women." *The New England Journal of Medicine* 327 (1992): 1637-1642.

Gass, M., and B. Dawson-Hughes. "Preventing osteoporosis-related fractures: an overview." *American Journal of Medicine* 119 (2006): S3-S11.

Giovannucci E. "The epidemiology of vitamin D and cancer incidence and mortality: a review." *Cancer Causes and Control* 16 (2005): 83-95.

Goulding A., et al. "Children who avoid drinking cow's milk are at increased risk for prepubertal bone fractures." *Journal of the American Dietetic Association* 104 (2004): 250-253.

Guarner F., et al. "Should yoghurt cultures be considered probiotic?" *British Journal of Nutrition* 93 (2005): 783-786.

Gueguen, L., et al. "The Bioavailability of Dietary Calcium." *Journal of the American College of Nutrition* 19 (2000): 119S-136S.

Holick, M. "High prevalence of vitamin D inadequacy and implications for health." *Mayo Clinic Proceedings* 81 (2006): 353-373.

Huth P., et al. "Major scientific advances with dairy foods in nutrition and health." *Journal of Dairy Science* 89 (2006): 1207-1221.

Johnson, R., et al. "The nutritional consequences of flavoured-milk consumption by school-aged children and adolescents in the United States." *Journal of the American Dietetic Association* 102 (2002): 853-856.

Marshall, T. A., et al. "Diet quality in young children is influenced by beverage consumption." *Journal of the American College of Nutrition* 24 (2005): 65-75.

McCarron D., and R. Heaney. "Estimated healthcare savings associated with adequate dairy food intake." *American Journal of Hypertension* 17 (2004): 88-97.

North American Menopause Society. "Management of osteoporosis in postmenopausal women: 2006 position statement of Menopause." May 2006.

Parvez, S., et al. "Probiotics and their fermented food products are beneficial for health." *Journal of Applied Microbiology* 100 (2006): 1171-1185.

Peterlik, M., and H. Cross. "Vitamin D and calcium deficits predispose for multiple chronic diseases." *European Journal of Clinical Investigation* 35 (2005): 290-304.

Popkin, B. M., et al. "A new proposed guidance system for beverage consumption in the United States." *American Journal of Clinical Nutrition* 83 (2006): 529-542.

Schrager, S. "Dietary calcium intake and obesity." *Journal of the American Board of Family Practice* 18 (2005): 205-210.

Vess, T., et al. "Lactose Intolerance." *Journal of the American College of Nutrition* 19 (2000): 165S-175S.

Weaver, C., et al. "Choices for achieving adequate dietary calcium with a vegetarian diet." *American Journal for Clinical Nutrition* 70 (1999): 543S-548S.

Weinberg L.G., et al. "Nutrient contributions of dairy foods in the United States, Continuing Survey of Food Intakes by Individuals, 1994-1996, 1998." *Journal of the American Dietetic Association* 104 (2004): 895-902.

More Beans, Please!

Allred, C., et al. "Soy processing influences growth of estrogen-dependent breast cancer tumors." *Carcinogenesis* 25 (2004): 1649-1657.

Anderson, J., and A. Major. "Pulses and lipaemia, short- and long-term effect: potential in the prevention of cardiovascular disease." *British Journal of Nutrition* 88 (2002): S263-S271.

Badger, T., et al. "Soy protein isolate and protection against cancer." *Journal of the American College of Nutrition* 24 (2005): 146S-149S.

Beninger, C., and G. Hosfield. "Antioxidant Activity of Extracts, Condensed Tannin Fractions, and Pure Flavonoids from Phaseolus vulgaris L. Seed Coat Colour Genotypes." *Journal of Agriculture and Food Chemistry* 51 (2003): 7879–7883.

Blackberry, I., et al. "Legumes: the most important dietary predictor of survival in older people of different ethnicities." *Asia Pacific Journal of Clinical Nutrition* 13 (2004): 217-220.

Boyapati, S., et al. "Soyfood intake and breast cancer survival: a followup of the Shanghai Breast Cancer Study." *Breast Cancer Research and Treatment* 92 (2005): 11-17.

Trock, B., et al. "Meta-analysis of soy intake and breast cancer risk." *Journal of the National Cancer Institute* 98 (2006): 459-471.

Messina, M., and G. Redmond. "Effects of soy protein and soybean isoflavones on thyroid function in healthy adults and hypothyroid patients: a review of the relevant literature." *Thyroid* 16 (2006): 249-258.

Omoni, A., and R. Aluko. "Soybean foods and their benefits: potential mechanisms of action." *Nutrition Reviews* 63 (2005): 272-283.

Sacks, F., et al. "Soy protein, isoflavones, and cardiovascular health: an American Heart Association Science Advisory for professionals from the Nutrition Committee." *Circulation* 113 (2006): 1034-1044.

Schäfer, G., et al. "Comparison of the effects of dried peas with those of potatoes in mixed meals on postprandial glucose and insulin concentrations in patients with type 2 diabetes." *American Journal of Clinical Nutrition* 78 (2003): 99-103.

Shu, X., et al. "Soyfood intake during adolescence and subsequent risk of breast cancer among Chinese women." *Cancer Epidemiology Biomarkers and Prevention* 10 (2001): 483-488.

Yan, L. and E. Spitznagel. "Meta-analysis of soy food and risk of prostate cancer in men." *International Journal of Cancer* 117 (2005): 667-669.

Yang, G., et al. "Longitudinal study of soy food intake and blood pressure among middle-aged and elderly Chinese women." *American Journal of Clinical Nutrition* 81 (2005): 1012-1017.

Zhang, X., et al. "Prospective cohort study of soy food consumption and risk of bone fracture among postmenopausal women." *Archives of Internal Medicine* 165 (2005): 1890-1895.

Zhang, X. "Soy food consumption is associated with lower risk of coronary heart disease in Chinese women." *Journal of Nutrition* 133 (2003): 2874-2878.

Fatty Fish Is Fabulous

Brouwer, I., et al. "N-3 Fatty acids, cardiac arrhythmia and fatal coronary heart disease." *Progressive Lipid Research* 45 (2006): 357-367.

Bouzan, C., et al. "A quantitative analysis of fish consumption and stroke risk." *American Journal of Preventive Medicine* 29 (2005): 347-352.

Cohen, J., et al. "A Quantitative Risk-Benefit Analysis of Changes in Population Fish Consumption." *American Journal of Preventive Medicine* 29 (2005): 325-334.

Dunstan, J., and S. Prescott. "Does fish oil supplementation in pregnancy reduce the risk of allergic disease in infants?" *Current Opinion in Allergy and Clinical Immunology* 5 (2005): 215-221.

Hamazaki, K., et al. "Fish oil reduces tooth loss mainly through its anti-inflammatory effects?" *Medical Hypotheses* 5 (2006): Epub ahead of print.

Hilakivi-Clarke, L., et al. "Mechanisms mediating the effects of prepubertal (n-3) polyunsaturated fatty acid diet on breast cancer risk in rats." *Journal of Nutrition* 135 (2005): 2946S-2952S.

Hu, F. B., et al. "Fish and long-chain omega-3 fatty acid intake and risk of coronary heart disease and total mortality in diabetic women." *Circulation* 107 (2003): 1852-1857.

Hu, F. B., et al. "Fish and omega-3 fatty acid intake and risk of coronary heart disease in women." *Journal of the American Medical Association* 287 (2002): 1815-1821.

Huang, T., et al. "Benefits of fatty fish on dementia risk are stronger for those without APOE epsilon4." *Neurology* 65 (2005): 1409-1414.

Iso, H., et al. "Intake of Fish and Omega-3 Fatty Acids and Risk of Stroke in Women." *Journal of the American Medical Association* 285 (2001): 304-312.

Leaf, A., et al. "Prevention of fatal arrhythmias in high-risk subjects by fish oil n-3 fatty acid intake." *Circulation* 112 (2005): 2762-2768.

Marchioli, R., et al. "Antiarrhythmic mechanisms of n-3 PUFA and the results of the GISSI-Prevenzione trial." *Journal of Membrane Biology* 206 (2005): 117-128.

Maroon, J., and J. Bost. "Omega-3 fatty acids (fish oil) as an anti-inflammatory: an alternative to nonsteroidal anti-inflammatory drugs for discogenic pain." *Surgical Neurology* 65 (2006): 326-331.

Mori, T., and R. Woodman. "The independent effects of eicosapentaenoic acid and docosahexaenoic acid on cardiovascular risk factors in humans." *Current Opinion in Clinical Nutrition and Metabolic Care* 9 (2006): 95-104.

Nettleton, J., and R. Katz. "N-3 long-chain polyunsaturated fatty acids in type 2 diabetes: a review." *Journal of the American Dietetic Association* 105 (2005): 428-440.

Oomen, C., et al. "Fish consumption and coronary heart disease mortality in Finland, Italy, and The Netherlands." *American Journal of Epidemiology* 151 (2000): 999-1006.

Pauletto P., et al. "Blood Pressure and Atherogenic Lipoprotein Profiles of Fish-Diet and Vegetarian Villagers in Tanzania: The Lugalawa Study." *Lancet* 348 (1996): 784-788.

Peet, M., and C. Stokes. "Omega-3 fatty acids in the treatment of psychiatric disorders." *Drugs* 65 (2005): 1051-1059.

Rees, A., et al. "Role of omega-3 fatty acids as a treatment for depression in the perinatal period." *Australian Journal of Psychiatry* 39 (2005): 274-280.

Romieu, I., et al. "Omega-3 Fatty Acid Prevents Heart Rate Variability Reductions Associated with Particulate Matter." *The American Journal of Respiratory and Critical Care Medicine* 172 (2005): 1534-1540.

Smith, W., et al. "Dietary fat and fish intake and age-related maculopathy." *Archives of Ophthalmology* 118 (2000): 401-404.

Sontrop, J., and M. Campbell. "Omega-3 polyunsaturated fatty acids and depression: a review of the evidence and a methodological critique." *Preventive Medicine* 42 (2006): 4-13.

Terry, P., et al. "Fatty fish consumption and risk of prostate cancer." *Lancet* 357 (2001): 1764-1766.

Wong, K. "Clinical efficacy of n-3 fatty acid supplementation in patients with asthma." *Journal of the American Dietetic Association* 105 (2005): 98-105.

Xiao, Y., et al. "The antiarrhythmic effect of n-3 polyunsaturated fatty acids: modulation of cardiac ion channels as a potential mechanism." *Journal of Membrane Biology* 206 (2005): 141-154.

Young, G., and J. Conquer. "Omega-3 fatty acids and neuropsychiatric disorders." *Reproductive Nutrition and Development* 45 (2005): 1-28.

More Chicken, Less Beef, & Eggs Are Okay

Chao, A., et al. "Meat Consumption and Risk of Colourectal Cancer." *Journal of the American Medical Association* 293 (2005): 172-182.

Cross, A., et al. "A prospective study of meat and meat mutagens and prostate cancer risk." *Cancer Research* 65 (2005): 11779-11784.

Fernandez, M. "Dietary cholesterol provided by eggs and plasma lipoproteins in healthy populations." *Current Opinion in Clinical Nutrition & Metabolic Care* 9 (2006): 8-12.

Fung, T. "Dietary Patterns, Meat Intake, and the Risk of Type 2 Diabetes in Women." *Archives of Internal Medicine* 164 (2004): 2235-2240.

Greene, C., et al. "Maintenance of the LDL cholesterol: HDL cholesterol ratio in an elderly population given a dietary cholesterol challenge." *Journal of Nutrition* 135 (2005): 2793-2798.

Hu, F., et al. "A Prospective Study of Egg Consumption and Risk of Cardiovascular Disease in Men and Women." *Journal of the American Medical Association* 281 (1999): 1387-1394.

Hu, F., et al. "Dietary saturated fats and their food sources in relation to the risk of coronary heart disease in women." *American Journal of Clinical Nutrition* 70 (1999): 1001-1008.

Glei, M., et al. "Hemoglobin and hemin induce DNA damage in human colon tumor cells HT29 clone 19A and in primary human colonocytes." *Mutation Research* 594 (2006): 162-171.

Key, T., et al. "Mortality in vegetarians and nonvegetarians: detailed findings from a collaborative analysis of 5 prospective studies." *American Journal of Clinical Nutrition* 70 (2000): 516S-524S.

Kritchevsky, S. "A review of scientific research and recommendations regarding eggs." *Journal of the American College of Nutrition* 23 (2004): 596S-600S.

Larsson, S., et al. "Processed meat consumption, dietary nitrosamines and stomach cancer risk in a cohort of Swedish women." *International Journal of Cancer* 119 (2006): 915-919.

Larsson, S., et al. "Red meat consumption and risk of cancers of the proximal colon, distal colon and rectum: the Swedish Mammography Cohort." *International Journal of Cancer* 113 (2005): 829-834.

Lee, A., and B. Griffin. "Dietary cholesterol, eggs and coronary heart disease risk in perspective." *Nutrition Bulletin* 31 (2006): 21-27.

Lewin, M., et al. "Red meat enhances the colonic formation of the DNA adduct O6-carboxymethyl guanine: implications for colourectal cancer risk." *Cancer Research* 66 (2006): 1859-1865.

Li, D., et al, "Lean meat and heart health." *Asia Pacific Journal of Clinical Nutrition* 14 (2005): 113-119.

Nerurkar, P., et al. "Effects of Marinating with Asian Marinades or Western Barbecue Sauce on PhIP and MeIQx formation in Barbecued Beef." *Nutrition and Cancer* 34 (1999): 147-152.

Newby, P., et al. "Risk of overweight and obesity among semi-vegetarian, lactovegetarian, and vegan women." *American Journal of Clinical Nutrition* 81 (2005): 1267-1274.

Norat, T., et al. "Meat, fish, and colourectal cancer risk: the European Prospective Investigation into cancer and nutrition." *Journal of the National Cancer Institute* 97 (2005): 906-916.

Song, Y., et al. "A Prospective Study of Red Meat Consumption and Type 2 Diabetes in Middle-Aged and Elderly Women." *Diabetes Care* 27 (2004): 2108-2115.

Steffen, L., et al. "Associations of plant food, dairy product, and meat intakes with 15-y incidence of elevated blood pressure in young black and white adults: the Coronary Artery Risk Development in Young Adults (CARDIA) Study." *American Journal of Clinical Nutrition* 82 (2005): 1169-1177.

Weggemans, R. "Dietary cholesterol from eggs increases the ratio of total cholesterol to high-density lipoprotein cholesterol in humans: a meta-analysis." *American Journal of Clinical Nutrition* 73 (2001): 885-991.

Zheng, W., et al. "Well-done meat intake and the risk of breast cancer." *Journal of the National Cancer Institute* 90 (1998): 1724-1729.

Go Nuts!

Alper, C., and R. Mattes. "Peanut consumption improves indices of cardiovascular disease risk in healthy adults." *Journal of the American College of Nutrition* 22 (2003): 133-141.

Chen, C., et al. "Flavonoids from almond skins are bioavailable and act synergistically with vitamins C and E to enhance hamster and human LDL resistance to oxidation." *Journal of Nutrition* 135 (2005): 1366-1373.

Chung-Jyi, T., et al. "A Prospective Cohort Study of Nut Consumption and the Risk of Gallstone Disease in Men." *American Journal of Epidemiology* 160 (2004): 961-968.

Chung-Jyi, T., et al. "Frequent nut consumption and decreased risk of cholecystectomy in women." *American Journal of Clinical Nutrition* 80 (2004): 76-81.

Hu, F., et al. "Frequent nut consumption and risk of coronary heart disease in women: prospective cohort study." *British Medical Journal* 317 (1998): 1341-1345.

Jaceldo-Siegl, K., et al. "Long-term almond supplementation without advice on food replacement induces favourable nutrient modifications to the habitual diets of free-living individuals." *British Journal of Nutrition* 92 (2004): 533-540.

Jiang, R., et al. "Nut and peanut butter consumption and risk of type 2 diabetes in women." *Journal of the American Medical Association* 288 (2002): 2554-2560.

Lovejoy, J. "The impact of nuts on diabetes and diabetes risk." *Current Diabetes Reports* 5 (2005): 379-384.

Maras, J., et al. "Intake of alpha-tocopherol is limited among US adults." *Journal of the American Dietetic Association* 104 (2004): 567-575.

Phillips, K., et al. "Phytosterol composition of nuts and seeds commonly consumed in the United States." *Journal of Agriculture and Food Chemistry* 53 (2005):

Mukuddem-Petersen, J., et al. "A systematic review of the effects of nuts on blood lipid profiles in humans." *Journal of Nutrition* 135 (2005): 9436-9445.

Seddon, J., et al. "Progression of age-related macular degeneration: association with dietary fat, transunsaturated fat, nuts, and fish intake." *Archives of Opthamology* 121 (2003): 1728-1737.

Strahan, T., et al. "Nuts for cardiovascular protection." *Asia Pacific Journal of Clinical Nutrition* 13 (2004): S33.

Fantastic Flax

Bloedon, L., and P. Szapary. "Flaxseed and cardiovascular risk." *Nutrition Reviews* 62 (2004): 18-27.

Boccardo, F., et al. "Enterolactone as a risk factor for breast cancer: a review of the published evidence." *Clinica Chimica ACTA* 365 (2006): 58-67.

Chen, J., et al. "Dietary flaxseed enhances the inhibitory effect of tamoxifen on the growth of estrogen-dependent human breast cancer (mcf-7) in nude mice." *Clinical Cancer Research* 10 (2004): 7703-11.

Chen, J., et al. "Exposure to flaxseed or its purified lignan during suckling inhibits chemically induced rat mammary tumorigenesis." *Experimental Biology and Medicine* 228 (2003): 951-958.

Dabrosin, C., et al. "Flaxseed inhibits metastasis and decreases extracellular vascular endothelial growth factor in human breast cancer xenografts." *Cancer Letters* 185 (2002): 31-37.

Demark-Wahnefried, W., et al. "Pilot study to explore effects of low-fat, flaxseed-supplemented diet on proliferation of benign prostatic epithelium and prostate-specific antigen." *Urology* 63 (2004): 900-904.

Demark-Wahnefried, W., et al. "Pilot study of dietary fat restriction and flaxseed supplementation in men with prostate cancer before surgery: exploring the effect on hormonal levels, prostate-specific antigen and histopathologic features." *Urology* 58 (2001): 47-52.

Harper, C., et al. "Flaxseed Oil Increases the Plasma Concentrations of Cardioprotective (n-3) Fatty Acids in Humans" *Journal of Nutrition* 136 (2006): 83-87.

Kuijsten, A., et al. "The Relative Bioavailability of Enterolignans in Humans Is Enhanced by Milling and Crushing of Flaxseed." *Journal of Nutrition* 135 (2005): 2812-2816.

Lemay, A., et al. "Flaxseed dietary supplement versus hormone replacement therapy in hypercholesterolemic menopausal women." *Obstetrical Gynecology* 100 (2002): 495-504.

Lin, X., et al. "Effect of flaxseed supplementation on prostatic carcinoma in transgenic mice." *Urology* 60 (2002): 919-924.

Mandasescu, S., et al. "Flaxseed supplementation in hyperlipidemic patients." *Revista Medico-Chiruricala A Societatii de Medici si Naturalisti Din Iasi* 109 (2005): 502-506.

Piller, R., et al. "Plasma enterolactone and genistein and the risk of premenopausal breast cancer." *European Journal of Cancer Prevention* 15 (2006): 225-232.

Rajesha, J., et al. "Antioxidant potentials of flaxseed by in vivo model." *Journal of Agriculture and Food Chemistry* 54 (2006): 3794-3799.

Thompson, L. "Dietary flaxseed alters tumor biological markers in postmenopausal breast cancer." *Clinical Cancer Research* 11 (2005): 3828-3835.

Wang, L., et al. "The inhibitory effect of flaxseed on the growth and metastasis of estrogen receptor negative human breast cancer xenograftsis attributed to both its lignan and oil components." *International Journal of Cancer* 111 (2005): 793-798.

Ditch the Soft Drinks, Drink Water, & Take Time for Tea

Bandyopadhyay, D. "In vitro and in vivo antimicrobial action of tea: the commonest beverage of Asia." *Biological Pharmacy Bulletin* 28 (2005): 2125-2127.

Bastianetto, S. "Neuroprotective effects of green and black teas and their catechin gallate esters against beta-amyloid-induced toxicity." *European Journal of Neuroscience* 23 (2006): 55-64.

Cabrera, C., et al. "Beneficial effects of green tea: a review." *Journal of the American College of Nutrition* 25 (2006): 79-99.

De Bacquer, D., et al. "Epidemiological evidence for an association between habitual tea consumption and markers of chronic inflammation." *Atherosclerosis* (2006): Epub.

Fukino, Y., et al. "Randomized controlled trial for an effect of green tea consumption on insulin resistance and inflammation markers." *Journal of Nutrition Science and Vitaminology* 51 (2005): 335-342.

Haqqi, T. "Prevention of collagen-induced arthritis in mice by a polyphenolic fraction from green tea." *Proceedings of the National Academy of Sciences* 96 (1999): 4524-4529.

Higdon, J., and B. Frei. "Coffee and health: a review of recent human research." *Critical Reviews in Food Science and Nutrition* 46 (2006): 101-123.

Kao, Y., et al. "Tea, obesity, and diabetes." *Molecular Nutrition and Food Research* 50 (2006): 188-210.

Kuriyama, S., et al. "Green tea consumption and cognitive function: a cross-sectional study from the Tsurugaya Project 1." *American Journal of Clinical Nutrition* 83 (2006): 355-361.

Lee, A., et al. "Protective effects of green tea against prostate cancer." *Expert Reviews in Anticancer Therapy* 6 (2006): 507-513.

Ludwig, D., et al. "Relation between consumption of sugar-sweetened drinks and childhood obesity: a prospective, observational analysis." *Lancet* 357 (2001): 505-508.

Nelson, M., and J. Poulter. "Impact of tea drinking on iron status in the UK: a review." *Journal of Human Nutrition and Dietetics* 46 (2006): 43-54.

Peters, U., et al. "Does tea affect cardiovascular disease? A meta-analysis." *American Journal of Epidemiology* 154 (2001): 495-503.

Reddy, V., et al. "Addition of milk does not alter the antioxidant activity of black tea." *Annals of Nutrition and Metabolism* 49 (2005): 189-195.

Rezai-Zadeh, K., et al. "Green tea epigallocatechin-3-gallate (EGCG) modulates amyloid precursor protein cleavage and reduces cerebral amyloidosis in Alzheimer transgenic mice." *Journal of Neuroscience* 25 (2005): 8807-8814.

Schulze, M., et al. "Sugar-sweetened beverages, weight gain, and incidence of type 2 diabetes in young and middle-aged women." *Journal of the American Medical Association* 292 (2004): 927-934.

Stangl, V. "The role of tea and tea flavonoids in cardiovascular health." *Molecular Nutrition and Food Research* 50 (2006): 218-228.

Sun, C., et al. "Green tea, black tea and breast cancer risk: a meta-analysis of epidemiological studies." *Carcinogenesis* (2005): Epub.

Wolfram, S., et al. "Anti-obesity effects of green tea: from bedside to bench." *Molecular Nutrition Food Research* 50 (2006): 176-187.

Zaveri, N. "Green tea and its polyphenolic catechins: medicinal uses in cancer and noncancer applications." *Life Sciences* 78 (2006): 2073-2080.

Red Wine for Good Health?

Arendt, B., et al. "Single and repeated moderate consumption of native or dealcoholized red wine show different effects on antioxidant parameters in blood and DNA strand breaks in peripheral leukocytes in healthy volunteers: a randomized controlled trial." *Nutrition Journal* 4 (2005): 33.

Cho, E., et al. "Alcohol Intake and Colourectal Cancer: A Pooled Analysis of 8 Cohort Studies." *Annals of Internal Medicine* 140 (2004): 603-613.

Coimbra, S., et al. "The action of red wine and purple grape juice on vascular reactivity is independent of plasma lipids in hypercholesterolemic patients." *Brazilian Journal of Medical and Biological Research* 38 (2005): 1339-1147.

Giles, T., et al. "Alcohol – A Cardiovascular Drug?" *The American Journal of Geriatric Cardiology* 14 (2005): 154-158.

Gronbaek, M. "Factors influencing the relation between alcohol and cardiovascular disease." *Current Opinions in Lipidology* 17 (2006): 17-21.

Hill, J. "In vino veritas: alcohol and heart disease." *American Journal of Medical Sciences* 329 (2005): 124-135.

Howard, A., et al. "Effect of Alcohol Consumption on Diabetes Mellitus." *Annals of Internal Medicine* 140 (2004): 211-219.

Karatzi, K., et al. "Red wine acutely induces favorable effects on wave reflections and central pressures in coronary artery disease patients." *American Journal of Hypertension* 18 (2005): 1161-1167.

Mukamal, K. "Drinking frequency, mediating biomarkers, and risk of myocardial infarction in women and men." *Circulation* 112 (2005): 1406-1413.

Mukamal, K., et al. "Prospective study of alcohol consumption and risk of dementia in older adults." *Journal of the American Medical Association* 289 (2003): 1405-1413.

Reynolds, K., et al. "Alcohol consumption and risk of stroke: a meta-analysis." *Journal of the American Medical Association* 289 (2003): 579-598.

Leaving Room for Chocolate

Ariefdjohan, M., and D. Savaiano. "Chocolate and cardiovascular health: is it too good to be true?" *Nutrition Reviews* 63 (2005): 427-430.

Ding, E., et al. "Chocolate and prevention of cardiovascular disease: a systematic review." *Nutrition & Metabolism* 3 (2006): 1-12.

Engler, M., and M. Engler. "The emerging role of flavonoid-rich cocoa and chocolate in cardiovascular health and disease." *Nutrition Reviews* 2006 (64): 109-118.

Fisher, N., and N. Hollenberg. "Flavanols for cardiovascular health: the science behind the sweetness." *Journal of Hypertension* 23 (2005): 1461-1463.

Grassi, D., et al. "Cocoa reduces blood pressure and insulin resistance and improves endothelium-dependent vasodilation in hypertensives." *Journal of the American Heart Association* 46 (2005): 398-405.

Keen, C., et al. "Cocoa antioxidants and cardiovascular health." *American Journal of Clinical Nutrition* 81 (2005): 298S-303S.

Kurosawa, T., et al. "Suppressive effects of cacao liquor polyphenols (CLP) on LDL oxidation and the development of atherosclerosis in Kurosawa and Kusanagi-hypercholesterolemic rabbits." *Atherosclerosis* 179 (2005): 237-246.

Wu, X., et al. "Lipophilic and hydrophilic antioxidant capacities of common foods in the United States." *Journal of Agriculture & Food Chemistry* 52 (2004): 4026-4037.

Pill Popping for Ultimate Health

Boonen, S., et al. "Calcium and vitamin D in the prevention and treatment of osteoporosis: a clinical update." *Journal of Internal Medicine* 259 (2006): 539-552.

Coulter, I., et al. "Antioxidants vitamin C and vitamin E for the prevention and treatment of cancer." *Journal of General Internal Medicine* 21 (2006): 735-744.

Douglas, R., et al. "Vitamin C for preventing and treating the common cold." *Cochrane Database System Reviews* 4 (2004): CD000980.

Dragsted, L., et al. "The 6-a-day study: effects of fruit and vegetables on markers of oxidative stress and antioxidative defense in healthy nonsmokers." *American Journal of Clinical Nutrition* 79 (2004): 1060-1072.

Giovannucci, E., et al. "Multivitamin Use, Folate, and Colon Cancer in Women in the Nurses' Health Study." *Annals of Internal Medicine* 129 (1998): 517-524.

Heaney, R. "Barriers to optimizing vitamin D3 intake for the elderly." *Journal of Nutrition* 136 (2006): 1123-1125.

HOPE and HOPE-TOO Trial Investigators. "Effects of Long-term Vitamin E Supplementation on Cardiovascular Events and Cancer." *Journal of the American Medical Association* 293 (2005): 1338-1347.

Jacobs, E., et al. "Multivitamin use and colourectal cancer incidence in a US cohort: does timing matter?" *American Journal of Epidemiology* 58 (2003): 621-628.

Lee, D., et al. "Heme iron, zinc and upper digestive tract cancer: the Iowa Women's Health Study." *International Journal of Cancer* 20 (2005): 643-647.

Martinez, M., et al. "Folate fortification, plasma folate, homocysteine and colourectal adenoma recurrence." *International Journal of Cancer* (2006): Epub ahead of print.

Morris, C., and S. Carson. "Routine vitamin supplementation to prevent cardiovascular disease: a summary of the evidence for the U.S. Preventive Services Task Force." *Annals of Internal Medicine* 139 (2003): 56-70.

Penniston, K., and S. Tanumihardjo. "The acute and chronic toxic effects of vitamin A." *The American Journal of Clinical Nutrition* 83 (2006): 191-201.

Rimm, E., et al. "Folate and vitamin B6 from diet and supplements in relation to coronary heart disease among women." *Journal of the American Medical Association* 5 (1998): 359-364.

Van Leeuwen, R., et al. "Dietary Intake of Antioxidants and Risk of Age-Related Macular Degeneration." *Journal of the American Medical Association* 294 (2005): 3101-3107.

Vieth, R. "Critique of the considerations for establishing the tolerable upper intake level for vitamin D: critical need for revision upwards." *Journal of Nutrition* 136 (2006): 1117-1122.

Get Off the Couch!

Dempsey, J., et al. "Prospective Study of Gestational Diabetes Mellitus Risk in Relation to Maternal Recreational Physical Activity before and during Pregnancy." *American Journal of Epidemiology* 159 (2004): 663-670.

Fleshner, M., et al. "Physical activity and stress resistance: sympathetic nervous system adaptations prevent stress-induced immunosuppression." *Exercise and Sport Sciences Reviews* 33 (2005): 120-126.

Hu, F., et al. "Adiposity as Compared with Physical Activity in Predicting Mortality among Women." *New England Journal of Medicine* 351 (2004): 2694-2703.

Hu, F., et al. "Television watching and other sedentary behaviors in relation to risk of obesity and type 2 diabetes mellitus in women." *Journal of the American Medical Association* 289 (2003): 1785-1791.

Hu, F., et al. "Walking compared with vigorous physical activity and risk of type 2 diabetes in women: a prospective study." *Journal of the American Medical Association* 282 (1999): 1433-1439.

Jakicic, J., and A. Otto. "Treatment and prevention of obesity: what is the role of exercise?" *Nutrition Reviews* 64 (2006): S57-S61.

Holcomb, C., et al. "Physical activity minimizes the association of body fatness with abdominal obesity in white, premenopausal women: Results from the Third National Health and Nutrition Examination Survey." *Journal of the American Dietetic Association* 104 (2004): 1859-1862.

Karmisholt, K., et al. "Physical activity for primary prevention of disease. Systematic reviews of randomised clinical trials." *Danish Medical Bulletin* 52 (2005): 86-89.

Laaksonen, D., et al. "Physical Activity in the Prevention of Type 2 Diabetes." *Diabetes* 54 (2005): 158-165.

Stewart, K. "Physical activity and aging." *Annals of the New York Academy of Sciences* 1055 (2005): 193-206.

Volek, J., et al. "Diet and exercise for weight loss: a review of current issues." *Sports Medicine* 35 (2005): 1-9.

Warburton, D., et al. "Health benefits of physical activity: the evidence." *Canadian Medical Association Journal* 174 (2006): 801-809.

Weuve, J., et al. "Physical activity, including walking, and cognitive function in older women." *Journal of the American Medical Association* 292 (2004): 1454-1461.

Zhang, C., et al. "A prospective study of pregravid physical activity and sedentary behaviors in relation to the risk for gestational diabetes mellitus." *Archives of Internal Medicine* 166 (2006): 543-538.

NUTRITION INFORMATION INDEX

Antioxidants, 16, 21–22, 25, 27, 30, 33, 34, 41, 75, 82, 86, 91, 92, 93, 98, 101, 103, 112

Alcohol (beer, wine, spirits), 36, 94, 97–99, 128, 135

Aging, 27, 29, 41, 64, 112, 120

Allergies, 27, 53, 54, 64, 67

Alzheimer's disease, 16, 21, 22, 28, 29, 35, 57, 64, 65, 69, 81, 92, 93, 112, 117

Arthritis, 10, 16, 30, 34, 64, 67, 70, 92, 93, 111, 117

Asthma, 27, 53, 54, 64, 67, 68, 92

Beans (legumes), 39, 43, 54, 56–62, 74, 76, 77, 78, 98, 99, 101, 106, 108, 126, 129, 133, 134, 135
    Beano (gas), 62
    Bean salads, 61, 133
    Canned, 36, 61, 62, 132, 139
    Chick-pea recipe, 60
    Hummus, 60, 61, 126, 133, 134
    Recommended intake, 61, 126

Blood Pressure, 10, 12, 22, 23, 24, 30, 31, 33, 35, 36, 37, 40, 41, 48, 50, 52, 58, 60, 75, 76, 81, 101, 102, 116, 119, 120, 312

Blood Sugar, 34, 39, 41, 45, 58, 59, 81, 88, 92, 98, 116

Bone Health, 28, 35, 48–50, 51, 52, 55, 57, 58, 59, 60, 66, 70, 81, 91, 95, 108, 111, 116, 117, 121

Brain Health, 15, 22, 27, 28, 29, 30, 35, 64, 65, 68, 69, 77, 92, 93, 98, 99, 116

Butter, 16, 17, 19, 24

Calories, 14, 21, 23, 24, 27, 30, 44, 45, 46, 53, 61, 74, 77, 83, 93, 94, 95, 99, 103, 118, 119, 121–22, 134–35, 137, 138

Cancer, 10, 14, 16, 17, 21, 22, 25, 27, 28, 29, 30, 33, 34, 35, 39, 40, 45, 57, 58, 73, 75–76, 80, 81, 83, 89, 91, 92, 97, 98, 101, 107, 112
    Breast, 12, 27, 28, 34, 58, 59, 60, 61, 62, 64, 66, 75, 86–87, 91, 98, 99, 111, 116
    Colon, 12, 28, 34, 41, 46, 51, 52, 53, 57, 58, 64, 66, 73, 76, 77, 81, 91, 98, 99, 108, 111, 116
    Mouth/Throat/Esophagus, 92, 98
    Lung, 27, 28, 34, 91, 113
    Ovarian, 28, 91
    Prostate, 27, 28, 30, 34, 58, 59, 64, 66, 75, 81, 86–87, 88, 91, 111
    Skin, 113
    Stomach, 28, 35, 53, 73, 76

Calcium, 25, 39, 42, 48–50, 51, 52, 53, 54, 55, 58, 80, 82, 109, 111, 139
    Calcium supplements, 52, 108, 111, 113, 128

Canola Oil, 14–15, 17, 18, 19, 64, 66, 68, 113, 124

Caffeine, 91, 92–93, 103

Carbohydrates, 14, 39, 43, 58, 59, 84
    Fermentable carbohydrates, 40

Carotenoids, 14, 22, 28, 30

Chicken—see Poultry

Children, 8, 10, 11, 22, 24, 25, 26, 27, 29, 45, 49, 50, 51, 53, 65, 67, 68, 69, 95, 122, 129, 136

Chocolate, 11–12, 25, 49, 53, 62, 100–04, 133, 135
    Cocoa, 98, 101, 102, 103, 104
    Recommended intake, 103, 128

Cholesterol, 16, 17, 129, 312
    In food, 17, 66, 77, 78
    HDL, 16–17, 41, 97, 312
    LDL, 15, 16, 18, 19, 22, 27, 30, 34, 40, 43, 44, 45, 58, 62, 80, 81, 86, 87, 88, 102, 104, 116, 312

Choline, 77

Coconut (coconut oil), 16, 83

Cod liver oil, 70

Coffee, 10, 53, 91, 92, 103, 135

Constipation, 40, 53, 58, 94

Corn oil, 66

DASH diet, 23, 50

Deep-Fried Foods, 14, 17, 78, 134

Dental health, 52, 53, 69, 92, 94, 95

Depression, 12, 48, 57, 65, 66, 69, 70, 71, 116, 120, 126, 136

Diabetes, 8, 10, 11, 16, 17, 18, 21, 22, 28, 33, 34, 35, 39, 40, 41, 43, 45, 57, 58, 59, 67, 70, 73, 77, 78, 80, 81, 88, 91, 92, 94, 95, 97, 107, 111, 113, 116, 119, 121, 122, 134, 312

Diet Soft Drinks, 94, 95

Dinner, 25, 36, 45, 69, 76, 77, 132, 133, 136, 138

Dining Out, 17, 24, 74, 94, 134–35

Eggs, 66, 74, 76, 77–78, 126, 127
    Omega-3 eggs, 77, 78, 113

Exercise—see Physical Activity

Eye Health, 15, 28, 64, 67, 68
    Cataracts, 21, 22, 28, 34, 64, 67, 77
    Macular Degeneration, 22, 28, 64, 67, 77, 80, 81, 112

Fat, 13–19, 31, 44, 45, 46, 74, 75, 83, 103, 134, 135
    Low Fat, 14, 16, 17, 18, 19, 21, 24, 25, 29, 31, 50, 52, 53, 55, 60, 66, 74, 76, 77, 78, 80, 119, 124, 125, 132, 134, 135, 137, 138
    Monounsaturated, 14, 15, 16, 19, 24, 80, 138
    Omega-3 Fats (fish source), 14, 15, 63–71, 78
    Omega-3 Fats (plant source), 14–15, 17, 64, 66, 68, 78, 82, 87, 88, 124
    Omega-6 Fats, 15, 17, 66
    Polyunsaturated, 14, 15, 19, 80, 138
    Ratio of omega-6 to omega-3 fats, 15, 17, 66,
    Recommended intake, 18–19, 124, 138
    Saturated, 14, 15, 16, 17, 18, 19, 44, 50, 52, 53, 59, 62, 66, 74, 77, 78, 80, 83, 87, 124, 134, 135, 137, 138, 139
    Trans, 14, 15, 16–17, 18, 19, 68, 77, 78, 80, 83, 87, 124, 134, 135, 137, 138, 139

Fast Food, 10, 24, 35, 36, 37, 44, 68, 84, 119, 124, 133, 134, 135, 136, 138

Fibre, 21, 22, 23, 27, 29, 39, 40, 41, 42, 43, 44, 45, 46, 58, 76, 77, 80, 81, 82, 83, 84, 86, 87–88, 89, 125, 129, 134, 137, 138, 139

Fish, 14, 15, 36, 48, 63–71, 73, 74, 75, 76, 77, 78, 99, 112, 126, 133, 134, 135, 139
    Contaminants (mercury, PCBs), 68–70

Fish oil supplements, 65, 67, 68, 69–70, 71, 126
    Omega-3 content of seafood, 71
    Recommended intake, 68, 71, 126
    Salmon, 64, 67, 68, 69, 70, 71, 78, 112, 126, 132, 133, 135

Fish oil supplements (*cont'd*)
  Tuna, 68, 69, 71
Flavonoids/Flavanols, 22, 26, 27, 33, 35, 41, 58, 59, 67, 81, 84, 91, 92, 93, 98, 99, 101–04
Flax, 15, 17, 18, 43, 64, 66, 68, 78, 85–89, 129
  Recommended intake, 89-88, 127
Free Radicals, 21–22, 27, 28, 33, 34, 41, 76, 86, 106, 108, 112
Frozen Dinners, 36, 132–33, 138
Fruit, 9, 21–31, 36, 39, 43, 50, 74, 76, 77, 78, 98, 99, 101, 106, 102, 113, 124, 129, 132, 133, 134, 135, 136, 139
  Apples, 21, 23, 26, 27, 28, 31, 34, 67, 84, 101, 124, 132, 133
  Apricots, 26
  Avocado, 19, 24, 25
  Bananas, 23, 24, 25, 44, 62, 84, 108, 133
  Berries, 21, 25, 26, 27, 29, 30, 31, 43, 62, 67, 76, 101, 103, 113, 124, 132, 135
  Cantaloupe, 24, 26, 108, 113
  Carrots, 23, 24, 26, 31, 113, 132, 133
  Cherries, 21, 26
  Dried fruit (dates, plums, prunes, raisins), 21, 23, 24, 26, 27, 44, 76, 84, 124
  Frozen/canned, 23, 24, 25, 29, 43, 62, 124, 132, 133, 139
  Fruit juice, 22, 23, 24, 25, 27, 28, 29, 30, 31, 36, 44, 45, 49, 50, 54, 55, 75, 76, 91, 94, 98, 101, 108, 112, 113, 124, 132, 135, 139
  Grapefruit, 26, 30, 108
  Grapes/grape juice, 24, 25, 26, 45, 98, 101, 133
  Guava, 30, 108, 113
  Kiwi, 24, 26, 76, 84, 108, 113
  Mango, 26
  Olives, 19
  Oranges/orange juice, 23, 24, 25, 26, 31, 54, 55, 76, 98, 108, 112, 113, 124, 132, 133
  Papaya, 26, 30, 113
  Peaches/nectarines, 23, 26
  Pears, 23, 26, 133
  Pineapple, 26
  Plum, 21, 26, 27
  Pomegranate juice, 24, 25, 27, 29–30, 31, 98, 124, 132, 133
  Prune juice, 24, 108
  Watermelon, 26, 30, 108

Gallstones, 81, 117
Garlic, 24, 33, 34–35, 36, 37, 75, 124
Genetically Modified Food, 61
Glycemic Index, 39, 58, 59
Grains, 38–48
  Bagels, 24, 41, 42, 45, 125, 135
  Barley, 39, 40, 41, 42, 45, 125, 139
  Bran, 39, 40, 41, 43, 44, 45, 46, 87
  Bread, 19, 24, 39, 41, 42, 43, 45–46, 89, 93, 125, 133, 134
  Bulgur, 41, 42, 125, 139
  Cereal, 41, 42–44, 45, 46, 76, 84, 89, 93, 98, 112, 125, 133, 138
  Crackers, 17, 36, 41, 42, 46, 125, 138
  Couscous, 46
  Germ, 39, 41, 42, 139
  Muffins, 41, 44, 45, 46, 87, 89, 103, 104, 125, 128, 133, 135

  Oats/Oatmeal, 34, 39, 40, 42, 43, 44, 139
  Pancakes, 41, 44, 45, 103, 104, 125, 128, 133
  Pasta, 36, 41, 42, 45, 46, 84, 125, 132, 133, 135
  Quinoa, 41, 42, 45, 125, 139
  Recommended intake, 41, 46, 125
  Refined grains, 39, 40, 41, 43, 45–46, 125
  Rice, 36, 39, 41, 42, 44, 46, 61, 62, 84, 125, 132, 136, 139
  Rye, 40, 42, 139
  Whole grains, 38–46, 62, 74, 76, 77, 78, 89, 99, 103, 106, 113, 125, 128, 129, 132, 133, 134, 139
Grapeseed Oil, 17

Heart Disease, 8, 11, 14, 15, 16, 18, 21, 22, 27, 28, 29, 30, 31, 33, 34, 35, 36, 39, 40, 41, 43, 45, 57, 58, 59, 60, 62, 64, 65, 66, 67, 69, 70, 71, 77, 78, 80, 81, 83, 84, 86, 91, 97, 98, 107, 112, 113, 122, 126, 312
  Arrhythmias, 15, 87
  Blood clots, 22, 27, 28, 35, 65, 97, 98, 99
  Blood vessel health, 15, 16, 22, 40, 50, 51, 81, 98, 102, 116
  Heart attack, 10, 15, 16, 22, 35, 41, 61, 64, 65, 70, 73, 76, 80, 87, 91, 97, 98, 102, 115, 119, 121
  Nitric Oxide, 16, 81, 102
Hemp Oil, 17
Herbs and Spices, 24, 32–37, 74, 93, 109, 124
  Cinnamon, 24, 27, 34, 37, 67, 93, 101, 124
  Cloves, 34, 37, 93, 124
  Oregano, 34, 37, 75, 124
  Turmeric, 34, 35, 37, 75, 124
Homocysteine, 81

Immune System, 22, 30, 33, 34, 53, 54, 81, 92, 111, 116
Inflammation, 15, 16, 22, 27, 29, 30, 34, 65, 66, 67, 68, 69, 81, 92, 97, 102, 116
Inflammatory Disorders (Crohn's, ulcerative colitis, psoriasis), 30, 34, 53, 64, 66–67, 69, 70, 71, 126
Isoflavones, 59

Japanese Diet, 14, 57, 59, 60, 64, 66, 74

Kidney Disease, 11, 35, 57, 69
Kidney Stones, 58, 94

Label Reading, 18, 35, 42, 44, 45, 46, 68, 74, 102, 132, 137–39
Lactose Intolerance, 53, 55
Lard, 16
Lignans, 41, 86, 87, 88, 89
Lunch, 49, 61, 133
Lutein, 22, 24, 28, 29, 30, 40, 77, 78, 108
Lycopene, 14, 22, 26, 30–31, 107, 108

Margarine, 15, 17–18, 18, 112, 113, 124
Mayonnaise, 18, 19, 66, 124
Meat, 14, 16, 17, 34, 36, 66, 72–78, 107, 113, 133, 135, 139
  Beef, 62, 66, 73, 74, 76, 135, 139
  Barbecued/Grilled, 35, 75–76
  Lamb, 73, 75
  Hamburgers, 16, 35, 62, 74, 75, 76, 134
  Pork, 73, 74

Processed meats (cold cuts, bacon, sausages, hot dogs), 16, 36, 73, 74, 75, 76, 77, 78, 126, 134
Recommended intake, 73, 78, 126, 129
Red meat, 73, 75, 76–77, 78, 107, 126
Veal, 73, 74
Mediterranean Diet, 14, 16, 19, 24, 33, 74
Menopause, 45, 50, 88, 107
Metabolic Syndrome, 41
Milk Products, 14, 16, 17, 47–55, 78, 111, 113, 125, 128, 129, 139
Cheese, 16, 24, 27, 28, 36, 50, 51, 52, 53, 54, 55, 112, 125, 134, 135
Chocolate milk, 49, 53, 103, 135
Ice cream, 16, 51, 53, 112, 125
Milk, 14, 25, 42, 44, 47–55, 73, 91, 92, 93, 95, 112, 125, 133, 134, 135, 136, 139
Recommended intake, 51, 52, 55, 125
Yogurt, 25, 29, 51, 52–53, 54, 55, 89, 112, 125, 132, 133, 135, 138
Minerals, 21, 27, 40, 46, 48, 50, 57, 80, 105–13, 128, 134, 137, 139
Copper, 39, 58, 66, 80, 107, 110
Iron, 40, 43, 44, 58, 66, 73, 74, 76–77, 80, 83, 93, 107, 108, 109, 110, 139
Magnesium, 36, 40, 41, 49, 50, 51, 55, 58, 80, 81, 82, 83, 108, 110
Potassium, 22, 23, 24, 25, 29, 36, 39, 50, 51, 52, 58, 70, 81, 82, 83, 95, 108
Recommended intakes, 109–10
Selenium, 39, 41, 66, 70, 73, 81, 83, 107, 109, 110, 112, 113, 128
Zinc, 39, 50, 58, 66, 73, 74, 80, 81, 82, 83, 106, 107, 108, 109, 110, 112
Multiple Sclerosis, 67, 111

Neural Tube Defects, 28, 77
Nitrates/nitrites/nitrosamines, 76, 82
Nitric Oxide, 16, 81, 102
Nuts and Seeds, 18, 19, 31, 36, 78, 79–84, 99, 113, 126, 132, 135, 138, 139
Almonds, 54, 82, 83, 84, 113
Brazil nuts, 82, 83, 113
Cashews, 82
Hazelnuts, 82, 113
Macadamia nuts, 82, 83
Pecans, 82
Peanuts, 82, 98
Peanut butter, 19, 80, 82, 83, 84, 89, 127, 132, 133
Pine nuts, 82
Pistachios, 82
Recommended intake, 82–84, 126, 127
Walnuts, 15, 64, 82

Obesity, 10, 12, 21, 39, 41, 57, 94, 95, 122
Olive Oil, 14, 16, 17, 18, 19, 45, 75, 113, 124
Organic, 25–26
Osteoporosis, 12, 48, 50, 52

Palm Oil, 16, 17
Parkinson's Disease, 34, 91
Pesticides, 25, 26, 61
Pizza, 30, 135, 136
Poultry, 36, 72–77, 78, 113, 126, 139
Chicken, 16, 17, 74, 76, 77, 78, 126, 132, 133, 134, 135, 136, 139
Turkey, 74, 134, 136
Prebiotic, 58
Pregnancy, 28, 30, 50, 53, 57, 66, 67, 68, 109, 110, 119
Probiotics, 52, 53, 54, 125
Processed Foods, 14, 16, 17, 30, 35, 36, 37, 39, 54, 59, 124, 138, 139
Protein, 14, 49, 50, 51, 55, 57, 58, 66, 70, 73, 77, 80, 81, 82, 83, 84, 134
Phenols, 16, 29, 33, 41, 46, 58, 93
Physical Activity, 9, 12, 36, 39, 48, 49, 50, 94, 114–22, 129, 138
Benefits, 115–17
Resistance exercise (lifting weights), 121, 122, 129
Walking, 118, 121, 122, 129
Phytates, 41
Phytoestrogens, 59, 86
Plant Sterols, 18, 24, 82, 83, 104
Psyllium, 40, 45

Red Wine, 30, 97, 98–99, 101
Resistant Starch, 40, 58

Safflower Oil, 15, 66
Salad Dressing, 14, 15, 18, 19, 24, 25, 29, 34, 36, 66, 124, 132, 134, 135
Salt (sodium), 23, 24, 25, 31, 33, 35–37, 54, 61, 62, 68, 76, 83, 91, 95, 124, 132, 133, 134, 136, 137, 138, 139
Seeds, 76, 79–84, 127, 135, 139
Pumpkin seeds, 82, 83
Sesame seeds, 82, 83, 86
Sunflower seeds, 82, 83, 116
Shellfish, 66, 71, 78
Smoothies, 25, 29, 34, 62, 89, 133, 135
Snacks, 23, 27, 31, 36, 43, 44, 60, 62, 84, 133, 135, 137, 138
Spices—see Herbs
Soft Drinks, 44, 49, 50, 91, 94–95, 135, 138
Soup, 26, 36, 45, 60, 62, 135, 136, 138
Soy, 57, 58–62, 76, 108, 126
Edamame, 62
Hummus, 60, 61, 126, 133, 134
Soybean Oil, 15, 66
Soy milk, 25, 52, 55, 60, 61, 62, 107, 111, 112, 113, 125, 126, 128, 135
Soy Nuts, 60, 61, 126
Tofu, 54, 61, 62, 126
Other soy products, 61, 62, 76, 126
Stress, 116
Stroke, 8, 10, 11, 16, 21, 22, 27, 28, 29, 34, 37, 39, 40, 58, 64, 65, 73, 76, 78, 81, 97, 98, 99, 102, 115, 117
Sugar, 10, 23, 25, 27, 30, 44, 53, 54, 58, 83, 91, 93, 94, 95, 134, 135, 137, 138, 139

Sugar Substitutes, 44, 95
Sunflower Oil, 66
Sushi, 62, 69, 133

Tea, 34, 67, 75, 91–93, 95, 98, 101, 103, 127, 132, 135
    Black tea, 75, 91, 92, 93, 95, 127, 135
    Green tea, 75, 91, 92, 93, 95, 127, 135
    Herbal tea, 93
    Oolong tea, 93
    Recommended intake, 92, 95, 127
    White tea, 93
Teenagers, 51, 136
Triglycerides, 34, 41, 43, 62, 65, 69, 70, 71, 86, 116, 126, 129, 312
Turkey—see Poultry

Urinary Tract Infection, 30

Vegetables, 14, 20–31, 36, 39, 40, 42, 43, 50, 57, 60, 74, 77, 78, 98, 99, 101, 106, 112, 113, 124, 129, 132, 134, 136, 139
    Artichokes, 21, 26, 61
    Asparagus, 24, 25, 26, 98
    Bok choy, 27, 54
    Broccoli, 25, 26, 27–28, 29, 31, 54, 76, 98, 113, 124, 132
    Broccoli sprouts, 29
    Brussels sprouts, 26, 27
    Cabbage, 26, 27
    Cauliflower, 25, 26, 27
    Cooking vegetables, 26, 28
    Corn, 26, 42
    Cruciferous vegetables, 27–28
    Dark leafy greens, 26, 28, 29, 77, 108, 113, 134
    Frozen/canned, 23, 24, 25, 124, 132, 139
    Iceberg lettuce, 29, 134
    Kale, 26, 27–28, 29, 54
    Onions, 24, 26, 33, 34–35, 36, 37, 124, 134
    Peas, 23, 25, 26
    Peppers (red/green), 25, 26, 76, 113, 133
    Potatoes, 21, 24, 26, 59, 108, 133
    Pumpkin, 26, 113
    Recommended intake, 22, 23, 27, 31, 124, 129
    Romaine, 26, 29, 134
    Spinach, 24, 26, 27, 28–29, 31, 42, 54, 98, 124, 132, 134
    Squash, 24, 26, 108
    Sweet potatoes, 24, 26, 108, 113
    Tomatoes/Tomato-based foods, 23, 24, 26, 27, 30–31, 36, 42, 43, 45, 108, 124, 132, 133, 134, 135
    Vegetable juice, 23, 24, 30, 31, 36, 91, 94, 132, 133
Vegetable Oils, 14, 15, 113
Vegetarian, 65, 73, 74, 76, 80, 134
Vitamins, 14, 21, 27, 40, 46, 57, 80, 105–13, 128, 134, 136, 139
    B vitamins, 28, 40, 57, 70, 73, 81, 82, 98, 107, 109
    Beta-Carotene, 14, 22, 26, 28, 30, 107, 109, 112, 113, 128
    Folate (folic acid), 22, 24, 25, 26, 28, 29, 40, 57, 58, 80, 81, 82, 83, 98, 99, 107, 108, 109
    Recommended intakes, 109
    Vitamin A, 14, 29, 70, 107
    Vitamin B12, 70, 73, 107, 109

Vitamin D, 14, 17, 42, 48, 49, 50, 51, 52, 53, 55, 70, 108, 109, 111–12, 113, 128, 139
Vitamin C, 22, 24, 25, 26, 27, 29, 44, 76, 102, 109, 112, 113, 128
Vitamin E, 14, 17, 29, 40, 41, 78, 80, 81, 82, 83, 84, 102, 107, 108, 109, 112, 113, 128
Vitamin K, 14, 24, 28, 29, 82, 108, 109
Vitamin & Mineral Supplements, 51, 52, 59, 105–13, 128
    Multivitamin, 106–10, 113, 128

Waist Circumference (abdominal fat), 41, 45, 116, 312
Water, 91, 93, 94, 95, 127, 129, 135
Weight Control (weight loss), 9, 10, 14, 18, 19, 21, 22, 36, 39, 40, 41, 42, 45, 46, 48, 51, 53, 62, 73, 78, 83, 92, 94, 99, 102, 103, 104, 116, 118, 119, 122, 129, 134, 136, 138
    Healthy weight guidelines (body mass index), 313
Whole Grains—see Grains

Zeaxanthin, 22, 28, 29, 40, 77

RECIPE INDEX

A

Adults Only Pasta Sauce, 196
All Bran Buds
    Banana Walnut Bread Muffins, 284
    Pumpkin Chocolate Chip Muffins, 286
    Super Snackers, 304
    Ultimate Healthy Chocolate Treat, 308
Almonds
    Strawberry and Spinach Salad, 148
    Super Snackers, 304
Almost as Good as Grandma's Cole Slaw, 150
Amazing Black Bean Quesadillas, 217
Anchovies
    Adults Only Pasta Sauce, 196
Antioxidant All-Star Salad Dressing, 146
Apple Pancakes, 291
Apples
    Apple Pancakes, 291
    California Spinach Salad, 147
    Mulligatawny Soup, 161
    Wonderful Waldorf Wheat Berry Salad, 194
Apricots, canned
    Chicken with Mango and Apricots, 245
Apricots, dried
    Dried Fruit Compote, 261
    Super Snackers
Artichoke and Chickpea Salad, 223
Artichokes
    Artichoke and Chickpea Salad, 223
Asian Noodle Salad, 198
Asian-Style Eggplant, 165
Asian-Style Steamed Spinach, 175
Asparagus
    Asparagus Stir-Fry, 166
    Grilled Asparagus, 167
    Grilled Veggie Salad, 168
Asparagus Stir-Fry, 166
Avocado
    Fresh California Guacamole, 153
    Japanese Brown Rice Salad, 185
    Orange, Avocado, and Black Bean Salsa Salad, 218
Awesome Lentil and Rice Salad, 182

B

Baby Carrots—see Carrots
Baby Greens
    Baby Greens with Mandarins and Honey Mustard Salad
        Dressing, 152
Baby Spinach
    Asian-Style Steamed Spinach, 175
    Basic Family-Style Steamed Spinach, 174
    California Spinach Salad, 147
    Greek Pizza Frittata, 258
    Nutrition Packed Curried Lentils with Spinach, 219
    Spinach with Ricotta, 175
    Strawberry and Spinach Salad, 148
    Summer Fresh Puréed Pea and Mint Soup, 163

Tex Mex Turkey Skillet Dinner, 249
Baked Salmon with Fresh Citrus, 226
Banana Chocolate Chip Muffins, 278
Banana Pancakes, 289
Bananas
    Banana Chocolate Chip Muffins, 278
    Banana Pancakes, 289
    Banana Walnut Bread Muffins, 284
    Super Banana Chocolate Shake, 266
Banana Walnut Bread Muffins, 284
Barley
    Barley and Brown Rice Pilaf with Mushrooms, 188
    Barley Risotto, 191
Basic Brussels, 169
Basic Brussels with Maple Syrup, 169
Basic Cocoa, 269
Basic Family-Style Steamed Spinach, 174
Basil—see Fresh Basil
Beans—see also Black Beans, Chickpeas, Kidney Beans, or Lentils
    Amazing Artichoke and Chickpea Salad, 223
    Amazing Black Bean Quesadillas, 217
    Blazin' Black Bean Chili, 207
    Cheater Refried Beans, 212
    Greek Salad with Chickpeas, 221
    Hummus Peanut Butter Sandwich Filling, 220
    Hummus with Roasted Red Peppers, 222
    Japanese-Style Edamame and Corn Salad, 204
    Jazzy Beans, 213
    Jerk Black Beans, 216
    Kindergarten Curry, 214
    Marvellous Mexican Beans, 215
    Nutrition-Packed Curried Lentils with Spinach, 219
    Orange, Avocado, and Black Bean Salsa Salad, 218
    Out-of-this-World Chili, 206
    Remarkable Refried Beans, 211
    Summer Fiesta Chickpea Salad, 208
    Totally Terrific Taco-Taco Salad, 209
    Quickie Quesadillas that your family will love, 210
Beef
    Beef Bourguignonne, 251
    Jamaican Spiced Marinade for Beef and Pork, 254
Beef Bourguignonne, 251
Berries—see Blueberry, Raspberry, or Fruit
Best Ever Berry Crisp, 260
Beverages
    Basic Cocoa, 269
    Iced Tea, 273
    Frozen Cocoa, 270
    Omega-3 Tropical Smoothie, 267
    Perfect Cup of Green Tea, 272
    Perfect Cup of Tea, 271
    Pomegranate Martini, 275
    Pomegranate Mocktini, 275
    Purple Pomegranate Smoothie, 268
    Super Banana Chocolate Shake, 266
    Super Soy Strawberry Smoothie, 266
Big Breakfast Cookies, 302–03

Black Beans
  Amazing Black Bean Quesadillas, 217
  Blazin' Black Bean Chili, 207
  Cheater Refried Beans, 212
  Jamaican Black Bean Pumpkin Soup, 158
  Jerk Black Beans, 216
  Marvellous Minestrone, 160
  Orange, Avocado, and Black Bean Salsa Salad, 218
  Out-of-this-World Chili, 206
  Remarkable Refried Beans, 211
  Totally Terrific Taco-Taco Salad, 209
  Blazin' Black Bean Chili, 207
Blueberries
  Best Ever Berry Crisp, 260
  Blueberry Pancakes, 290
  Blueberry Wheat Berry Salad, 192
  Frozen Blueberry Yogurt, 262
  Romaine with Feta and Blueberries, 149
  Wild Blueberry Muffins, 280
  Whole Wheat Blueberry Buttermilk Pancakes, 287
Blueberry Wheat Berry Salad, 192
Bran Buds—see All Bran Buds
Breakfast Burrito, 257
Broccoli
  Asian Noodle Salad, 198
  Broccoli and Cheddar Cheese Soup, 156
Brown Rice
  Awesome Lentil and Rice Salad, 182
  Barley and Brown Rice Pilaf with Mushrooms, 188
  Brown Rice with Dried Cranberries and Orange, 186
  Japanese Brown Rice Salad, 185
  Make It Once, Eat It All Week Brown Rice, 181
  Sensationally Simple Stir Fried Rice, 183
  Short-grain Brown Rice Risotto with Kale and Squash, 187
  Smith's House Recipe for the Harried Mother, 184
Brown Rice with Dried Cranberries and Orange, 186
Brussels Sprouts
  Basic Brussels, 169
  Brussels with Maple Syrup, 169
Build a Better Bowl (of cereal), 293
Buttermilk
  Banana Chocolate Chip Muffins, 278
  Cranberry Orange Muffins, 285
  Double Chocolate Muffins, 283
  Pumpkin Chocolate Chip Muffins, 286
  Super Nutritious Bran Muffins, 282
  Whole Wheat Blueberry Buttermilk Pancakes, 287
Butternut Squash
  Butternut Squash with Brown Sugar and Cinnamon, 170
  Short-Grain Brown Rice Risotto with Kale and Squash, 187
Butternut Squash with Brown Sugar and Cinnamon, 170

C
Cabbage
  Almost as Good as Grandma's Coleslaw, 150
  Asian Noodle Salad, 198
Cake
  Don't Forget to Leave Room for Chocolate Cake, 310–11

California Spinach Salad, 147
Canned Tomatoes—see Diced Tomatoes
Carrots
  Carrots with Raisins and Orange Juice, 172
  Honey-Glazed Carrots, 171
Carrots with Raisins and Orange Juice, 172
Cashews
  Barley and Brown Rice Pilaf with Mushrooms, 188
  Chicken with Lime Garlic and Cashews, 244
  Sensationally Simple Stir Fried Rice, 183
Cheater Refried Beans, 212
Cheese—see Cheddar, Light Feta, Light Ricotta, Monterey Jack
  Cheese, or Parmesan
Cheddar
  Breakfast Burrito, 257
  Broccoli and Cheddar Cheese Soup, 156
Cherry Tomatoes—see Grape Tomatoes
Chewy Chocolate Chip Cookies, 298
Chicken Breasts
  Chicken with Dried Cranberries and Orange, 243
  Chicken with Lime Garlic and Cashews, 244
  Chicken with Mango and Apricots, 245
  Grilled Herb Chicken, 247
  Honey Mustard Chicken Your Honey Will Love, 248
  Quick and Hearty Chicken Noodle Soup, 162
Chicken Thighs
  Grilled Herb Chicken, 247
  Mulligatawny Soup, 161
  Polynesian-Style Slow Cooker Chicken, 246
Chicken with Dried Cranberries and Orange, 243
Chicken with Lime Garlic and Cashews, 244
Chicken with Mango and Apricots, 245
Chickpeas
  Artichoke and Chickpea Salad, 223
  Greek Salad with Chickpeas, 221
  Hummus Peanut Butter Sandwich Filling, 220
  Hummus with Roasted Red Peppers, 222
  Summer Fiesta Chickpea Salad, 208
Chili
  Blazin' Black Bean Chili, 207
  Out-of-this-World Chili, 206
Chocolate
  Banana Chocolate Chip Muffins, 278
  Chewy Chocolate Chip Cookies, 298
  Cocoa Crisps, 297
  Decadent Brownies, 306–07
  Don't Forget to Leave Room for Chocolate Cake, 310–11
  Pumpkin Chocolate Chip Muffins, 286
  Super Banana Chocolate Shake, 266
  Super Nutritious Chocolate Chip Bran Muffins, 282
  Super Snackers, 304
  Ultimate Healthy Chocolate Treat, 308
Chocolate Soy Beverage—see Soy Beverages
Cilantro—see Fresh Cilantro
Cocoa Crisps, 297
Cocoa Powder
  Basic Cocoa, 269
  Cocoa Crisps, 297

Don't Forget to Leave Room for Chocolate Cake, 310–11
Frozen Cocoa, 270
Super Banana Chocolate Shake, 266
Company's Comin' Salmon, 227
Cookies
    Big Breakfast Cookies, 302–03
    Chewy Chocolate Chip Cookies, 298
    Cocoa Crisps, 297
    Oatmeal Raisin Cookies, 300
    Peanut Butter Cookies, 299
    Snappy Gingersnaps, 301
Corn
    Blazin' Black Bean Chili, 207
    Corn and Diced Red Peppers, 173
    Japanese-Style Edamame and Corn Salad, 204
    Tex Mex Turkey Skillet Dinner, 249
    West Coast Salmon Chowder, 240
Corn and Diced Red Peppers, 173
Cranberries, dried
    Awesome Lentil and Rice Salad, 182
    Big Breakfast Cookies, 302–03
    Brown Rice with Dried Cranberries and Orange, 186
    Chicken with Dried Cranberries and Orange, 243
    Cranberry Orange Muffins, 285
    Creamy Rice Pudding, 309
    Dried Fruit Compote, 261
    Super Snackers, 304
    Wonderful Waldorf Wheat Berry Salad, 194
Cranberries, whole fresh or frozen
    Cranberry Orange Muffins, 285
    Roasted Sweet Potatoes with Cranberries, 179
Creamy Rice Pudding, 309
Crunchy Cinnamon Granola, 264
Cucumber—see English Cucumber
Currants
    Awesome Lentil and Rice Salad, 182
    Build a Better Bowl (of cereal), 293
Curry
    Kindergarten Curry, 214
    Mulligatawny Soup, 161
    Nutrition Packed Curried Lentils with Spinach, 219

D
Dates
    Old-Fashioned Date Squares, 305
    Super Nutritious Bran Muffins, 282
Decadent Brownies, 306–07
Diced Tomatoes
    Adults Only Pasta Sauce, 196
    Blazin' Black Bean Chili, 207
    Jamaican Black Bean Pumpkin Soup, 158
    Kid Friendly Spaghetti Sauce, 197
    Mairlyn's Amazing Tomato Sauce, 200
    Marvellous Minestrone, 160
    Nutrition-Packed Curried Lentils with Spinach, 219
    Out-of-this-World Chili, 206
    Rotini with Plum Tomatoes and Lentils, 201

Dijon Mustard
    Antioxidant All-Star Salad Dressing, 146
    Everyday House Dressing, 145
    Honey Mustard Salad Dressing, 145
    Jazzy Beans, 213
    Unbelievably Delicious Raspberry Salad Dressing, 144
Don't Forget to Leave Room for Chocolate Cake, 310–11
Double Chocolate Muffins, 283
Dried Fruit Compote, 261

E
Edamame
    Japanese Style Edamame and Corn Salad, 204
Eggs
    Breakfast Burrito, 257
    Greek Pizza Frittata, 258
Eggplant
    Asian-Style Eggplant, 165
English Cucumber
    Greek Salad with Chickpeas, 221
    Japanese Brown Rice Salad, 185
Evaporated Milk—see Fat-Free Evaporated Milk
Everyday House Dressing, 145

F
Fantastic Frozen Yogurt Times Four, 262
Fat-Free Evaporated Milk
    Broccoli and Cheddar Cheese Soup, 156
    West Coast Salmon Chowder, 240
Feta Cheese—see Light Feta Cheese
Flaxseed, Ground
    Banana Chocolate Chip Muffins, 278
    Banana Walnut Bread Muffins, 284
    Big Breakfast Cookies, 302–03
    Mairlyn's Pancake Mix, 288
    Pumpkin Chocolate Chip Muffins, 286
    Super Banana Chocolate Shake, 266
    Super Nutritious Bran Muffins, 282
    Super Snackers, 304
    Ultimate Healthy Chocolate Treat, 308
French Toast, 294
French Vanilla Yogurt—see Low-Fat French Vanilla Yogurt
Fresh Basil
    Amazing Artichoke and Chickpea Salad, 223
    Grape Tomato Salad, 151
    Greek Pizza Frittata, 258
    Greek Salad with Chickpeas, 221
    Grilled Herb Chicken, 247
    Mairlyn's Amazing Tomato Sauce, 200
    Marvellous Minestrone, 160
    Rotini with Feta and Tomatoes, 202
    Summer Fiesta Chickpea Salad, 208
    Walnut Pesto, 154
Fresh California Guacamole, 153
Fresh Cilantro
    Amazing Black Bean Quesadillas, 217
    Asian Noodle Salad, 198

Fresh Cilantro (*cont'd*)
    Grilled Salmon with Raspberries, 229
    Hummus Peanut Butter Sandwich Filling, 220
    Spicy Salmon Cakes, 234
Fresh Parsley
    Amazing Artichoke and Chickpea Salad, 223
Frozen Bananas—*see* Bananas
Frozen Blueberry Yogurt, 262
Frozen Cocoa, 270
Frozen Concentrated Orange Juice—*see* Orange Juice Concentrate
Frozen Mango Yogurt, 262
Frozen Mixed Berry Yogurt, 262
Frozen Raspberry Yogurt, 262
Fruit and Berries, fresh or frozen
    Basic Fantastic Frozen Yogurt, 262
    Best Ever Berry Crisp, 260
    Dried Fruit Compote, 261
    Frozen Blueberry Yogurt, 262
    Frozen Mango Yogurt, 262
    Frozen Mixed Berry Yogurt, 262
    Frozen Raspberry Yogurt, 262
    Grilled Salmon with Raspberries, 229
    My Very Own Fast Food Berry Parfait, 263
    Omega-3 Tropical Smoothie, 267
    Pomegranate Martini, 275
    Purple Pomegranate Smoothie, 268
    Super Banana Chocolate Shake, 266
    Super Soy Strawberry Smoothie, 266

G

Garbanzo beans—*see* Chickpeas
Garlic Lover's Lemon Shrimp, 228
Garlic Pork with Stir-Fried Peppers, 252
Grains
    Awesome Lentil and Rice Salad, 182
    Barley and Brown Rice Pilaf with Mushrooms, 188
    Barley Risotto, 191
    Blueberry Wheat Berry Salad, 192
    Brown Rice with Dried Cranberries and Orange, 186
    Japanese Brown Rice Salad, 185
    Make It Once, Eat It All Week Brown Rice, 181
    Quinoa 101, 189
    Quinoa Pilaf, 190
    Sensationally Simple Stir-Fried Rice, 183
    Short-grain Brown Rice Risotto with Kale and Squash, 187
    Smith's House Recipe for the Harried Mother, 184
    Wonderful Waldorf Wheat Berry Salad, 194
Granola
    Crunchy Cinnamon Granola, 264
Grape Juice
    Kid Friendly Spaghetti Sauce, 197
Grape Tomatoes
    Grape Tomato Salad, 151
    Summer Fiesta Chickpea Salad, 208
    Grape Tomato Salad, 151
Greek Salad with Chickpeas, 221
Greek Pizza Frittata, 258
Grilled Herb Chicken, 247
Grilled Salmon with Raspberries, 229
Grilled Veggie Salad, 168
Ground Flaxseed—*see* Flaxseed

H

Honey
    Honey Glazed Carrots, 171
    Honey Mustard Chicken Your Honey Will Love, 248
    Honey Mustard Salad Dressing, 145
    Wild Blueberry Muffins, 280
Honey Glazed Carrots, 171
Honey Mustard Chicken Your Honey Will Love, 248
Honey Mustard Salad Dressing, 145
Hot Pepper Jelly
    Chicken with Dried Cranberries and Orange, 243
Hummus Peanut Butter Sandwich Filling, 220
Hummus with Roasted Red Peppers, 222

I

Iced Blackcurrant Tea, 274
Iced Cinnamon Mint Green Tea, 274
Iced Green Tea, 274
Iced Spiced Black Tea, 274
Iced Tea, 273
Immune Enhancing Shiitake Mushroom Soup, 157
Irish Oats
    Overnight Oats, 292

J

Japanese Brown Rice Salad, 185
Japanese-Style Edamame and Corn Salad, 204
Jamaican Black Bean Pumpkin Soup, 158
Jamaican Spiced Marinade for Beef and Pork, 254
Jazzy Beans, 213
Jerk Black Beans, 216

K

Kale
    Immune Enhancing Shiitake Mushroom Soup, 157
    Marvellous Minestrone, 160
    Quick and Hearty Chicken Noodle Soup, 162
    Short-Grain Brown Rice Risotto with Kale and Squash, 187
Kid Friendly Spaghetti Sauce, 197
Kidney Beans
    Marvellous Minestrone, 160
    Out of This World Chili, 206
Kindergarten Curry, 214

L

Leek and Lemon Soup, 159
Leeks
    How to Clean, 159
    Leek and Lemon Soup, 159
    Mulligatawny Soup, 161
Lemon and Lemon Juice
    Baked Salmon with Fresh Citrus, 226
    Garlic Lovers Lemon Shrimp, 228

Grilled Herb Chicken, 247
Leek and Lemon Soup, 159
Lentils
    Awesome Lentil and Rice Salad, 182
    Nutrition Packed Curried Lentils with Spinach, 219
    Rotini with Plum Tomatoes and Lentils, 201
Light Feta Cheese
    Blueberry Wheat Berry Salad, 192
    Greek Pizza Frittata, 258
    Greek Salad with Chickpeas, 221
    Romaine with Feta and Blueberries, 149
    Rotini with Feta and Tomatoes, 202
Light Ricotta
    Spinach with Ricotta, 175
Lime and Lime Juice
    Baked Salmon with Fresh Citrus, 226
    Company's Comin' Salmon, 227
    Orange Avocado Black Bean Salsa Salad, 218
    Poached Salmon with Mairlyn's World Famous Lime Mayo,
        230
    Sensational Salmon with Mango Salsa, 232
Low-Fat French Vanilla Yogurt
    Fantastic Frozen Yogurt Times Four, 262
    My Very Own Fast Food Berry Parfait, 263
    Omega-3 Tropical Smoothie, 267
    Purple Pomegranate Smoothie, 268
Low-Fat Mayonnaise
    Spicy Salmon Cakes, 234
    Totally Kid Friendly Salmon Cakes, 238

M
Mairlyn's Amazing Tomato Sauce, 200
Mairlyn's Pancake Mix, 288
Make It Once, Eat It All Week Brown Rice, 181
Mango
    Chicken with Mango and Apricots, 245
    Frozen Mango Yogurt, 262
    Mango Chutney, 245
    Sensational Salmon with Mango Salsa, 232
Maple Syrup
    Brussels with Maple Syrup, 269
    Roasted Sweet Potatoes and Cranberries, 179
Marmalade—Orange
    Chicken with Dried Cranberries and Orange, 243
Marshmallows
    Super Snackers, 304
Marvellous Mexican Beans, 215
Marvellous Minestrone, 160
Mini Chocolate Chips
    Banana Chocolate Chip Muffins, 278
    Chewy Chocolate Chip Cookies, 298
    Pumpkin Chocolate Chip Muffins, 286
    Super Nutritious Chocolate Chip Bran Muffins, 282
    Super Snackers, 304
Mint
    Blueberry Wheat Berry Salad, 192
    Summer Fresh Puréed Pea and Mint Soup, 163

Monterey Jack Cheese
    Amazing Black Bean Quesadillas, 217
    Quickie Quesadillas that your family will love, 210
Muffins, Pancakes, and French Toast
    Apple Pancakes, 291
    Banana Chocolate Chip Muffins, 278
    Banana Pancakes, 289
    Banana Walnut Bread Muffins, 284
    Blueberry Pancakes, 290
    Cranberry Orange Muffins, 285
    Double Chocolate Muffins, 283
    French Toast, 294
    Mairlyn's Pancake Mix, 288
    Pumpkin Chocolate Chip Muffins, 286
    Super Nutritious Bran Muffins, 282
    Whole Wheat Blueberry Buttermilk Pancakes, 287
    Wild Blueberry Muffins, 280
Mulligatawny Soup, 161
Mushrooms—see Portabello, Porcini, or Shiitake
My Very Own Fast Food Berry Parfait, 263

N
Nutrition-Packed Curried Lentils with Spinach, 219
Nuts—see specific nuts

O
Oat Bran
    Big Breakfast Cookies, 302–03
    Cranberry Orange Muffins, 285
    Wild Blueberry Muffins, 280
Oatmeal Raisin Cookies, 300
Oats, large flake or quick
    Best Ever Berry Crisp, 260
    Big Breakfast Cookies, 302–03
    Crunchy Cinnamon Granola, 264
    Mairlyn's Pancake Mix, 288
    Oatmeal Raisin Cookies, 300
    Old-Fashioned Date Squares, 305
    Overnight Oats, 292
Old-Fashioned Date Squares, 305
Old-Fashioned Iced Black Tea, 273
Olives
    Adults Only Pasta Sauce, 196
    Grape Tomato Salad, 151
    Greek Pizza Frittata, 258
    Greek Salad with Chickpeas, 221
    Rotini with Feta and Tomatoes, 202
Omega-3 Tropical Smoothie, 267
Orange
    Baked Salmon with Fresh Citrus, 226
    Orange Avocado Black Bean Salsa Salad, 218
Orange Juice
    Carrots with Raisins and Orange Juice, 172
    Omega-3 Tropical Smoothie, 267
    Poached Salmon with Mairlyn's World-Famous Lime Mayo,
        230
    Roasted Sweet Potatoes and Cranberries, 179

Orange Juice Concentrate, frozen
  Chicken with Dried Cranberries and Orange, 243
  Chicken with Mango and Apricots, 245
  Company's Comin' Salmon, 227
  Dried Fruit Compote, 261
  Old-Fashioned Date Squares, 305
  Poached Salmon with Mairlyn's World Famous Lime Mayo, 230
  Quickie Sweet Potatoes, 177
Orange Marmalade—see Marmalade
Out-of-this-World Chili, 206
Overnight Oats, 292

P

Pancakes
  Apple Pancakes, 291
  Banana Pancakes, 289
  Blueberry Pancakes, 290
  Mairlyn's Pancake Mix, 288
  Whole Wheat Blueberry Buttermilk Pancakes, 287
Parmesan
  Barley Risotto, 191
  Short-grain Brown Rice Risotto with Kale and Squash, 187
Pasta
  Asian Noodle Salad, 198–99
  Rotini with Feta and Tomatoes, 220
  Rotini with Plum Tomatoes and Lentils, 201
Peanut Butter Cookies, 299
Peanuts and Peanut Butter
  Asian Noodle Salad, 198–99
  Hummus Peanut Butter Sandwich Filling, 220
  Sensationally Simple Stir Fried Rice, 183
  Super Snackers, 304
  Smith's House Recipe for the Harried Mother, 184
Peas
  Barley and Brown Rice Pilaf with Mushrooms, 188
  Smith's House Recipe for the Harried Mother, 183
  Summer Fresh Puréed Pea and Mint Soup, 163
Peppers—see Red Peppers, fresh or roasted
Perfect Cup of Green Tea, 272
Perfect Cup of Tea, 271
Pesto—see Walnut Pesto
Pineapple, canned
  Polynesian-Style Slow Cooker Chicken, 246
Plum Tomatoes—see Diced Tomatoes
Poached Salmon with Mairlyn's World Famous Lime Mayo, 230
Polynesian-Style Slow Cooker Chicken, 246
Pomegranate Juice
  Blazin' Black Bean Chili, 207
  Jamaican Spiced Marinade for Beef and Pork, 254
  Pomegranate Martini, 275
  Pomegranate Mocktini, 275
  Purple Pomegranate Smoothie, 268
Pomegranate Martini, 275
Pomegranate Mocktini, 275
Porcini Mushrooms
  Barley and Brown Rice Pilaf with Mushrooms, 188

Pork
  Garlic Pork with Stir-Fried Peppers, 252
  Jamaican Spiced Marinade for Beef and Pork, 254
Portobello Mushrooms
  Barley Risotto, 191
Potatoes
  Roasted Garlic Potatoes, 176
Pot Barley—see Barley
Poultry—see Chicken Breast, Chicken Thighs, or Turkey
Prunes, strained or whole
  Big Breakfast Cookies, 302–03
  Don't Forget To Leave Room for Chocolate Cake, 310–11
  Dried Fruit Compote, 261
  Super Nutritious Bran Muffins, 282
Pumpkin Chocolate Chip Muffins, 286
Pumpkin Purée
  Double Chocolate Muffins, 283
  Jamaican Black Bean Pumpkin Soup, 158
  Pumpkin Chocolate Chip Muffins, 286
Purple Pomegranate Smoothie, 268

Q

Quick and Hearty Chicken Noodle Soup, 162
Quickie Quesadillas that your family will love, 210
Quickie Sweet Potatoes, 177
Quick Oats—see also Oats
  Mairlyn's Pancake Mix, 288
Quinoa 101, 189
Quinoa Pilaf, 190

R

Raisins
  Carrots with Raisins and Orange Juice, 172
Raspberries
  Frozen Raspberry Yogurt, 262
  Grilled Salmon with Raspberries, 229
  Strawberry and Spinach Salad, 148
  Unbelievably Good Raspberry Salad Dressing, 144
Really Great Salmon, 231
Red Cabbage—see Cabbage
Red Peppers, fresh
  Amazing Black Bean Quesadillas, 217
  Asian noodle Salad, 198
  Asparagus Stir Fry, 166
  Chicken with Lime, Garlic, and Cashews, 244
  Corn and Diced Red Peppers, 173
  Garlic Pork with Stir-Fried Peppers, 252
  Grilled Veggie Salad, 168
  Jazzy Beans, 213
  Marvellous Mexican Beans, 215
  Orange, Avocado, and Black Bean Salsa Salad, 218
  Summer Fiesta Chickpea Salad, 208
  West Coast Salmon Chowder, 240
Red Peppers, roasted
  Hummus with Roasted Red Peppers, 222
  Kid Friendly Spaghetti Sauce, 197
  Mairlyn's Amazing Tomato Sauce, 200

Rotini with Plum Tomatoes and Lentils, 201
Red Wine
    Adults Only Pasta Sauce, 196
    Beef Bourguignonne, 251
Remarkable Refried Beans, 211
Ribena
    Antioxidant All-Star Salad Dressing, 146
    Grilled Salmon with Raspberries, 229
Rice—see Brown Rice
Ricotta—see Light Ricotta
    Roasted Garlic Potatoes, 176
Roasted Sweet Potatoes, 178
Roasted Sweet Potatoes and Cranberries, 179
Romaine with Feta and Blueberries, 149
Rosemary, fresh or dried
    Beef Bourguignonne, 251
    Grilled Herb Chicken, 247
    Roasted Garlic Potatoes, 176
Rotini with Feta and Tomatoes, 202
Rotini with Plum Tomatoes and Lentils, 201

S

Salads and Salad Dressings
    Almost as Good as Grandma's Cole Slaw, 150
    Amazing Artichoke and Chickpea Salad, 223
    Awesome Lentil and Rice Salad, 182
    Antioxidant All-Star Salad Dressing, 146
    Baby Greens with Mandarins and Honey Mustard Salad
        Dressing, 152
    California Spinach Salad, 147
    Everyday House Dressing, 145
    Grape Tomato Salad, 151
    Greek Salad with Chickpeas, 221
    Honey Mustard Salad Dressing, 145
    Japanese Brown Rice Salad, 185
    Romaine with Feta and Blueberries, 149
    Strawberry and Spinach Salad, 148
    Summer Fiesta Chickpea Salad, 208
    Unbelievably Delicious Raspberry Salad Dressing, 144
    Wonderful Waldorf Wheat Berry Salad, 194
Salsa
    Amazing Black Bean Quesadillas, 217
    Breakfast Burrito, 257
    Marvellous Mexican Beans, 215
    Orange Avocado Black Bean Salsa Salad, 218
    Out-of-this-World Chili, 206
    Tex Mex Turkey Skillet Dinner, 249
Salmon—see Seafood
Sensationally Simple Stir-Fried Rice, 183
Sensational Salmon with Mango Salsa, 232
Seafood
    Baked Salmon with Fresh Citrus, 226
    Company's Comin' Salmon, 227
    Garlic Lovers Lemon Shrimp, 228
    Grilled Salmon with Raspberries, 229
    Poached Salmon with Mairlyn's World-Famous Lime Mayo,
        230
    Really Great Salmon, 231

Sensational Salmon with Mango Salsa, 232
Spicy Salmon Cakes, 234
Terrific Salmon Teriyaki, 233
Totally Kid Friendly Salmon Cakes, 238
Ultimate Salmon Sandwich Filling, 236
Wasabi Salmon, 239
West Coast Salmon Chowder, 240
Shiitake Mushrooms
    Barley and Brown Rice Pilaf with Mushrooms, 188
    Immune Enhancing Shiitake Mushroom Soup, 157
Short-grain Brown Rice Risotto with Kale and Squash, 187
Shrimp
    Garlic Lover's Lemon Shrimp, 228
Skim Milk Powder
    Frozen Cocoa, 270
    Mairlyn's Muffin Mix, 288
S33kinless, Boneless Chicken Breasts—see Chicken Breasts
Smith's House Recipe for the Harried Mother, 184
Snappy Gingersnaps, 301
Sockeye Salmon, canned
    Spicy Salmon Cakes, 234
    Totally Kid Friendly Salmon Cakes, 238
    Ultimate Salmon Sandwich Filling, 236
Soups
    Broccoli and Cheddar Cheese Soup, 156
    Immune Enhancing Shiitake Mushroom Soup, 157
    Jamaican Black Bean Pumpkin Soup, 158
    Leek and Lemon Soup, 159
    Marvellous Minestrone, 160
    Mulligatawny Soup, 161
    Quick and Hearty Chicken Noodle Soup, 162
    Summer Fresh Puréed Pea and Mint Soup, 163
Soy Beverages
    Don't Forget to Leave Room for Chocolate Cake, 310–11
    Super Banana Chocolate Shake, 266
    Super Soy Strawberry Smoothie, 266
Spiced Green Tea, 274
Spicy Salmon Cakes, 234
Spinach—see also Baby Spinach
    Spinach with Ricotta, 175
Steel Cut Oats—see also Oats
    Overnight Oats, 292
Strawberries
    Strawberry and Spinach Salad, 148
    Super Soy Strawberry Smoothie, 266
Strawberry and Spinach Salad, 148
Strawberry Soy Beverage—see Soy Beverages
Summer Fiesta Chickpea Salad, 208
Summer Fresh Puréed Pea and Mint Soup, 163
Super Banana Chocolate Shake, 266
Super Nutritious Bran Muffins, 282
Super Soy Strawberry Smoothie, 266
Sweet Potatoes
    Quickie Sweet Potatoes, 177
    Roasted Sweet Potatoes, 178
    Roasted Sweet Potatoes and Cranberries, 179
    Super Snackers, 304

T

Tahini
    Hummus with Roasted Red Peppers, 222
Tea, black and green
    Iced Blackcurrant Tea, 274
    Iced Cinnamon Mint Green Tea, 274
    Iced Green Tea, 274
    Iced Spiced Black Tea, 274
    Iced Tea, 273
    Liz's Spiced Green Tea, 274
    Old-Fashioned Iced Black Tea, 273
    Perfect Cup of Green Tea, 272
    Perfect Cup of Tea, 271
Teriyaki
    Terrific Salmon Teriyaki, 233
Tex Mex Turkey Skillet Dinner, 249
Tomatoes, fresh—*see also* Canned Tomatoes and Grape Tomatoes
    Rotini with Feta and Tomatoes, 202
Totally Kid Friendly Salmon Cakes, 238
Totally Terrific Taco-Taco Salad, 209
Turkey, ground and leftover
    Totally Terrific Taco-Taco Salad, 209
    Tex Mex Turkey Skillet Dinner, 249

U

Ultimate Healthy Chocolate Treat, 308
Ultimate Salmon Sandwich Filling, 236
Unbelievably Delicious Raspberry Salad Dressing, 144

V

Vanilla Yogurt—*see* Low-Fat French Vanilla Yogurt
Vegetables
    Asian Style Eggplant, 165
    Asian Style Steamed Spinach, 175
    Asparagus Stir-Fry, 166
    Basic Brussels, 169
    Basic Family-Style Steamed Spinach, 174
    Brussels with Maple Syrup, 169
    Butternut Squash with Brown Sugar and Cinnamon, 170
    Carrots with Raisins and Orange Juice, 172
    Corn and Diced Red Peppers, 173
    Grilled Asparagus, 167
    Grilled Veggie Salad, 168
    Honey Glazed Carrots, 171
    Quickie Sweet Potatoes, 177
    Roasted Garlic Potatoes, 176
    Roasted Sweet Potatoes, 178
    Roasted Sweet Potatoes and Cranberries, 179
    Spinach with Ricotta, 175

W

Walnut Pesto, 154
Walnuts
    California Spinach Salad, 147
    Cranberry Orange Muffin, 285
    Walnut Pesto, 154
    Wonderful Waldorf Wheat Berry Salad, 194

Wasabi Salmon, 239
West Coast Salmon Chowder, 240
Wheat Berry
    Blueberry Wheat Berry Salad, 192
    Wonderful Waldorf Wheat Berry Salad, 194
Wheat Bran
    Banana Chocolate Chip Muffins, 278
    Cranberry Orange Muffins, 285
    Pumpkin Chocolate Chip Muffins, 286
    Super Nutritious Bran Muffins, 282
    Whole Wheat Blueberry Buttermilk Pancakes, 287
Wheat Germ
    Pumpkin Chocolate Chip Muffins, 286
    Whole Wheat Blueberry Buttermilk Pancakes, 287
Whole Grain Cereal, Spoon size Shredded Wheat + Bran
    Spicy Salmon Cakes, 234
    Super Snackers, 304
    Totally Kid Friendly Salmon Cakes, 238
    Ultimate Healthy Chocolate Treat, 308
Whole Wheat Blueberry Buttermilk Pancakes, 287
Whole Wheat Flour
    Banana Chocolate Chip Muffins, 278
    Banana Walnut Bread Muffins, 284
    Big Breakfast Cookies, 302–03
    Chewy Chocolate Chip Cookies, 298
    Cocoa Crisps, 297
    Cranberry Orange Muffins, 285
    Decadent Brownies, 306–07
    Don't Forget to Leave Room for Chocolate Cake, 310–11
    Double Chocolate Muffins, 283
    Mairlyn's Pancake Mix, 288
    Oatmeal Raisin Cookies, 300
    Old-Fashioned Date Squares, 305
    Peanut Butter Cookies, 249
    Pumpkin Chocolate Chip Muffins, 286
    Snappy Gingersnaps, 301
    Super Nutritious Bran Muffins, 282
    Whole Wheat Blueberry Buttermilk Pancakes, 287
    Wild Blueberry Muffins, 280
Wild Blueberry Muffins, 280
Wonderful Waldorf Wheat Berry Salad, 194

Y

Yams—*see* Sweet Potatoes
Yogurt—*see* Low-Fat French Vanilla Yogurt
Yves Veggie Ground Round
    Out-of-this-World Chili, 206

ABOUT THE AUTHORS

LIZ PEARSON is a registered dietitian with a passion for peanut butter sandwiches and an undying love for chocolate. Liz's approach to healthy eating is sane and sensible. She communicates timely, relevant nutrition research, while emphasizing the need for fun food (like chocolate!) in moderation. Liz runs "The Pearson Institute of Nutrition," whose mission is to translate the often-confusing and ever-changing science of nutrition into practical, commonsense advice that people can follow in their busy lives. Liz's first book, *When in Doubt, Eat Broccoli! (but leave some room for chocolate)* received outstanding reviews from consumers and health professionals alike. Her second book, *The Ultimate Healthy Eating Plan (that still leaves room for chocolate!)* was a national bestseller and won a North American-wide award for best book in the health/nutrition category. Liz was the "Ask the Expert" nutrition columnist for *Chatelaine* magazine for almost seven years and continues to write feature articles for magazines and newspapers across Canada. She appears regularly on radio and television and has appeared on CTV's "Canada AM," City TV, the Life Network's "Health on the Line," TV Ontario's "More 2 Life," and CBC Radio. Liz is an award-winning, professional speaker. She speaks regularly at conventions and conferences across North America. She is also a consultant and media spokesperson for the food industry. For many years she played an active role in the 5-to-10-a-day fruit and vegetable campaign sponsored by the Heart and Stroke Foundation of Canada and the Canadian Cancer Society. Liz is married, lives in Toronto, and has two girls.

MAIRLYN SMITH first got hooked on cooking at the ripe old age of 4. Her mom let her make brownies; one lick of the batter and Mairlyn was a foodie for life. They say that when you're 10 years old, you really know what you want to be when you grow up. At 10 she wanted to be an actress, a cooking show host, a cookbook author, a teacher, and really thin. She become a home ec and drama teacher in the late '70s, an actress in the early '80s, a cooking show host in the early '90s, and a cookbook author in the mid-1990s. She's still working on that thin thing.

Mairlyn has appeared on television morning and lunchtime news shows, cooking up a storm from Vancouver to Halifax, as well as on the "Vicki Gabereau Show," CBC's "Midday" and "Newsworld," City TV's "Breakfast TV," CTV's "Canada AM," and Balance Television.

She is the only home economist who is also an alumnus of The Second City Comedy Troupe. Her versatility in acting and cooking with a comedic flair landed her a cooking segment on Discovery Channel's "Harrowsmith Country Life" and a Gemini nomination for Best Host.

Mairlyn lives in Toronto with her fifteen-year-old son, who loves kidney beans, broccoli, and the Maple Leafs, her partner Scott, who has eaten everything in all of her books, and their dog Bailey.